## DATE DUE

| JAN 0 8 1997 | |
| NOV 7 2000 | |
| JUN 2 5 2002 | |
| | |
| | |
| | |
| | |
| | |
| | |
| | |
| | |
| | |
| | |
| | |
| | |

GAYLORD                                    PRINTED IN U.S.A.

# Tuberculosis

Piglet sidled up to Pooh from behind,
'Pooh,' he whispered. 'Yes, Piglet?'
'Nothing,' said Piglet, taking Pooh's paw.
'I just wanted to be sure of you.'

A.A. Milne


This book is dedicated to those whom
I always want to be sure of:
Suzanne
Rachel
Zach
Arielle
Jonina

# Tuberculosis

**Edited by Larry I. Lutwick**

## CHAPMAN & HALL MEDICAL

London · Glasgow · Weinheim · New York · Tokyo · Melbourne · Madras

**Published by Chapman & Hall, 2–6 Boundary Row, London SE1 8HN, UK**

Chapman & Hall, 2–6 Boundary Row, London SE1 8HN, UK

Blackie Academic & Professional, Wester Cleddens Road, Bishopbriggs, Glasgow G64 2NZ, UK

Chapman & Hall GmbH, Pappelallee 3, 69469 Weinheim, Germany

Chapman & Hall USA, One Penn Plaza, 41st Floor, New York NY 10119, USA

Chapman & Hall Japan, ITP-Japan, Kyowa Building, 3F, 2-2-1 Hirakawacho, Chiyoda-ku, Tokyo 102, Japan

Chapman & Hall Australia, Thomas Nelson Australia, 102 Dodds Street, South Melbourne, Victoria 3205, Australia

Chapman & Hall India, R. Seshadri, 32 Second Main Road, CIT East, Madras 600 035, India

First edition 1995

© 1995 Chapman & Hall

Typeset in Times 10/12 pt by Florencetype Ltd, Stoodleigh Court, Devon
Printed in Great Britain at the University Press, Cambridge

ISBN 0 412 60740 9

A catalogue record for this book is available from the British Library

♾ Printed on permanent acid-free text paper, manufactured in accordance with ANSI/NISO Z39.48-1992 and ANSI/NISO Z39.48-1984 (Permanence of Paper).

# Contents

# Contributors

*Elfatih I.M. Abter*
Division of Infectious Diseases, Beth Israel Medical Center, 1st Avenue and 16th Street, New York, NY 10003, USA

*Peter G. Barber*
Department of Pharmacy, Maimonides Medical Center, 4802 Tenth Avenue, Brooklyn, NY 11219, USA

*Ronald L. Barbour*
Division of Infectious Diseases, Maimonides Medical Center, 4802 Tenth Avenue, Brooklyn, NY 11219, USA

*Kenneth G. Castro*
Division of Tuberculosis Elimination, National Center for Prevention Services, Centers for Disease Control and Prevention, Public Health Service, United States Department of Health and Human Services, 1600 Clifton Road, E–10, Atlanta, GA 30333, USA

*Edward K. Chapnick*
Division of Infectious Diseases, Department of Medicine, Maimonides Medical Center, 4802 Tenth Avenue, Brooklyn, NY 11219, USA

*Jeneane Chirico*
Department of Pharmacy, Maimonides Medical Center, 4802 Tenth Avenue, Brooklyn, NY 11219, USA

*William M. Goldman*
Department of Pharmacy, Maimonides Medical Center, 4802 Tenth Avenue, Brooklyn, NY 11219, USA

*Jeremy D. Gradon*
Division of Infectious Diseases, Department of Medicine, Sinai Hospital, 2401 West Belvedere Avenue, Baltimore, MD 21215, USA

*Joyce R. Grossman*
Division of Infectious Diseases, Department of Medicine, Maimonides Medical Center, 4802 Tenth Avenue, Brooklyn, NY 11219, USA

*Amin Hakim*
Division of Infectious Diseases, Department of Pediatrics, Maimonides Medical Center, 4802 Tenth Avenue, Brooklyn, NY 11219, USA

*Livette S. Johnson*
Infectious Diseases Service, Memorial Sloan-Kettering Cancer Center, 1275 York Avenue, New York, NY 10021, USA

*Joseph H. Kent*
Division of Tuberculosis Elimination, National Center for Prevention Services, Centers for Disease Control and Prevention, Public Health Service, United States Department of Health and Human Services, 1600 Clifton Road, E–10, Atlanta, GA 30333, USA

*Sheldon H. Landesman*
Division of Infectious Diseases, Department of Medicine, State University of New York, Health Science Center at Brooklyn, 450 Clarkson Avenue, Brooklyn, NY 11203, USA

*Michael H. Levi*
Division of Microbiology and Immunology, Department of Pathology, Montefiore Medical Center, Albert Einstein College of Medicine, 111 East 210th Street, Bronx, NY 10467, USA

*Larry I. Lutwick*
Division of Infectious Diseases, Maimonides Medical Center, 4802 Tenth Avenue, Brooklyn, NY 11219, USA

*Suzanne M. Lutwick*
Department of Infection Control, Maimonides Medical Center, 4802 Tenth Avenue, Brooklyn, NY 11219, USA

*Constance Mangone*
Department of Pharmacy, Maimonides Medical Center, 4802 Tenth Avenue, Brooklyn, NY 11219, USA

*Octavio Maragni*
Department of Pharmacy, Maimonides Medical Center, 4802 Tenth Avenue, Brooklyn, NY 11219, USA

*Ida M. Onorato*
Surveillance and Epidemiologic Investigation Branch, Division of Tuberculosis Elimination, National Center for Prevention Services, Centers for Disease Control and Prevention, Public Health Service, United States Department of Health and Human Services, 1600 Clifton Road, E–10, Atlanta, GA 30333, USA

*Edward L. Pesanti*
Medical Service Veterans Administration Medical Center, Newington, CT, and Division of Infectious Diseases, University of Connecticut Health Center School of Medicine, Farrington, CT, USA

*Neal Rairden*
Department of Pharmacy, Maimonides Medical Center, 4802 Tenth Avenue, Brooklyn, NY 11219, USA

*Orlando Schaening*
Division of Infectious Diseases, Maimonides Medical Center, 4802 Tenth Avenue, Brooklyn, NY 11219, USA

*Douglas V. Sepkowitz*
Maimonides Medical Center, 4802 Tenth Avenue, Brooklyn, NY 11219, USA

*Kent A. Sepkowitz*
Infectious Diseases Service, Memorial Sloan-Kettering Cancer Center, 1275 York Avenue, New York, NY 10021, USA

*Rosemary Smith*
Department of Pharmacy, Maimonides Medical Center, 4802 Tenth Avenue, Brooklyn, NY 11219, USA

*Annette J. Stahl Avicolli*
Department of Pharmacy, Maimonides Medical Center, 4802 Tenth Avenue, Brooklyn, NY 11219, USA

# Acknowledgements

Infectious disease is one of the great tragedies of living things – the struggle for existence between different forms of life. Man sees it from his own prejudiced point of view, but clams, oysters, insects, fish, flowers, tobacco, potatoes, tomatoes, fruit, shrubs, trees, have their own varieties of smallpox, measles, cancer or tuberculosis. Incessantly, the pitiless war goes on, without quarter or armistice – a nationalism of species against species.

But however secure and well-regulated civilized life may become, bacteria, Protozoa, viruses, infected fleas, lice, ticks, mosquitoes and bedbugs will always lurk in the shadows ready to pounce when neglect, poverty, famine, or war lets down the defenses. Even in normal times they prey on the weak, the very young and the very old, living along with us, in mysterious obscurity waiting their opportunities. About the only genuine sporting proposition that remains unimpaired by the relentless domestication of a once free-living human species is the war against these ferocious little creatures, which lurk in the dark corners and stalk us in the bodies of rats, mice and all kinds of domestic animals; which fly and crawl with the insects, and waylay us in our food and drink and even in our love.

Hans Zinsser (1934) *Rats, Lice and History*. Little, Brown and Co., Boston, MA, pp. 7, 13–14.

The literary example of Hans Zinsser is gratefully acknowledged by the editor. Dr Zinsser's ability to communicate medical information in an easily readable form sets an example of what should be aimed for, to generate a product which can be read, not just studied.

The authors wish to thank the following individuals for their collective assistance in the preparation of the chapters in this book: Nilda Barberi, Joyce Harris, Maria Rodriguez, Toby Sahm, Rosie Sanchez, Patricia Scurvin and Sanell Sickles. Acknowledgement must also be given to Lydia Friedman, James Verlander, Richard Patrimonio and Mary Doherty for their help in finding old journals and confirming citations and to Willie

Wood, the Maimonides Medical Center staff photographer, for all his assistance with many of the figures. Dr Valerie Altavas and Catherine Rice also deserve acknowledgement for their help and advice in various aspects of this work.

Thanks are due to Dr Timothy Brewer of the Infectious Diseases Unit of the Department of Medicine of Harvard Medical School, Boston, for reading the manuscript in advance of publication.

Finally, every project has its Atlas, carrying it on his back towards completion. The editor acknowledges this book's Atlas, Geri Rich, who almost singlehandedly brought all of the chapters into a form suitable for publication. Her visual and verbal input into this book were invaluable.

# Introduction

Larry I. Lutwick

. . . there is always some little thing that is too big for us . . . [1]

Every reader has a favorite source for quotations. For me, it is a small cockroach named Archy whose thoughts, adventures and interactions with a cat called Mehitabel are chronicled by Don Marquis. The observation in the opening quotation about 'always some little thing' is the quintessential statement for the infectious disease clinician. Although some pathogens are visible with the naked eye, some with the light microscope, some only with the electron microscope and others remain visually elusive (such as the hepatitis C agent), all are by necessity smaller than the infected or infested host.

One of these little things, *Mycobacterium tuberculosis*, has since early days been exacting a substantial toll of morbidity and mortality on humanity. Suspected tuberculous disease has been found in the bony remains of a Stone Age individual who lived about 6000 years ago [2]. Indeed, the disease is mentioned in the scriptures describing plagues that could afflict humanity:

The Lord will smite thee with consumption, and with fever, and with inflammation, and with fiery heat . . . and they shall pursue thee until thou perish [3].

The Industrial Revolution, bringing an increasing population into crowded cities, caused the infection to become epidemic. As described by Ryan in his excellent book, *The Forgotten Plague: How the Battle Against Tuberculosis was Won and Lost* [4], the London Bills of Mortality recorded that one in five deaths was caused by tuberculosis (TB) in the mid 1600s. By the turn of the 19th century, the worldwide death rate was 7 million with 50 million people openly infected. Numerous artists, writers, composers and statesmen were reported by Ryan [4] to have been afflicted with TB, including Chopin, Paganini, Rousseau, Goethe, Chekhov, Schiller, Keats, Shelley, Cardinal Richelieu and Sir Walter Scott. Indeed, the association between TB and creativity was such that it was thought that the disease could inspire genius, referred to as *spes phthisica* [4]. The disease inspired opera as well with the heroines of *La Bohème* and *La Traviata* based on consumptive beauties.

A recent interview with Paul Sledzik, a curator at the National Museum of Health and Medicine in Washington, DC, illustrated the role of TB in superstition [5]. Folklore in New England existing as late as 1892 led relatives of persons who died of TB to mutilate the corpses in their graves. This practice was based on the belief that tuberculous individuals, wasting away with their consumption, were victims of vampires. After death, the remains were mutilated to prevent the 'vampires' from draining life force from the living. The 'stake through the heart' methodology was apparently a European tradition not practiced in the USA.

This book has been developed in direct response to the current rise in TB and the increase in multi-drug-resistant infection in the developed world. It is aimed to be not only a primer in TB for the primary care physician but also a reference for the internist and infectious disease clinician. The areas covered include: history; epidemiology; clinical disease in adults, children and HIV-infected patients; microbiology; tuberculin skin testing; infection control and prevention; drugs and treatment for standard and resistant disease; and infection with nontuberculous mycobacteria.

The time required to assemble a book may mean that by the date of publication the information may be incomplete or out of date. This is likely to occur in the present case because the changes in the epidemiology and resistance patterns of *M. tuberculosis* have caused a recent extraordinary increase in attention on the infection. Examples of recent publications regarding microbiology include reports of the description of the molecular basis of isoniazid effect and resistance [6] and the identification of *M. tuberculosis* genome fragments which confer intracellular entry and increased macrophage survival [7]. Reports of new technology for the detection of drug susceptibilities include the use of recombinant mycobacteriophages that introduce the luciferase gene into mycobacteria which then produce light if not drug inhibited [8] and the automated detection of rifampin resistance using polymerase chain reaction and single strand conformation polymorphism analysis [9].

Osler and McCrae's textbook of medicine [10] has a message to the practitioner regarding TB which is still quite applicable decades later:

> The leadership of the battle against this scourge is in your hands. Much has been done, much remains to do. By early diagnosis and prompt, systematic treatment of individual cases, by striving in every possible way to improve the social condition of the poor, by joining actively in the work of the local and national antituberculosis societies you can help in the most important and the most hopeful campaign ever undertaken by the profession.

It is clear that prompt and strict attention to appropriate TB isolation and control methodology is the most important factor in the control of the epidemic. Increasing the funds from governmental agencies to TB control is paramount for achieving this goal. It has been pointed out [11] that, curiously, it was not the world public health institutions that revived the global recognition of TB but rather the World Bank. Despite the fact that 12% of the US gross national product is spent on health care [11], the amount spent on prevention is disappointingly small. The World Health Organization estimates that if the amount of aid spent on TB treatment programs could be increased from 15 to 100 million dollars yearly, then 1.2 million deaths every year could be avoided [12].

In the end, as Bloom and Murray [11] so aptly state, the fundamental principle of infectious disease control was best articulated in 1513 by the political scientist Machiavelli:

It happens then as it does to physicians in the treatment of Consumption which in the commencement is easy to cure and difficult to understand; but when it has neither been discovered in due time nor treated upon a proper principle, it becomes easy to understand and difficult to cure. The same thing happens in state affairs; by foreseeing them in a distance, which is only done by men of talents, the evils which might arise from them are soon cured; but when, from want of foresight, they are suffered to increase to such a height that they are perceptible to everyone, there is no longer any remedy.

N. Machiavelli, *The Prince.*

I sincerely hope that those who make the decisions regarding the allocation of funds for TB control at all levels (global, national and local, including each individual health care delivery system) do not continue the short sighted thought processes that have brought TB to the height at which it now exists.

## REFERENCES

1. Marquis, D. (1929) *Archy and Mehitabel.* Doubleday, Doran and Co., Garden City, New York.
2. Formicola, V., Milanesi, Q. and Scarsini, C. (1987) Evidence of spinal tuberculosis at the beginning of the fourth millenium BC from Arene Candide Cave (Liguria, Italy). *Am J Phys Anthropol,* **72**, 1–6.
3. *Deuteronomy* XXVIII:22.
4. Ryan, F. (1992) *The Forgotten Plague: How the Battle against Tuberculosis was Won and Lost.* Little, Brown, and Co., Boston, MA.
5. Associated Press (1993) New Englanders 'killed' corpses, experts say. *New York Times,* 31 October 1993, p. 36.
6. Banerjee, A., Dubnau, E., Quemard, A. *et al.* (1994) *inhA*, a gene encoding a target for isoniazid and ethionamide in *Mycobacterium tuberculosis. Science,* **263**, 227–30.

7. Arruda, S., Bomfim, G., Knights, R. *et al.* (1993) Cloning of an *M. tuberculosis* DNA fragment associated with entry and survival inside cells. *Science*, **261**, 1457–7.

8. Jacobs, W.R., Barletta, R.G., Udani, R. *et al.* (1993) Rapid assessment of drug susceptibilities of *Mycobacterium tuberculosis* by means of luciferase reporting phages. *Science*, **260**, 819–22.

9. Telenti, A., Imboden, P., Marchesi, F. *et al.* (1993) Direct, automated detection of rifampin-resistant *Mycobacterium tuberculosis* by polymerase chain reaction and single-strand conformation polymorphism analysis. *Antimicrobial Agents Chemotherap*, **37**, 2054–8.

10. Osler, W. and McCrae, T. (1922) Tuberculosis, in *The Principles and Practice of Medicine*, D. Appleton and Co., New York, pp. 231.

11. Bloom, B.R. and Murray, C.J.L. (1992) Tuberculosis: commentary on a re-emergent killer. *Science*, **257**, 1055–64.

12. Reuters (1993) Agency cites urgent need to fight increase in TB. *New York Times*, 16 November 1993, p. C8.

# A history of tuberculosis  |  2

Edward L. Pesanti

'Tis called the evil:
A most miraculous work in this good king;
Which often since my here-remain in England
I have seen him do. How he solicits heaven,
Himself best knows; but strangely visited people,
All swollen and ulcerous, pitiful to the eye,
The mere despair of surgery, he cures,
Hanging a golden stamp about their necks,
Put on with holy prayers; and 'tis spoken,
To the succeeding royalty he leaves
The healing benediction.

*Macbeth*, IV, iii, 146

## 2.1 THE KING'S TOUCH (TUBERCULOUS LYMPHADENITIS)

Thus did Shakespeare describe the medieval healing of scrofulous subjects by the kings of England. The 'king's touch', supplemented in earlier years with the issuance of a gold coin, was an old tradition at the time of Shakespeare, variously attributed to Edward the Confessor or Clovis the Great (depending on whether the writer lived on the English or French side of the English Channel). Queen Anne (1665–1714) is said to have discontinued the custom though the rite remained in the *English Book of Common Prayer* for another half century [1]. While there may have been trepidations at discontinuance of the custom, it appears that the gold coin was quite as important as the royal touch because '. . . many that have been touched, have upon loss of their Gold felt returns of their Malady, which upon recovery of that have vanished' [2]. While Wiseman, in 1696, went to great pains to establish the pre-eminence of the English monarch in this therapeutic endeavor [2], Lowe, in 1597, failed to mention the royal cure in his chapter on scrofula [3]. It is difficult to imagine that the author of the first surgical text written in English was unfamiliar with the custom. It is more likely that prudence and the adage suggesting that silence is preferable to derogatory comments were the main influences on Lowe.

Royal families did not attempt to cure other forms of tuberculosis (TB). At the time, scrofula and phthisis were not recognized as related illnesses. Of all forms of TB, scrofula is the one most likely to give the appearance of having been cured by the king's touch. This form of TB occurred mostly in those with intact cellular immunity [4,5]. After the advent of effective TB therapy, the need for therapy after excision of scrofulous nodes still needed to be addressed [6,7]. In the 1950s, excision of the nodes was considered by some to be curative. Indeed, like the king's touch, excision did cure scrofula. That a large fraction of patients went on to develop and, before effective drugs, die of TB would not have been thought relevant to treatment of the initial condition. It is likely that in most patients scrofula did not recur.

Dubos noted that 'the persistence for several centuries of this treatment is at once testimony to the power of the placebo effect, the gullibility of patients, physicians (and monarchs), and the deep human need to feel that we can modify nature's course' [8]. It is, on a positive note, testimony to careful observation. Although they may have erred in assigning causality to royal intervention, the medieval physicians and royalty did recognize a disease process that could be brought into remission. It was not until after the discovery of the tubercle bacillus that consumption and scrofula were accepted as being related conditions with the same causation.


## 2.2 HISTORICAL PERSPECTIVES

Many excellent surveys of the history of TB have been published, with the classic *The White Plague* [8] having been recently reprinted. An attempt to condense in this single chapter what more adept authors have stated in books would be fruitless. Thus, I will attempt to review, for the general reader, the approach to TB therapy through the ages, with a focus on the evolution of current therapy.

The treatment of phthisis or consumption has been a major concern throughout the history of medicine. Hippocrates discussed phthisis in *The Epidemics* [9]. While it is likely that many of the patients did indeed have TB, it is equally likely that most did not. Most cases were of an acute illness, with prominent delirium, terminating within a few days. Such a course can occur in TB, but cannot be considered typical. Without a known causative agent, it must be assumed that only some patients considered by Hippocrates (and most of his successors until the current century) to have consumption really had illness caused by *Mycobacterium tuberculosis*.

## 2.3 IMPACT OF TUBERCULOSIS ON MORTALITY

Before discussing the approaches to the cure of TB, it is worthwhile to review the magnitude of its impact on human mortality. Sydenham in 1682 stated that phthisis kills 'two thirds of those who die of chronic diseases' [10]. At the beginning of the 19th century, approximately 20% of the deaths in cities in Massachusetts were attributed to TB [11]. The TB mortality rate in European cities of that era was 500–800/100 000/year [12]. In 1892, Osler quotes a German saying 'jedermann hat am Ende ein bischen Tuberculose' (every man at the end has a little tuberculosis) and goes on to review his data indicating that 22% of patients died of TB and another 6% died of other causes with active TB [13]. On both sides of the Atlantic Ocean, TB was the leading cause of non-accidental death. It appears that in cities, if skin tests were available, almost all would have been positive. Grigg has estimated that such a prevalence of infected persons would have been needed for the death rate seen in 1800–1850 [12]. Throughout the 20th century, the number of cases and the death rate have declined dramatically in the USA (Figure 2.1) and Europe [8,14,15].

The rate of decline was roughly exponential, but follows more closely a curve defined by a Gompertz equation, which is used by actuaries to estimate life expectancy (Figure 2.2) [17]. It is not clear that any medical interventions had an impact on prevalence [12], as has been noticed for several major infectious diseases [15]. Certainly, sanatorium supporters could have pointed to the decline in death rate between 1900 and 1950 as evidence of the efficacy of the treatment, a decline that is much more striking when plotted on a simple arithmetic scale (Figure 2.3).

## 2.4 HISTORY OF TUBERCULOSIS THROUGH TREATMENT

It is perhaps simplest to divide the approach to TB treatment into three eras. At all times, the current fashionable concepts of disease pathogenesis were blended into the approach. For the sake of simplicity, the periods may be considered as follows.

1. The classical approach. Various sensible and nonsensical, but always dogmatic, approaches were combined. Bloodletting had a central role from Hippocrates [9] until the 20th century. When chemistry became a thriving enterprise, these approaches were combined with 'specifics', most of which are, from our current vantage point, frightening and ridiculous.
2. Sanatoria. Intertwined with this therapy was an aggressive surgical approach typified by thoracoplasty and other, usually disfiguring, operative interventions.
3. Chemotherapy. Although chemical intervention was available long before effective chemotherapy, this era may be considered to have

begun with the discovery that sulfanilamide was active against TB infection in 1938 [18]. It should be noted that discovery of truly effective chemotherapy occurred over 50 years after the identity of the organism was established by Koch in 1882 [19].

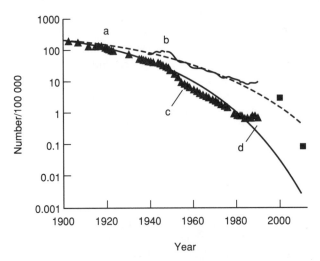

**Figure 2.1** The decline in US morbidity and mortality due to TB during the 20th century. The calculated values (extrapolated back from the earliest national estimates for morbidity available to the author) were calculated by the Gompertz equation to give the best fit to the morbidity and mortality during the non-war years. Note that (a) World War I and/or the influenza pandemic of 1917 and (b) World War II led to increased morbidity and mortality, even in the USA, in which there was no actual combat. Also evident is (c) the decline in TB mortality with the advent of chemotherapy and (d) the rise in mortality above the calculated curve with the appearance of AIDS. If the Gompertz curves are reasonable ways to plot the data, it is also evident that availability of chemotherapy had no noticeable impact on the incidence of the disease. The ACET goals (solid squares) [16] are the goals of the Advisory Committee for the Elimination of Tuberculosis. If the calculated curves are reasonable estimates of the natural decline of the disease, the 'goals' will probably be met. HIV infection can be expected to thwart attempts to eradicate tuberculosis. Deaths: solid triangle, published; solid line, calculated. Cases: solid line, published; dotted line, calculated.

### 2.4.1 Classical approach

The treatment of TB patients relied for centuries on various combinations of dietary restrictions, choice of proper climate and cough palliation. Hippocrates treated febrile patients with a combination of purgatives, bloodletting and his mainstay of therapeutics, ptisan, a thin barley mash. Although not mentioned in any source of which I am aware, such a mash may have supported fermentation in the warm Aegean climate. The feeling of well being derived from ingestion of suitably fermented barley is still widely appreciated.

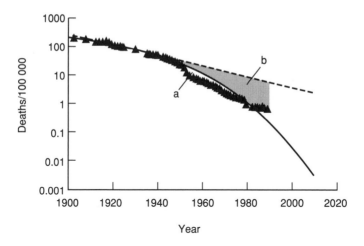

**Figure 2.2** This figure is included to illustrate the dependence of estimates of the impact of chemotherapy of TB statistics on the method chosen to estimate the trends of change in incidence or, in this figure, deaths. If a simple exponential decline (dashed line) is assumed, the impact of therapy is greatly exaggerated (b) compared with the apparent effect when (a) the actuarial formula, the Gompertz equation (solid line), is used. Both curves fit the observed data well, but the less complex equation may overestimate the impact of therapy on mortality. Published data are represented by solid triangles.

Lowe succinctly summarizes the classical approach to the TB cure with 'the cure consisteth in remedies universals and perticuler as in good regiment, eate litle of light digestion, abstaine from such things as ingender grosse humors, purge oft, blede in both thy armes, haunt no humide places . . .' and drink a herbal tea [3]. All therapeutic approaches were founded on the physician's view of the cause of the disease. When phthisis was viewed as derived from atmospheric imbalances, climatic interventions were stressed. When imbalance of bodily humors was emphasized, restoration of balance, usually by bloodletting (today we might use plasmapheresis or leukopheresis), was emphasized.

A common dietary admonition was avoidance of meat and alcohol, presumably based on the well known effects of those compounds on the critical balance of the humours. Hippocrates agreed that beef was harmful in most acute infections, but felt that properly cooked pork was highly salutary [9]. The wasting characteristic of chronic infections was long recognized as a bad prognostic sign. Some physicians, including Osler, felt that therapy should be directed primarily toward reversing the nutritional decline, even to the point of tube feeding if the patient could not cooperate [13]. With the increasing use of bloodletting in medical therapeutics, most of the renowned 18th and 19th century physicians advocated vigorous, and presumably in many cases lethal, bloodletting.

Some aspects of TB therapy, while of dubious efficacy, were at least

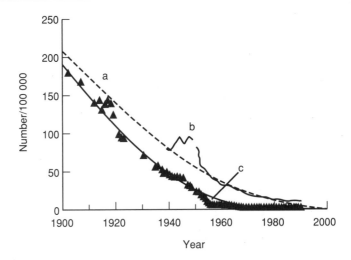

**Figure 2.3** This figure contains the same data depicted in Figures 2.1 and 2.2, but plotted on a linear scale. While the rate of TB decline has probably been relatively constant throughout the 20th century, the decline in numbers of cases is far smaller in the chemotherapy era than it had been at the beginning of the century. (It is easy to notice that 5% of 1000 is a larger number than 5% of 10.) Far fewer people were dying of TB at the beginning of the chemotherapy era than were dying of the disease in 1900, even accounting for the growing population. On this scale, the impact of (a) World War I and (b) World War II on mortality and morbidity are more evident and (c) the impact of chemotherapy and AIDS much less evident than in the previous plots. Deaths: solid line, published data; dashed line, calculated values. Cases: solid triangles, published data; solid line, calculated values.

pleasant. The beneficial effects of a pleasant climate had been generally accepted. Most doctors recommended some combination of mild, sanguine climates with clear mountain or salt air and pine forests. Since the authors (British, French, German and even Persian [20]), generally lived in crowded, malodorous urban centers – the gutters of the streets laden with the 'morning toast' [21] from emptied chamber pots – it seemed obvious to them that the air was not favorable to the healing of a lung affliction. Retirement to a salubrious climate was recommended widely. One of the most appealing, if similarly ineffective, cures was proposed by Sydenham [10], who stated variously that 'of all the remedies that I know, nothing so cherishes and strengthens the blood and spirits, as riding on horseback, long distances, every day . . . Riding is as good in a decline or in a phthisis as in hypochondriasis'. It is difficult to imagine how such an astute clinician would have concluded that 'bark is no surer a cure for ague, than riding for phthisis'.

By 1800, TB therapy appeared to be based on 'removal to a warm climate', abstention from 'spiritous liquors' and meat, and symptomatic treatment of cough with sweet concoctions, supplemented, if necessary, with 'tinctura opia camphorata' [22]. Except for bloodletting, this summarized the 18th century approach, little changed from that applied in ancient Greece.

With the development of chemistry as a science in the 19th century, a variety of specific treatments were introduced to the therapeutic armamentarium. Merely perusing the table of contents in Louis' book [23] illustrates the variety of therapeutic options:

'I. Protioduret of Iron; II. Chloride of Sodium; III. Subcarbonate of Potass; IV. Sal ammoniac; V. Chloride of Lime; VI. Chlorine gas; VII. Digitalis; VIII. Hydrocyanic Acid; IX. Creosote; X. Iodine'.

While the author is appropriately skeptical about the value of the remedies, he devotes considerable text to them, suggesting widespread use.

While most of the remedies proposed as specifics have fallen into disuse for the treatment of respiratory infections, the use of creosote, a derivative of wood tar, has persisted for almost 200 years. Although native creosote is not readily available as a medicine, one of the first creosote phenols to be synthesized, guaiacol, is widely available as the glycerin ester guaifenesin or glycerol guaiacolate (Figure 2.4). The compound is still used for its original purpose of easing chronic coughs. I have not found a clinical trial that documents that the compound does anything for a cough, but I have not walked into a drug store that did not have several brands of guafenesin-containing syrup prominently displayed.

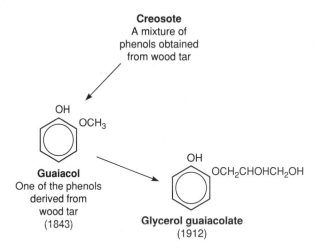

**Creosote**
A mixture of
phenols obtained
from wood tar

**Guaiacol**
One of the phenols
derived from
wood tar
(1843)

**Glycerol guaiacolate**
(1912)

**Figure 2.4** The persistence of creosote derivatives in the medical armamentarium is either a tribute to their effectiveness as cough remedies or in Dubos' words, 'testimony to the power of the placebo effect, the gullibility of patients, physicians (and monarchs), and the deep human need to feel that we can modify nature's course' [8]. The route from a popular remedy for TB (creosote) to a more refined version for the same indication (guaiacol) to a widely used cough syrup ingredient (guaifenesin or glycerol guaiacolate) is a short one, with no side trails. The acceptability of wood tar distillates in therapy is unfettered by the usual controlled trials that have characterized the chemotherapy era in TB treatment.

### 2.4.2 Sanatoria

With the development of drug therapy and advancements in medical technology, came the movement to provide the benefits of nutrition, rest and clean air for as many TB patients as possible in sanatoria. In 1854, Brehmer founded a sanatorium in Germany that came to be emulated by numerous others [1]. Dettweiler, in 1876, founded a sanatorium which emphasized the value of fresh air and rest. He also felt that wine and cognac were of value in the therapy of TB patients.

This type of sanatorium, situated in the Alps, with elegant rooms and meals was the scene for Mann's *The Magic Mountain*. The young protagonist in the story, Hans Castorp, spent seven years recovering sufficiently from TB to be last seen running through the cannon fire on a World War I battleground. A daily ritual at the Davos, Switzerland sanatorium was rest in the fresh air, warm or cold.

'As he lay there above the glittering valley, lapped in the bodily warmth preserved to him by fur and wool, in the frost night illumined by the brilliance from a lifeless star, the image of life displayed itself to young Hans Castorp' [24].

Herr Castorp's cure was based entirely on an effort to stimulate the natural healing powers, as pharmaceuticals were thought to be of little import. Work was not permitted, but, judging from Herr Castorp's skiing, exercise was permitted.

The American sanatorium began with Trudeau, who went to the Adirondacks expecting to die from TB two years after graduation from medical school. He improved, worsened again on moving back to the city, and improved again at Saranac Lake. By 1885, Dr Trudeau was able to admit the first two patients to the cottages he had constructed. The current Trudeau Institute, a research facility, uses the same grounds that served as the sanatorium until well into the modern chemotherapy era. In 1891, Bowditch established a sanatorium in Massachusetts, in a location that offered neither mountain air nor pine forests. Similarly, in the 1890s, sanatoria were opened in Great Britain, with facilities being located in Edinburgh (1894) and at the Brompton Hospital in London (1904). At the latter hospital, unlike the facility in *The Magic Mountain*, the treatment involved graded amounts of manual labor, probably to the benefit of the patients and certainly to the benefit of the institution. What detrimental effect the enforced inactivity in other institutions may have had on the patients' recovery was never considered. With minor, and usually inconsequential variations, these sanatoria were mimicked throughout the world (Figure 2.5) and served as the sites of treatment of TB until recently. During the period of sanatorium treatment, US TB mortality declined precipitously (Figure 2.1). In absolute numbers, the decline in death rate during the sanatorium era was substantial and much greater than subsequent improvements.

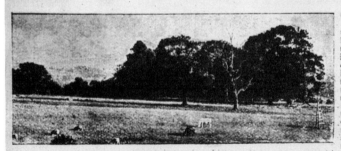

## VALE OF CLWYD SANATORIUM.

THIS Sanatorium is established for the treatment of Tuberculosis of the Lungs and of the Pleural Cavities. It is situated in the midst of a large area of parkland at a height of 450 feet above sea level, on the south-west slopes of mountains rising to over 1,800 feet, which protect it from north and east winds and provide many miles of graduated walks with magnificent views.

**Fully-trained Nurses.** Nurse on duty all night. X-Ray apparatus newly installed. Every facility for treatment by Artificial Pneumothorax. Electric lighting in every room. Heating by Radiators. For particulars apply to Medical Superintendent, H. MORRISTON DAVIES, M.D.Cantab., F.R.C.S., Llandebr Hall, Ruthin, N. Wales.

**Figure 2.5** An advertisement for a tuberculosis sanatorium published in *Tubercle*, Volume 1, 1919.

In the period during which sanatoria flourished, major advances in medical technology appeared. It was during this period that *M. tuberculosis* was found to be the causative agent of all forms of TB and X-rays were discovered. Although not therapeutically valuable, as Koch had initially declared [13,14], tuberculin was found to be a useful aid in diagnosing infection with the bacterium [25]. Aided by X-rays, surgeons were brought into the efforts to assist recovery from TB [1,26]. Following original attempts in the 19th century, pneumothorax and pneumoperitoneum (Figure 2.6) became almost invariable accompaniments to the sanatorium treatment of TB. These and subsequent attempts were based on the intuitively obvious observation that the negative intrathoracic pressure of breathing contributed to, or caused, the development and growth of cavities. At best pneumothorax was associated with sustained improvement in less than half the patients. No trial was performed comparing pneumothorax with placebo [26].

During the same period, phrenic nerve paralysis was employed, using a variety of techniques. This approach never gained the stature of pneumothorax. Faced with the less than spectacular results of simple instillation of gas into the thoracic space, more aggressive surgical approaches were developed. Plombage, collapse of the lungs by instillation of gas, paraffin, bone, rubber bags, muscle, or oil, into an extrapleural space to collapse the entire thoracic cavity, was also employed.

During this time, surgical techniques were rapidly improving such that thoracoplasty and, eventually, pulmonary resection displaced simple pneumothorax or pneumoperitoneum [1,26]. With experience, thoracoplasty was associated with an operative mortality said to be less than 2% and cure rates said to be greater than 80%. Again, I can find no mention of studies that rigorously establish the efficacy of the procedure and, as is often the case in such surgical procedures, long-term data are not available. In

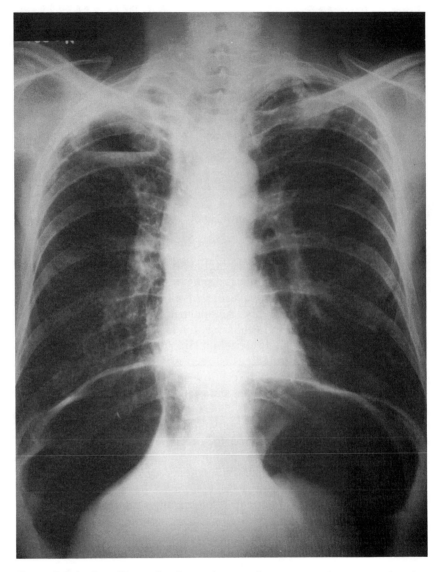

**Figure 2.6** A chest X-ray showing a therapeutic pneumoperitoneum and active upper lobe pulmonary TB.

1936, the first successful lobectomy and first successful pneumonectomy for TB were reported [26]. These procedures were accomplished by tourniquet ligation of the hilum. According to a nurse of the period quoted by Gaensler, 'either the patient suddenly turned blue and died because the bronchial stump had blown, or the patient suddenly turned white and died when the artery had blown' [26].

The procedure for individually ligating the various components of the hila was developed during the 1940s. These methods greatly reduced the hazards of the operations, permitting extension of operative intervention to a wider population of patients. Plombage did not, however, disappear quickly. With the availability of plastics in the 1950s, extraperiosteal plombage using hollow plastic spheres (ping-pong balls) became a preferred procedure. Thus, by the time that effective chemotherapy appeared, attempts to reduce the burden of *M. tuberculosis* by mechanical means had reached a high state of sophistication. Subsequently, surgery for pulmonary TB become rare and is reserved for unique cases which cannot be dealt with by drugs. The current increase in multi-drug-resistant TB may increase the role for surgery in pulmonary TB.

### 2.4.3 Chemotherapy

Medicine has long sought a specific treatment for phthisis. It seems a safe conclusion that anything that worked for some febrile illness was heralded by someone as a cure for TB. At various times, digitalis, quinine, mercury, iodine and creosote were thought to have specific action against TB. Even Koch, caught up in the political and media events surrounding his announcement of the discovery of *M. tuberculosis* appears to have fallen prey to this quest for a 'holy grail' treatment. He announced in 1890 that tuberculin dramatically improved tuberculous guinea pigs. He and many others quickly brought tuberculin into clinical medicine. Within a short time, both the *Lancet* and the *British Medical Journal* published negative editorials about tuberculin and Osler in the first edition of his textbook stated that 'of twenty-three cases in which we have used it at the Johns Hopkins Hospital, only three were benefitted; in the others the action was either negative or actually detrimental' [13]. The search for an effective agent continued.

The first article documenting convincing activity of a drug against *M. tuberculosis* was published in 1938 [18]. Rich and Follis showed that sulfanilamide inhibited the growth of *M. tuberculosis* in guinea pigs. None of the animals was cured, however, and those given the highest doses suffered lethal toxicity. Obviously, a cure for the disease was not found, but experiments had suggested that chemotherapy was an achievable goal. Subsequent progress was rapid with a report of the activity of dapsone in 1940 [27], and the discovery of the activity of streptomycin in 1945 [28,29]. With amazing speed after the introduction of streptomycin, p-aminosalicylic acid (PAS), isoniazid and pyrazinamide were introduced into clinical practice.

The introduction of streptomycin into anti-TB therapy led to fundamental changes, not only in treatment, but also in how the medical profession evaluated its therapeutic agents. The American Trudeau Society and the Veterans Administration each organized a cooperative trial of streptomycin, where data from many physicians could be compiled into a single summary [30]. In England, the idea of the cooperative trial was enhanced further by the inclusion of controls, assigned by random processes, in the trial of streptomycin [31]. Rather than waste a scarce compound of uncertain efficacy in a series of uncontrolled trials, with possibly inconclusive results, the British Medical Research Council (MRC) directed its first supplies of streptomycin into randomized trials. Within a short time, the efficacy (and limitations) of the drug were obvious.

The approach used by the MRC has established a standard by which all subsequent studies of drugs can be compared. It was used in most subsequent trials of anti-TB therapy conducted by a variety of groups which have demonstrated [32,33] that: addition of a second drug (PAS) prevented the emergence of resistance during therapy with streptomycin [34]; combination therapy, using two or more effective agents, one of which was isoniazid, was almost universally effective [35]; when effective drugs were used, bed rest and sanatorium care were no longer necessary [33,36]; with effective therapy, it was not hazardous to send a TB patient home with acid-fast bacillus (AFB) positive sputum smears [37]; TB can be prevented by isoniazid (INH) use in patients whose only sign of the infection is a reactive tuberculin test [38]; effective therapy did not require that the drugs be given in divided doses [39] or even daily [40]; rifampin was more effective, and easier to administer, than streptomycin [41]; and the duration of therapy could be shortened from 2 years to as little as 6 months [42,43].

At each step, the proposed new regimen was directly compared with the previous 'best' regimen. Thus, although the trials were difficult to design and execute, they yielded unequivocal results and rapid progress in the design of drug regimens. TB treatment regimens are discussed in more detail in Chapter 12.

With the development of effective therapy, surgery for pulmonary TB was almost eliminated and most sanatoria closed. TB had been transformed from a relentlessly progressive, often fatal illness to an infection which responded to appropriate drugs. With the appearance of HIV infection, the decline in incidence and death rate caused by TB has stopped. In areas where HIV infection is widespread, a resurgence in TB morbidity and mortality is evident [16,44,45]. Complicating this is the appearance of multiple drug-resistant strains of *M. tuberculosis* [46–49], which make TB more difficult to cure with drugs, even in experienced centers [50]. These developments have forced society and medicine once again to deal with TB as a serious problem.

## REFERENCES

1. Keers, R.Y. (1978) *Pulmonary Tuberculosis. A Journey down the Centuries*, Baillière Tindall, London.
2. Major, R.H. (1965) *Classic Descriptions of Disease*, 3rd edn, Charles C. Thomas, Springfield, IL.

3. Lowe, P. (1597; reprinted 1981) *The Whole Course of Chirurgerie*, The Classics of Medicine Library, Birmingham, AL.
4. Iles, P.B. and Emerson, P.A. (1974) Tuberculous lymphadenitis. *Brit Med J*, **1**, 143–5.
5. Lenzini, L., Rottoli, P. and Rottoli, L. (1977) The spectrum of human tuberculosis. *Clin Exp Immunol*, **27**, 230–7.
6. Byrd, R.B., Kopp, R.K., Gracey, D.R. and Puritz, E.M. (1971) The role of surgery in tuberculous lymphadenitis in adults. *Am Rev Respir Dis*, **103**, 816–20.
7. Kent, D.C. (1967) Tuberculous lymphadenitis: not a localized disease process. *Am J Med Sci*, **254**, 866–73.
8. Dubos, R. and Dubos, J. (1952; reprinted 1992) *The White Plague. Tuberculosis, Man, and Society*, Rutgers University Press, New Brunswick, NJ.
9. Adams, F. (1849; reprinted 1985) *The Genuine Works of Hippocrates*, The Classics of Medicine Library, Birmingham, AL.
10. Latham, R.G. (1848; reprinted 1979) *The Works of Thomas Sydenham, M.D.*, The Classics of Medicine Library, Birmingham, AL.
11. Holmberg, S.D. (1990) The rise of tuberculosis in America before 1820. *Am Rev Respir Dis*, **142**, 1228–32.
12. Grigg, E.R.N. (1958) The arcana of tuberculosis. Part I–II. *Am Rev Tuberc Pulm Dis*, **78**, 151–72.
13. Osler, W. (1892; reprinted 1978) *The Principles and Practice of Medicine*. The Classics of Medicine Library, Birmingham, AL.
14. Lowell, A.M. (1966) A view of tuberculosis morbidity and mortality fifteen years after the advent of the chemotherapeutic era 1947–1962. *Adv Tuberc Res*, **15**, 55–124.
15. Gordis, L. (1985) The virtual disappearance of rheumatic fever in the United States: lessons in the rise and fall of disease. *Circulation*, 72, 1155–62.
16. Centers for Disease Control (1989) A strategic plan for the elimination of tuberculosis in the United States. *MMWR*, **38** (S-3), 1–25.
17. Batschelet, E. (1979) *Introduction to Mathematics for Life Sciences*, Springer, New York, pp. 301–33.
18. Rich, A.R. and Follis, R.H. (1938) The inhibitory effect of sulfanilamide on the development of experimental tuberculosis in the guinea pig. *Bull Johns Hopk Hosp*, **52**, 77–84.
19. Koch, R. (1961; reprinted 1975) The etiology of tuberculosis, in *Milestones in Microbiology*, American Society for Microbiology, Washington, DC, pp. 109–15.
20. Gruner, O.C. (1593; reprinted 1984) *A Treatise on the Canon of Medicine of Avicenna*, The Classics of Medicine Library, Birmingham, AL.
21. Dryden, J. (1970) Mac Flecknoe, in *The Norton Anthology of Poetry*, WW Norton, New York, pp. 160–5.
22. Heberden, W. (1802; reprinted 1982) *Commentaries on the History and Cure of Diseases*, The Classics of Medicine Library, Birmingham, AL.
23. Louis, P.C.A. (translated by W.H. Walshe) (1844; reprinted 1986) *Researches on Phthisis. Anatomical Pathological and Therapeutical*. The Classics of Medicine Library, Birmingham, AL.
24. Mann, T. (1955) *The Magic Mountain*, The Modern Library, Random House, New York, p. 276.
25. Von Pirquet, C.E. (1911) Allergy. *Arch Intern Med*, **7**, 383–436.

26. Gaensler, E.A. (1982) The surgery for pulmonary tuberculosis. *Chest*, **125S**, 73–84.
27. Rist, N., Bloch, F. and Hamon, V. (1940) Action inhibitrice du sulfamide et d'une sulfone sur la multiplication in vitro et in vivo du Bacille tuberculeux aviaire. *Ann Inst Pasteur*, **64**, 203–37.
28. Feldman, W.H., Hinshaw, H.C. and Mann, F.C. (1945) Streptomycin in experimental tuberculosis. *Am Rev Tuberc*, **52**, 269–98.
29. Hinshaw, H.C., Feldman, W.H. and Pfuetze, K.H. (1946) Treatment of tuberculosis with streptomycin: a summary of observations on one hundred cases. *JAMA*, **132**, 778–82.
30. Comroe, J.H. (1978) Pay dirt: the story of streptomycin. Part II. Feldman and Hinshaw, Lehman. *Am Rev Respir Dis*, **117**, 957–68.
31. British Medical Research Council. (1948) Streptomycin treatment of pulmonary tuberculosis. *Br Med J*, **2**, 769–82.
32. D'Esopo, N.D. (1982) Clinical trials in pulmonary tuberculosis. *Chest*, **125S**, 85–93.
33. Fox, W. (1968) The John Barnwell Lecture: Changing concepts in the chemotherapy of pulmonary tuberculosis. *Am Rev Respir Dis*, **97**, 767–90.
34. British Medical Research Council. (1950) Treatment of pulmonary tuberculosis with streptomycin and para-amino-salicylic acid. A Medical Research Council investigation. *Br Med J*, **2**, 1073–85.
35. British Medical Research Council (1952) The treatment of pulmonary tuberculosis with isoniazid. An interim report to the Medical Research Council by their Tuberculosis Chemotherapy Trials Committee. *Br Med J*, **2**, 735–46.
36. Hirsch, J.G., Schaedler, R.W., Pierce, C.H. and Smith, I.M. (1957) A study comparing the effects of bed rest and physical activity on recovery from pulmonary tuberculosis. *Am Rev Tuberc Pulm Dis*, **75**, 359–409.
37. Kamat, S.R., Dawson, J.J.Y., Devadatta, S. *et al.* (1966) A controlled study of the influence of segregation of tuberculous patients for one year on the attack rate of tuberculosis in a five year period in close family contacts. *Indian J Tuberc*, **14**, 11–23.
38. Ferebee, S.H. and Mount, F.W. (1962) Tuberculous morbidity in a controlled trial of the prophylactic use of isoniazid among household contacts. *Am Rev Respir Dis*, **85**, 490–521.
39. Wilson, J.L. and Lampe, W.T. (1964) Single daily dose regimen in the treatment of pulmonary tuberculosis. *Am Rev Respir Dis*, **89**, 756–9.
40. Sbarbaro, J.A. and Johnson, S. (1968) Tuberculous chemotherapy for recalcitrant outpatients administered directly twice weekly. *Am Rev Respir Dis*, **97**, 895–903.
41. Newman, R., Doster, B.E., Murray, F.J. and Woolpert, S.F. (1974) Rifampin in initial treatment of pulmonary tuberculosis. A U.S. Public Health Service tuberculosis therapy trial. *Am Rev Respir Dis*, **109**, 216–32.
42. East African/British Medical Research Councils (1972) Controlled clinical trial of short-course (6 month) regimens of chemotherapy for treatment of pulmonary tuberculosis. *Lancet*, **1**, 1079–85.
43. Fox, W. and Mitchison, D.A. (1975) Short-course chemotherapy for pulmonary tuberculosis. *Am Rev Respir Dis*, **111**, 325–53 (corrections 845–8).
44. Bloom, B.R. and Murray, C.J.L. (1992) Tuberculosis: commentary on a re-emergent killer. *Science*, **257**, 1055–64.

45. Slutkin, G., Leowski, J. and Mann, J. (1988) The effects of the AIDS epidemic on the tuberculosis problem and tuberculosis programmes. *Bull Int Union Tuberc Lung Dis*, **63**, 21–4.
46. Edlin, B.R., Tokars, J.I., Grieco, M.H. *et al.* (1992) An outbreak of multidrug-resistant tuberculosis among hospitalized patients with the Acquired Immunodeficiency Syndrome. *N Engl J Med*, **326**, 1514–21.
47. Shafer, R.W., Chirgwin, K.D., Glatt, A.E. *et al.* (1991) HIV prevalence, immunosuppression, and drug resistance in patients with tuberculosis in an area endemic for AIDS. *AIDS*, **5**, 399–405.
48. Pitchenik, A.E., Russell, B.W., Cleary, T. *et al.* (1982) The prevalence of tuberculosis and drug resistance among Haitians. *N Engl J Med*, **307**, 162–5.
49. Freiden, T.R., Sterling, T., Pablos-Mendez, A. *et al.* (1993) The emergence of drug-resistant tuberculosis in New York City. *N Engl J Med*, **328**, 521–6.
50. Goble, M., Iseman, M.D., Madsen, L.A. *et al.* (1993) Treatment of 171 patients with pulmonary tuberculosis resistant to isoniazid and rifampin. *N Engl J Med*, **328**, 527–32.

# 3 | Epidemiology of tuberculosis

Ida M. Onorato, Joseph H. Kent, Kenneth G. Castro

## 3.1 INTRODUCTION

At the beginning of this century, tuberculosis (TB) was the leading cause of death in the USA. The incidence of TB has declined steadily since the middle of the 19th century (Figure 3.1) owing to the isolation of patients in sanatoria, improved ventilation and nutrition. This decline led to predictions that TB would be eliminated in the USA. The first was by Wade Hampton Frost who believed that natural dynamics would eliminate transmission. In 1937, he said that 'under present conditions of human resistance and environment the tubercle bacillus is losing ground and the eventual eradication of tuberculosis requires only that the present balance against it be maintained' [1].

With the introduction of streptomycin in 1947 and para-aminosalicylic acid in 1949, the downward trend in morbidity and mortality continued. With the subsequent discovery in 1952 of isoniazid (INH), used for treatment and chemoprophylaxis, the incidence of TB had dropped by 75% in the 1950s and specific TB hospitals became unnecessary. Participants in the 1959 Arden House Conference felt that the new anti-TB drugs were the 'magic bullet' that would eliminate the infection [2]. In fact, over the years the number of US counties that had reported no cases of TB had increased from 20% in 1964 to 39% in 1991 [National Centers for Disease Control and Prevention (CDC), unpublished data].

In 1984, Dr James Mason, then Director of the CDC, challenged the public health community to eliminate TB [3]. The elimination was felt to be a realistic goal because '(1) tuberculosis is retreating into geographically and demographically defined pockets; (2) biotechnology now has the potential for generating better diagnostic, treatment, and prevention modalities; and (3) computer, telecommunications, and other technologies can enhance technology transfer'. An Advisory Committee was formed and in 1989 the

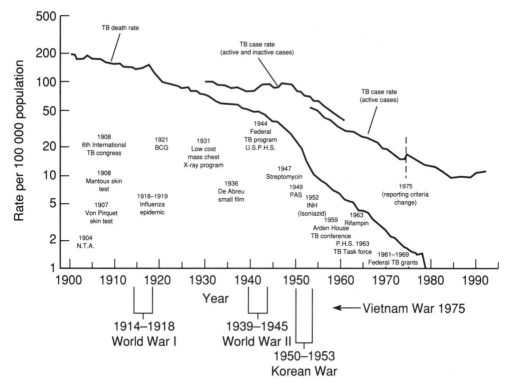

**Figure 3.1** TB case rates and death rates in the USA since 1990.

committee put forth a plan that was felt to be realistic for the elimination of TB by the year 2010 [3]. Elimination was defined as an incidence of less than 1 case per million population, or approximately 300 cases per year. An interim target of 35 cases per million population was set for the year 2000. Support for the plan was substantial with major professional groups endorsing the idea. Many indicators suggested that TB elimination was feasible.

In 1985, however, the long standing decline in incidence ceased and the number of cases of TB began to increase. This increase has continued and heralds a new era in the US history of the infection. In this new era, the demography of TB infected persons has changed and new risks for acquiring the tubercle bacillus and for adverse clinical outcomes have appeared.

## 3.2 THE NATIONAL TUBERCULOSIS SURVEILLANCE SYSTEM

### 3.2.1 Surveillance development

In the USA national surveillance for TB is carried out by the CDC under the Public Health Service Act. TB is a reportable disease in all states and territories of the US, the District of Columbia and Puerto Rico. The CDC considers the modern era of TB surveillance to have begun in 1951 when the Public Health Service convened a committee to study the problems of disease reporting and to decide on a plan for standardized national reporting [4]. Although TB had been reportable for almost 30 years, there had been so little agreement on definitions of reportability or uniformity in reporting practices that data obtained had been of little use in determining trends or in planning control programs. The committee devised a standard case definition for reporting and this definition was adopted by all state health departments in the next two years. Since 1953, there have been two other major modifications in the definition of a reportable case of TB. These changes were also accepted by all health departments. Therefore, TB surveillance trends have been calculated from 1953 onward based on standardized case reporting.

### 3.2.2 Case definition

The following case definition for surveillance was published recently [5]. A confirmed case of TB is one that is laboratory confirmed or, in the absence of laboratory confirmation, a case that meets the clinical case definition. Laboratory criteria for diagnosis include one of the following:

- *Mycobacterium tuberculosis* isolation from a clinical specimen
- demonstration of *M. tuberculosis* from a clinical specimen by DNA probe or mycolic acid pattern on high pressure liquid chromatography
- demonstration of acid-fast bacillus (AFB) in a clinical specimen when a culture has not been or cannot be obtained.

For cases that lack bacteriologic confirmation, all elements of the clinical case definition must be met:

- a positive tuberculin skin test
- other signs and symptoms compatible with TB, such as an abnormal, unstable (worsening or improving) chest X-ray, or clinical evidence of current disease
- treatment with two or more anti-TB medications and completed diagnostic evaluation.

Persons who have had TB diagnosed more than one year previously and who have recurred are counted as new cases.

In the USA, persons suspected of having TB are reported by physicians, laboratories, hospitals, schools, nursing homes and other reporting sources to the local health departments [6,7]. Persons and agencies required by law to report suspected cases vary in different states. Suspected cases are then investigated by the local health department and, if confirmed, are reported to the CDC. Since 1985, an individual case report form (Report of a Verified Case of Tuberculosis (RVCT form)) has been submitted to CDC for each confirmed case. In 1993, in response to the increase in TB cases and the need for better epidemiologic data to determine the causes of this rise, the surveillance system was expanded and the RVCT form was revised to include other data. Data elements collected since January 1993 include risks for acquisition of TB, such as HIV test results, alcoholism, drug use, residence in a chronic care facility or prison, homelessness, and certain occupations (migrant agricultural worker, health care worker, correctional facility personnel). The new RVCT form also collects information about drug susceptibility testing, treatment regimens and the form and outcome of therapy.

### 3.2.3 Reporting mechanisms

In practice, TB surveillance in the USA has been largely by passive methods. The most common reporting source in most states is the public health laboratory. Among all adult TB cases reported to the CDC in 1991, 85% were confirmed by culture (Table 3.1) [CDC, unpublished data]. Another 3% of cases had a positive AFB smear or a pathologic diagnosis of infection. Of adult cases, 9% met the clinical case definition [5]. Of the cases reported to the CDC, 2% did not meet the published case definition but were diagnosed as TB by a care provider. For pediatric cases, only 23% were culture positive, reflecting the difficulties in obtaining specimens from children. The majority of cases in children met the clinical case definition, with 17% of cases not meeting any definition. It is not possible to evaluate whether cases that did not meet the definition failed to do so because they did not have TB or because insufficient information was submitted to the CDC to verify the case.

The completeness of reporting of TB cases is not known. A systematic survey of the completeness of reporting nationally has not been conducted. In the past, individual states and cities evaluated their own surveillance systems for completeness of case reporting. One study showed that 63% of TB cases were reported to the health department in Washington, DC in 1971, based on reviews of hospital discharge diagnoses [8]. Estimates by other local health departments ranging from 40% to 81% of cases were reported [9,10].

**Table 3.1** Case definitions of tuberculosis cases reported to the CDC from 53 reporting areas[a], 1991

| Case definition | Cases meeting case definition (%) | |
| --- | --- | --- |
| | *Adult* | *Pediatric* |
| Culture positive | 85 | 23 |
| Acid-fast bacillus smear positive or pathology diagnosis | 3 | 2 |
| Clinical case | 9 | 58 |
| Do not meet definition | 2 | 17 |

[a] Fifty states, District of Columbia, New York City and Puerto Rico.

## 3.3 TUBERCULOSIS INCIDENCE, 1985–1992

In 1953, 84 304 cases of TB were reported in the USA with an annual incidence of 53.0 cases per 100 000 population [11]. Since then, reported cases have declined substantially. The lowest number of cases occurred in 1985 when 22 201 were reported with an incidence of 9.3 cases per 100 000 population (Table 3.2) [12]. Annual rates have risen each year since 1985, so that in 1992, 26 673 cases were reported from the 50 states and the District of Columbia for an incidence of 10.5 cases per 100 000 population [13]. The overall increase of 4472 cases is a 20.1% increase since 1985 (Figure 3.2). From 1991 to 1992, cases increased by 1.5% (390 cases) [13]. In addition, in 1992, 312 cases were reported from Puerto Rico and 58 cases from American Samoa, the US Virgin Islands and other US territories. These cases are traditionally not included in the US case totals.

Another method of measuring the magnitude of the changes in the TB epidemic is to estimate the difference between the current number of cases observed and the number of cases predicted to occur if the declines of recent decades had continued. If the observed decline from 1981 to 1984 of an average annual decrease of 1706 cases or a decrease of 6.7% per year is assumed to be the trend that would have continued [14], then an excess of 51 700 TB cases has occurred since 1985 (Figure 3.3) [13]. The reasons for the change in trends are complex and require analysis of the demographic and risk factors of recent TB cases.

### 3.3.1 Geographic distribution

In 1992, as in 1985, cases were reported from all 50 states, the District of Columbia, Puerto Rico and the territories [13]. Increases in the number of cases reported were observed from 1991 to 1992 in 22 states and Puerto Rico, while decreased numbers of cases were seen in 27 states and the District of Columbia. Nebraska reported 28 cases in each year. Incidence rates ranged from a high of 25.2 cases per 100 000 population in North Carolina to a low of 1.2 in Vermont. Since 1985, the changes in the TB epidemic have been very focal, geographically. Significant increases in the number of reported cases occurred in only nine states (Georgia, Florida, New York, New Jersey, Texas, California, Washington, Nevada, Arizona). In these states, the changes have been dramatic, with nearly a doubling of cases in New York and New Jersey and a 54% increase in California (Table 3.3). Significant decreases occurred in 16 states.

TB is a disease of urban areas. Of cities with populations of 250 000 inhabitants or more, the highest number of cases (3811 cases) was reported from New York City with 52 cases per 100 000 population in 1992. The highest rate was reported from Atlanta, Georgia, with 78.2 cases per 100 000, followed by Newark, New Jersey, with 68.3 cases per 100 000 population. The lowest incidences reported for large cities were 1.5–2.3 cases per

**Table 3.2** Reported cases and rates of tuberculosis in the USA by sex, age group, race/ethnicity, and country of origin, 1985 and 1992

| Characteristic | Cases | | | Rate[a] | | |
|---|---|---|---|---|---|---|
| | 1985 | 1992 | Change (%) | 1985 | 1992 | Change (%) |
| Total | 22 201 | 26 673 | +20.1 | 9.3 | 10.5 | +12.9 |
| **Sex** | | | | | | |
| Male | 14 496 | 17 433 | +20.3 | 12.5 | 14.0 | +12.0 |
| Female | 7704 | 9236 | +19.9 | 6.3 | 7.1 | +12.7 |
| Unknown | 1 | 4 | –[b] | NA[c] | NA | |
| **Age group (years)** | | | | | | |
| 0–4 | 789 | 1074 | +36.1 | 4.4 | 5.5 | +25.0 |
| 5–14 | 472 | 633 | +34.1 | 1.4 | 1.7 | +21.4 |
| 15–24 | 1672 | 1974 | +18.1 | 4.2 | 5.5 | +31.0 |
| 25–44 | 6758 | 10 444 | +54.5 | 9.2 | 12.7 | +38.0 |
| 45–64 | 6138 | 6487 | +5.7 | 13.7 | 13.4 | –2.1 |
| ≥65 | 6356 | 6025 | –5.2 | 22.3 | 18.7 | –16.1 |
| Unknown | 16 | 36 | – | NA | NA | |
| **Race/Ethnicity** | | | | | | |
| White non-Hispanic | 8453 | 7618 | –9.9 | 4.5 | 4.0 | –11.1 |
| Black non-Hispanic | 7592 | 9623 | +26.8 | 23.0 | 31.7 | +37.8 |
| Hispanic | 3092 | 5397 | +74.5 | 21.4 | 22.4 | +4.7 |
| Asian/Pacific Islander | 2530 | 3698 | +46.2 | 41.6 | 46.6 | +12.0 |
| American Indian/ Alaskan Native | 397 | 305 | –23.2 | 18.9 | 16.3 | –13.8 |
| Unknown/Other[d] | 137 | 32 | – | NA | NA | |
| **Country of origin** | [e] | | | | | |
| Foreign born | 4925 | 7270 | +47.6 | NA | NA | |
| US born | 17 712 | 19 225 | +8.5 | NA | NA | |
| Unknown | 131 | 178 | – | NA | NA | |

[a] Per 100 000 population. Population by race/ethnicity are projections obtained from Bureau of Census (Source: Bureau of Census, Current Populations Reports Series, No. 1092, November 1992, p. 25).
[b] Not calculated.
[c] Denominator data not available.
[d] Includes Blacks and Whites of unknown ethnicity.
[e] Cases reported for 1986, the first year with uniform national reporting of country of origin for persons with TB.

100 000 population in cities in the Southwest and West. Compared with an overall US population TB case rate of 10.5 cases per 100 000 population, urban areas (defined as cities with 100 000 population or greater) had an incidence of 22 cases per 100 000 in 1992. In contrast, non-urban areas had a three-fold lower incidence of 6.5 cases per 100 000 population [13].

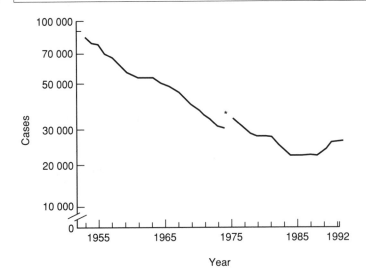

**Figure 3.2** Reported cases of TB in the USA 1953–1992.

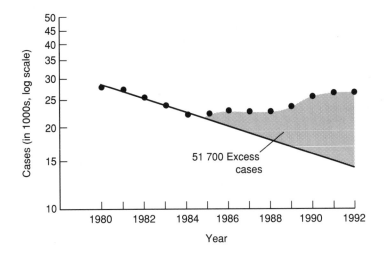

**Figure 3.3** Expected (solid line) and observed (solid circle) TB cases in the USA 1980–1992.

### 3.3.2 Age distribution

Since 1953, the age distribution of TB cases in the USA has increasingly shifted to peak in older age groups [15]. This cohort effect was consistent with the overall decline in case rates during this period. Decreasing primary transmission in younger age groups resulted in the majority of cases being due to reactivation. Infection was acquired by older persons

**Table 3.3** Reported tuberculosis cases by state, USA, 1985 and 1992

| State | Number of cases | | Change in cases | Percentage change |
|-------|------|------|------|------|
| | *1985* | *1992* | | *(%)* |
| New York | 2481 | 4574 | +2093 | +84.4 |
| California | 3491 | 5382 | +1891 | +54.2 |
| Texas | 1891 | 2510 | +619 | +32.7 |
| New Jersey | 545 | 984 | +439 | +80.6 |
| Florida | 1425 | 1707 | +282 | +19.8 |
| All others | 12 368 | 11 516 | −852 | −6.9 |
| Total | 22 201 | 26 673 | +4472 | +20.1 |

during their youth when TB was prevalent in the USA, reactivating later related to the longer life span of the population. By 1985, the median age of TB patients was 49 years. The elderly accounted for 29% of all cases (Table 3.2). Cases in young children (which signify recent TB acquisition) represented only 5.7% of the total.

As with most other epidemiologic trends, the age distribution of TB cases reversed from 1985 to 1992 (Table 3.2). While TB in the elderly continued to decrease, infections in younger age groups began to increase with the largest rise in persons 25–44 years of age. Since adults of child-bearing age have the most contact with their own and other children, a concomitant rise in cases was also seen in those 14 years of age and younger. In developing countries, annual surveys of tuberculin (PPD) skin test positivity in young children are used to estimate the annual risk of infection and are an index of the degree of transmission of TB in children [16,17]. Such surveys are not performed for this purpose in the USA. However, the occurrence of the disease in very young children signals recent acquisition of infection. From 1985 to 1992, TB cases in children 0–4 years of age have increased by 36% (Table 3.2) [13]. The greatest increases were in children born in the USA who were of Hispanic or Asian/Pacific Island origin. These cases may be a result of increased immigration of persons of childbearing age from countries where TB is highly endemic.

Differences exist in the age distribution of TB cases by race and ethnicity (Figure 3.4). In non-Hispanic Whites, the age group with the highest incidence in 1985 was the elderly but since then cases in elderly non-Hispanic Whites have continued to decline slowly while cases in 25–44 year olds have increased [CDC, unpublished data]. Among non-Hispanic Whites, the median age for TB cases fell from 62 years to 59 years from 1985 to 1992. The largest percentage increases in the number of reported cases have occurred in Blacks and Hispanics in the 25–44 age group. Reported cases have doubled in this age group since 1985 while remaining stable in the elderly. The median age of reported cases among Blacks decreased from 43 to 40 years from 1985 to 1992. Postulated reasons for this increase include the spread of HIV infection due to sexual transmission and parenteral drug use [18]. Among Hispanics, increased immigration of young adults is partially responsible for the downward trend in age distribution [19]. The median age of Hispanic TB patients born in the USA has been stable at 37 years, while the median age of foreign-born Hispanic cases is 32 years.

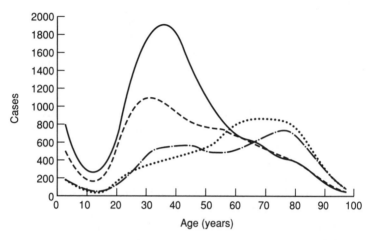

**Figure 3.4** TB cases among Blacks and Hispanics in 1985 (dashed line) and 1992 (solid line) compared with non-Hispanic Whites in 1985 (dotted line) and 1992 (dash dot dash line) in the USA.

### 3.3.3 Race and ethnicity

The dynamics of USA TB epidemiology have, in recent years, become increasingly divergent for different racial and ethnic groups [20–24]. In 1992, 71% of TB cases occurred in minorities [13]. Case rates were highest in Asians and Pacific Islanders. Compared with non-Hispanic Whites, case rates were seven times higher in Blacks and five times higher in Hispanics. Comparisons of case rates by different demographic groups are problematic because the population denominators do not include persons who have not legally immigrated to the country.

Since 1985, cases have decreased in non-Hispanic Whites by 9.9% overall, mostly owing to decreased cases in the elderly (Table 3.2). Cases in American Indians and Alaskan natives have decreased by 23.2% because more effective control programs have been implemented in these groups over the past decades and this has had an effect on disease incidence [25]. The greatest percentage increase in cases has been seen in Hispanics.

Cases in different racial and ethnic groups are not evenly distributed throughout the USA. TB in Blacks is clustered in urban centers in the south, along the north Atlantic seaboard and in southern California. Cases in

Hispanics are concentrated in Texas, California, New Mexico, Florida and in the northeast. Infections in American Indians are seen in the western states and in states with Indian reservations. These geographic patterns reflect patterns of immigration of these ethnic groups and of resettlement of Blacks into cities after World War II.

### 3.3.4 Gender

TB case rates have always been higher in adult males than in females. There are differences, however, based on racial and ethnic groups. In 1991, the male to female ratio of cases for non-Hispanic Whites, Blacks and Hispanics was 2.2, 2.4 and 1.8, respectively [CDC, unpublished data]. However, for Asians/Pacific Islanders and American Indians/Alaskan natives, the ratio was 1.2. Since 1985, cases in males have increased 17.7%, while cases in females have increased 19.6% ($p>0.05$). However, in the 25–44 year age group, cases in males have increased by 56% compared with 43% in females ($p<0.001$). One possible explanation is HIV-induced immunosuppression leading to active TB. In the USA, many more males than females are infected with HIV [26]. Indirect evidence for this is the increase in the male to female rate ratio for non-Hispanic Whites since 1985.

### 3.3.5 Place of birth

Persons who were born outside the USA and have immigrated to the USA account for a substantial portion of the current epidemic in the USA and the increased cases seen in recent years. Information about country of birth has been reported to the CDC for all TB cases since 1986. In 1986, 22% of all reported cases were born outside the USA [12]. In 1992, 27% of reported cases were foreign born, an increase of 2345 cases or a 47.6% increase (Table 3.2) [13]. During the same period, cases in persons born in the USA increased from 17 712 to 19 225 cases, or an 8.5% increase. Of the total increase in cases since 1986, 60% of the increase is in foreign born persons. An unknown proportion of these persons are also infected with HIV, making it difficult to determine directly the extent to which each factor is contributing to the TB epidemic. Neither immigration nor HIV infection alone accounts for the increases seen since 1985.

Cases in foreign born persons increased in all age groups but most increases were in the 25–44 year age group. This age group is likely to be seeking immigration to the USA for economic and political reasons. Cases in children 0–14 years of age almost doubled as families with young children were resettled in the USA.

Of the foreign born cases, 44% were born in Asia, 42% in Central or South America, 6% in the Caribbean, 5% in Europe and 3% in Africa [CDC, unpublished data]. Mexico, the Philippines, Indochina (Vietnam,

Kampuchea and Laos), South Korea, Haiti and the People's Republic of China accounted for the majority whose birth place was known. These are also the countries from which most immigrants enter the USA [27]. Foreign born cases made up over 90% of all cases among Asian and Pacific Islanders and half of all cases among Hispanics in 1992.

The differing and increasing rates of TB in various racial and ethnic groups in the USA can be explained, in part, by persons entering from other countries who reactivate their infection soon after entry. From 1986 to 1992, 29% of cases occurred in persons who had been in the USA for less than one year [CDC, unpublished data]. More than half (58%) occurred in persons who had immigrated within the last five years [13]. Case rates by state are also affected by their popularity as a destination for foreign born persons. Increases in this category have occurred in Hawaii, California, New York, Texas, Florida and Massachusetts.

## 3.4 SPECIAL POPULATIONS AT INCREASED RISK OF TUBERCULOSIS

### 3.4.1 HIV infection and AIDS

HIV infection is the strongest risk factor yet identified for progression to active TB [28]. Persons who are coinfected with *M. tuberculosis* and HIV develop active TB at a rate of approximately 8–10% per year compared with the estimated 5–10% lifetime TB risk in persons with intact immune systems [29,30]. In addition, HIV-infected individuals who acquire new infection with *M. tuberculosis* have an even higher risk of developing TB, often very rapidly following initial infection [31–34]. When the tubercle bacillus is introduced in this population, primary TB infection can progress rapidly to active disease (within 4–8 weeks) with high attack rates (39% and 37% in two reports) [31,32].

Prior to 1993, there was no direct measure of the number of USA TB cases that were attributable to HIV. Epidemiologic evidence existed, however, to link the epidemics of TB and AIDS. There was a clear temporal relationship between the AIDS epidemic and the resurgence of TB. After years of steady declines, from 1986 to 1992 there were 51 700 more TB cases reported to the CDC than expected. During this same period, the epidemic of AIDS that began in 1981 was increasing steadily. In 1992, over 250 000 AIDS cases were reported [35]. Additionally, the largest increases in TB occurred in areas with a high incidence of reported AIDS cases. Cantwell *et al.* [36] grouped states by their cumulative AIDS incidence rates by dividing the number of cumulative AIDS cases reported through June 1992 by the state's 1991 population. High AIDS incidence states had over 100 AIDS cases per 100 000 population, intermediate incidence states 48–100 AIDS cases per 100 000 and low incidence states had fewer than 48 cases per 100 000 population. The trend in TB cases was determined in each of these three groups from 1985 to 1991 by linear regression of the logarithm of the TB cases (Figure 3.5). For those areas with high AIDS incidence rates, TB increased by 8.3% per year. Areas with low AIDS rates actually had a decreasing number of TB cases (–3.3% per year). In states with intermediate AIDS incidence, there was no effect on case rates.

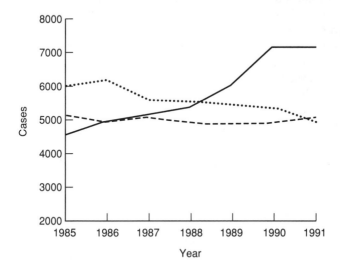

**Figure 3.5** Trends in US born patients with TB in states, stratified by cumulative AIDS incidence per 100 000 population, 1985–1991. High, over 100 (solid line); intermediate, 48–100 (dashed line); low, less than 48 (dotted line).

Using two surveillance systems for AIDS and TB, Burwan *et al.* [37] estimated the number of patients with both diseases. These registries were matched in each state and even with inherent limitations, 4–5% of AIDS patients were also on the TB registry. The percentage of TB patients who were also diagnosed with AIDS increased steadily from less than 1% in 1981 to 8% in 1990. These data suggest that a portion of the increase in TB that began in 1985 is due to the AIDS epidemic. The calculated fraction of excess TB cases that could be accounted for by identified dual registry matched cases was 31%. This proportion is a minimum estimate of the effect of HIV on TB because some persons who are diagnosed with one of the diseases will be diagnosed with the matching disease in later years or in another state and are thus not included.

HIV seroprevalence surveys conducted anonymously in 35 TB clinics in 18 metropolitan areas from 1988 to 1990 showed a median HIV prevalence rate of 5.9% with a range by clinic of 0–58.3% [38,39]. The highest rates were in clinics in New York City, Newark, Boston and Miami. Most HIV-infected patients had pulmonary TB, but HIV infections were more prevalent among patients with extrapulmonary TB than in pulmonary TB patients (19.8% compared with 10.2%, $p < 0.0002$).

### 3.4.2 Persons with certain medical conditions

Other medical conditions that produce immune suppression have been associated with TB, presumably by causing reactivation of latent infection. Hematologic malignancies, cancer chemotherapy, therapy with cortico-steroids and end stage renal failure have all been reported as risks for active TB [40]. The risk of active TB in persons with diabetes mellitus is thought to be two to four times that of the general population [41]. Severe weight loss or starvation increases the risk of active disease by affecting the immune system, while conditions associated with gastrectomy appear to have an increased risk even without weight loss [40]. Miners and potters who have pulmonary silicosis have both an increased TB incidence and increased severity of the disease [42,43]. Especially relevant to social conditions in US society, both alcoholism and drug addiction are associated with TB. In these situations, malnutrition, infection with HIV and increased exposure may all play a role in increasing the risk of both exposure and reactivation [29,30,44–46].

### 3.4.3 Migrant agricultural workers

Seasonal and migrant agricultural workers are thought to have a TB incidence six times greater than the general US population [47–49]. Rates of tuberculin positivity are also high, in one study 29% among US born Black workers and 55% among Haitian workers [50]. Rates vary by racial and ethnic group and probably reflect both infection acquired in the country of origin and primary transmission in camps associated with the farms. In a population based study, tuberculin positivity rates were 33% in Hispanic workers, 62% in Blacks and 76% in Haitians [51].

### 3.4.4 Homeless persons

Homelessness is associated with both the acquisition of TB and reactiva-tion of latent disease [52]. Prior to the revision of the RVCT form in January 1993, data were not available on the number of reported TB cases in homeless people. An evaluation of 1853 men living in a shelter in Manhattan over a 6 year period revealed 42.8% were tuberculin positive and 6% had active disease [53]. TB outbreaks have been reported from homeless shelters [54,55]. Drug use, alcoholism, HIV infection and non-adherence to therapy all contribute to reactivation of latent infection in the homeless [56–58].

### 3.4.5 Patients and health care workers

The aggregation of people in nursing homes and hospitals provides conditions for TB transmission. A survey of cases in 29 states found that

7.8% of patients older than 64 years were living in a nursing home at the time of diagnosis [59]. In these situations, residents are likely to have a high prior prevalence of infection owing to their previous living conditions. The potential for reactivation and subsequent spread to other residents is enhanced by immunosuppression in elderly, ill residents and/or HIV-infected patients and by the ventilation systems in such institutions which are often substandard. Outbreaks have been reported in hospitals and nursing homes [60,61].

Nosocomial TB transmission to hospital and other institutional workers has occurred most dramatically in the recent outbreaks of multi-drug-resistant TB [33,34,62–64]. However, outbreaks in hospitals were reported before the era of resistant disease and health care workers have long been known to have an increased risk of acquiring the infection [65–67]. In the pre-chemotherapy era, it was estimated that the average time to conversion of the tuberculin skin test among student nurses was 1.5 years [68]. More recently, surveys of tuberculin test conversions among hospital workers show rates ranging from 0.11 to 2.3% per year, depending on the background TB rate in the community [69,70]. Rates of tuberculin test conversion associated with hospital employment had been declining [71]. A recent tuberculin survey of house staff in a high TB incidence area, however, found that 2.4% of infectious disease fellows and 11% of pulmonary fellows converted their skin test during the two year training period [72].

### 3.4.6 Residents and workers in correctional facilities

TB has been a problem in correctional facilities for many years [73]. This problem has grown over the last decade because of an expanding prison population leading to overcrowded prisons, relatively high rates of HIV infection in prison inmates, and high TB rates in the communities from which the majority of inmates originate [74]. In a survey of reported TB cases from 29 states, 1.8% of patients 15–64 years of age were living in a correctional institution at the time of diagnosis [59]. In the New York State prison system, the incidence of active TB among inmates increased from 15.4 per 100 000 in 1976 through 1978 to 105.5 per 100 000 in 1986 [75].

### 3.5 EPIDEMIOLOGY OF DRUG-RESISTANT TUBERCULOSIS

### 3.5.1 Development of drug resistance

Against the backdrop of an increasing incidence of TB in the USA, a second problem, drug-resistant TB, has emerged. Resistant infection, especially multi-drug-resistance (MDR), is much more difficult and expensive to treat, thus greatly complicating control efforts for this disease [76,77]. MDR TB has a high mortality rate even with treatment [33,63,76,78,79]. Many of the same epidemiologic factors that have led to an increase in overall

TB also contribute to the increase in drug-resistant disease. The origins of drug resistance in TB have been understood since early in the chemotherapeutic era [80–84]. These mechanisms are discussed in Chapters 7 and 12.

Primary drug resistance is defined as resistance to one or more drugs in persons with TB who are not known to have had prior treatment with antituberculous medications [85]. Secondary or acquired drug resistance can be documented by increasing levels of resistance to one or more drugs in a strain recovered from a patient undergoing ineffectual therapy [85]. Transmitted drug resistance is said to have occurred when a single or multi-drug-resistant organism is recovered from patients who are high risk contacts of other individuals known to be shedding strains with comparable patterns of drug resistance [85].

Because drug-resistant *M. tuberculosis* strains showed attenuated pathogenicity in laboratory animals, it was postulated that these bacilli might be less able to establish human infection or disease [86,87]. However, studies of the prevalence of TB in contacts of persons with drug-resistant infection and multiple outbreaks of MDR TB document that drug-resistant organisms retain pathogenicity [33,62–64,78,79,88]. Thus, although drug-resistant TB has developed mainly as the result of inadequate management of patients with drug-susceptible infection who then developed acquired drug resistance, these drug-resistant strains can also be transmitted from person to person.

More recently, MDR TB has become a problem in the USA. There has been a dramatic increase in the number of outbreaks reported in the last few years involving HIV-infected patients in institutional settings [33,62–64,78,79]. Surveillance data also suggest an increase in the number of total cases [89]. Of great concern is the increase in combined resistance to INH and rifampin, the two most effective TB medications [89,90].

### 3.5.2 Risk factors for drug resistance

In the final analysis, drug resistance can ultimately be traced to poorly chosen medical therapy or noncompliance with treatment [90]. Any factor which increases the chance of inappropriate or incomplete treatment has the potential to cause resistant TB. Multiple risk factors for drug-resistant TB have been identified. Two of the main factors in the USA are previous treatment for active infection or being a native of a country with a high prevalence of drug-resistant organisms [91,92]. Other risk factors identified include the presence of cavitary lung disease and homelessness [68,93,94].

### (a) Previous treatment

The reasons why previous TB treatment is a risk factor for resistant infection are obvious. Either owing to noncompliance by the patient or improper prescribing by physicians, patients may receive inadequate treatment which selectively allows the low number of drug-resistant organisms found in all large populations of *M. tuberculosis* to expand [77,95,96]. As compared with most other infectious diseases, TB has to be treated for a long time (a minimum of 6 months) with multiple drugs. It is difficult for health care providers to predict who will be compliant with a regimen [97].

Although noncompliance has frequently been implicated as the main culprit in acquired TB resistance, errors in management by physicians have also contributed. When the TB sanatoria closed during the 1960s, the care of TB patients shifted from institutions and physicians with expertise in the field to general practitioners with little training in the area. Studies of treatment both early in the post-sanatorium period (1971–1975) and as recently as 1990 document frequent mistakes in the prescribing of anti-tuberculous medications by physicians [77,96]. Common errors are the use of an inadequate primary therapy regimen, addition of a single agent to a failing regimen, and failure to suspect or recognize initial drug resistance. These mistakes lead to increased drug resistance [77]. A third factor related to previous TB therapy that can affect the outcome of therapy even with proper prescribing and a compliant patient is malabsorption of medications. This has not been studied in the development of TB drug resistance but has been documented to occur in AIDS enteropathy and may be a factor in the development of resistance [76,98].

### (b) Immigrants

Drug-resistant TB is relatively common in developing countries, and being a recent immigrant from a country with high rates of drug resistance is a consistent risk factor for primary drug-resistant infection in the USA [85,91,92,99]. Many reports have documented higher rates of resistance in immigrants from Haiti, Latin America and Southeast Asia [91,92,99–103]. In Indochinese refugees, high rates of resistance to INH and streptomycin have been demonstrated but resistance to rifampin is uncommon [100]. Likewise in Haitian refugees, INH resistance was very common but resistance to rifampin low [102]. In developing nations, rates of drug resistance are higher than in developed countries for several reasons. In these nations, TB remains a common disease, so the number of persons being treated for TB and thus being at risk of developing resistance is high [91]. Ill tuberculous individuals may take medications until they feel better, then discontinue the medications for economic or convenience reasons [83]. Methodology to improve patient adherence to therapy is discussed in Chapter 9. TB medications are available without a prescription in many developing nations and may be included in proprietary medications such as antitussives [91]. Intermittent and unsupervised use of these medications can facilitate the development of resistance. In a first quarter survey of all US TB isolates, 20% from immigrants were resistant to at least one drug [89].

*(c) Cavitary tuberculosis*

In two recent studies, cavitary lung disease was found to be a risk factor for the development of drug resistance [92,93]. This factor was first noted by Howard in the late 1940s, and the enormous population of tubercle bacilli present in these cavitary pulmonary lesions was recognized by Canetti in 1965 as the key to the emergence of resistance [80,104]. Given the known proportion of resistant isolates in a large population of tubercle bacilli, there might be between 10 000 and 100 000 organisms resistant to one or another antituberculous drug present in a cavitary lesion at the beginning of therapy [83]. With this large number of resistant organisms present, the chances of resistance developing are increased if there is any inconsistency or inadequacies in therapy [80,92,93]. The presence of cavitary disease is an additive risk factor to prior treatment. In one study, 59% of patients with a history of prior treatment had resistant infection while 71% of patients with both a history of prior treatment and cavitary disease had a resistant isolate [93].

*(d) Coexisting HIV infection*

Infection with HIV reflects and magnifies some infectious diseases that are endemic in a particular area [105]. In one study from New York, HIV infection was found to be an independent risk factor for drug resistance in TB [90]. Another factor that has led to the recent propagation of these drug-resistant strains is the concurrence of TB in HIV-infected intravenous drug users [46]. This has created a large pool of persons at very high risk of developing active TB who are also at risk for nonadherence to therapy, leading to the development of drug resistance [29]. Just as HIV infection is contributing substantially to the excess of TB in the USA, it is also a factor in the increase of multi-drug-resistant cases [91,106].

In persons with HIV and drug-resistant TB, the combination of decreased immunity and the loss of the most effective antituberculous drugs, especially INH and rifampin, makes effective treatment difficult and lengthy if not impossible, and can lead to prolonged periods of infectivity [33,62,63,78,79].

*(e) Homelessness*

Homelessness is also a risk factor for drug-resistant TB [94,107]. Outbreaks of both susceptible and resistant infection in homeless shelters have been reported [54,55,108]. During a 14 month period in 1984–1985, an outbreak of TB resistant to INH and streptomycin was reported from a 350 bed homeless shelter in Boston [108]. Of 49 shelter related cases, 22 had resistance to these two drugs. These isolates were of the same phage type and this outbreak was thought to be due to recent transmission from a single index case with a 10 year history of INH and streptomycin-resistant TB.

The difficulties in treating this infection in the homeless population are enormous. Brudney and Dobkin prospectively studied 224 consecutive TB patients admitted to a public hospital in New York City [58]. Nearly 70% of these patients were homeless or had unstable housing. Of 178 patients discharged on antituberculous medications, 99 (56%) never returned for outpatient follow up or medication and overall 89% were lost to follow up and failed to complete therapy. Within 12 months of discharge, 48 were readmitted with active TB at least once, and of the 40 patients discharged a second time, 35 were lost to follow up. The experience described is a perfect scenario for the generation of drug resistance. The role of decreased public funding of TB programs is unclear but, in New York City in particular, cutbacks in funding of these programs have resulted in less supervision of active cases, thus increasing the likelihood of incomplete or erratic therapy which allows resistance to develop [58,109].

### 3.5.3 Community and hospital based surveys

Nationwide surveillance for drug-resistant TB has only recently begun in the USA. A number of surveys, however, that have included selected hospitals and health departments throughout the USA as well as regional and hospital based surveys, have been carried out since the early 1960s [89,90,93,110–119].

The CDC has conducted surveillance of primary drug resistance in a non-random sample of hospital, state and city laboratories over three time periods. Although the three surveys were not done in the same location or carried out in the same manner, they do allow some analysis of the trend over time. The first survey [113] conducted in 22 hospitals and sanatoria from 1961 to 1968, found a resistance rate to a single drug of 3.5% and to two or more drugs of 1%. Rates of resistance did not rise over the 8 years and were significantly higher in the younger than in the older age groups. A second survey of 20 laboratories from 1975 through 1982 revealed a rate of primary resistance to one drug of 6.9% and to two or more drugs of 2.3% [110]. Rates of resistance declined over the period of this survey and there were large differences in the rate by geographic area, race and ethnicity. As in the first survey, younger age groups had a significantly higher rate of resistance [110,115, CDC, unpublished data]. In the third survey of 31 health departments from 1982 through 1986, the rate of primary resistance was 9% and there was a significantly decreasing trend over the period of the study [115]. The resistance rate (9%) was higher than the previous survey (6.9%), but this was likely due to differences in methodology and not a true increase. Although the absolute rates differed among these three surveys, within each survey the rate remained stable or decreased, suggesting that nationwide rates of primary drug resistance remained stable or decreased during these periods.

Drug-resistance surveys of regions or population subgroups may reveal trends not detected in nationwide surveys. A study of drug resistance from a hospital in southern California from 1969 through 1984, as an example, revealed rates of primary resistance of 23% and rates of acquired resistance of 59% [93]. Surprisingly, these rates changed significantly over the 15 year study period, and as early as 1969–1972, documented rates of multi-drug-resistance as high as 12.3% were noted [114]. The majority of the patients served by this hospital were indigent and members of racial and ethnic minorities. The authors cautioned that these resistance rates were not typical of Los Angeles County as a whole, but reflected the patient population referred to their institution. Additionally, a 1965–1968 survey of a pediatric population in New York City showed an incidence of primary resistance to INH of 9.7% and an incidence of primary multi-drug-resistance of 6.7% [116]. These rates were higher than rates in adults in New York City at that time [120].

Patients with isolated INH resistance respond well to therapy, but the combination of INH and rifampin resistance presents more difficulties for treatment. Fortunately, even in the most recent CDC survey from 1982 to 1986, primary resistance to rifampin remained rare at 0.6% and showed a decreasing trend [115, CDC, unpublished data]. During this period, the report found only 0.5% of isolates tested had combined INH and rifampin resistance. Local studies revealed problems of growing rifampin resistance before they were reflected in national surveys. From 1971 through 1974, soon after rifampin began to be used, a significant increase in resistance among *M. tuberculosis* isolates from Massachusetts was found [119]. The majority of the resistant isolates were obtained from patients who had received more than one month of rifampin treatment and did not represent primary resistance, but these results revealed the potential for transmitted drug resistance to rifampin existed. All of these rifampin-resistant organisms were also resistant to other drugs. A continuing survey of a pediatric population in New York City revealed that for the period 1981–1984, there were significantly more isolates resistant to rifampin than from 1969–1980 [118]. Thus, although rifampin resistance remained rare in nationwide surveys as late as 1986, increasing levels of resistance to the drug were detected in local surveys before this time.

There are several important points that can be made from these studies. In the USA, the overall rate of single drug primary drug resistance remained low through the mid-1980s, but as early as the 1970s there were geographic regions, as well as racial and ethnic groups, with rates significantly higher than those for the entire country. In addition, rates have been consistently higher in young age groups [118]. TB in the young is a sentinel event demonstrating recent transmission of the infection, and the occurrence of primary drug resistance in the young is likely an indicator of recent transmission of resistant organisms from patients who have received inadequate therapy (transmitted drug resistance). Even though overall rates of primary drug resistance remained low and the resistance to rifampin very low as late as 1986, there were indications from smaller studies that drug resistance was increasing.

More recently, a national survey of all reported TB cases in the first quarter of 1991 revealed primary resistance to one or more drugs in 13.4% of isolates and to INH and rifampin in 3.2% [89]. For 1991, 67% of primary drug-resistant isolates were reported from five areas (New York City, California, Texas, New Jersey, Florida) and 61% of the isolates resistant to both INH and rifampin were from New York City. A hospital survey performed in 1992 found patients with isolates resistant to at least INH and rifampin have been admitted to hospitals in at least 40 states [112]. In April 1991, a New York City survey of every patient with a positive AFB culture revealed that 33% of patients had isolates resistant to at least one drug, 26% to INH, and 19% to both INH and rifampin [90]. Among patients who had never been treated, resistance to one or more medication was 23% compared with 10% in a New York City survey conducted in 1982–1984. A 1988–1989 survey of resistance at one hospital in New York City serving a mostly indigent population found primary drug resistance in 22.6% of isolates and acquired resistance in 49.2% [121]. The incidence of MDR TB was 17.5%, and of all isolates resistant to at least one medication, 56.6% were multi-drug-resistant. Overall, 12.6% of isolates were resistant to both INH and rifampin.

In summary, these studies suggest an increasing incidence of multi-drug-resistance, including strains with combined resistance to INH and rifampin. Although cases of resistant strains are found in diverse geographic areas, the large increases are concentrated in large urban areas and often involve indigent racial and ethnic minorities.

### 3.5.4 Outbreaks of drug-resistant tuberculosis

*(a) Outbreak descriptions*

Of the reported outbreaks of drug-resistant TB which occurred prior to 1990, three involved extended families and household contacts [122–124], one involved close contacts of a high school student [125], and one outbreak involved residents of a homeless shelter [108]. These outbreaks occurred over a 13 year period and did not cluster in any particular region of the country. In the two institutional outbreaks (the school and the homeless shelter), the organisms were resistant to INH and streptomycin and did not involve combined resistance to INH and rifampin [108,125].

Since 1990, nine outbreaks of MDR TB have been investigated by CDC in conjunction with local authorities. These outbreaks included eight hospitals and one prison, involving nearly 300 patients and health care workers (Table 3.4) [33,62–64,78,79, CDC, unpublished data]. Most of those infected were also HIV infected and mortality was high (Table 3.4). Nosocomial spread occurred in each of these outbreaks, as documented by

**Table 3.4** Nosocomial HIV related multi-drug-resistant tuberculosis outbreaks

| Facility[a] | Time period | Total cases | Resistance pattern* | HIV infection % | Deceased[b] % | Median time from tuberculosis diagnosis to death (weeks) |
|---|---|---|---|---|---|---|
| Hospital A, Miami | 1988–1991 | 65 | INH, RIF (EMB, ETA) | 93 | 72 | 7 |
| Hospital B[c], NYC | 1988–1991 | 51 | INH, SM (RIF, EMB) | 100 | 89 | 16 |
| Hospital C, NYC | 1989–1992 | 70 | INH, RIF, SM (EMB, ETA, KM, RBT) | 95 | 77 | 4 |
| Hospital D, NYC | 1990–1991 | 29 | INH, RIF (EMB, ETA) | 91 | 83 | 4 |
| Hospital E, NYS | 1991 | 7 | INH, RIF, SM (EMB, ETA, KM, RBT) | 14 | 43 | 4 |
| Hospital F, NYC | 1990–1991 | 16 | INH, RIF, SM (EMB, ETA, KM, RBT) | 82 | 82 | 4 |
| Hospital I, NJ | 1990–1992 | 14 | INH, RIF (EMB) | 100 | 86 | 4 |
| Hospital J, NYC | 1991–1992 | 28 | INH, RIF, SM (EMB, ETA, KM, RBT) | 96 | 93 | 4 |
| Prisons[d], NYS | 1990–1992 | 42 | INH, RIF (SM, EMB, ETA, KM, RBT) | 98 | 79 | 4 |

* Drugs not in parentheses displayed resistance in all cases; drugs in parentheses displayed resistance in most cases.
[a] NYC, New York City; NYS, New York State; NJ, New Jersey.
[b] Includes only cases for which outcome data has been ascertained.
[c] HIV infection was part of the case definition.
[d] Twenty-four prison cases are also counted with Hospital C.
INH, isoniazid; RIF, rifampin; SM, streptomycin; EMB, ethambutol; ETA, ethionamide; KM, kanamycin; RBT, rifabutin.

epidemiologic and laboratory investigations. All of the outbreaks in New York City and New York State were characterized by patients who had previously been in outbreak hospitals during a time when other patients were hospitalized with active MDR TB [33,62,63,78,79]. In the outbreak in Florida, patients had documented prior exposure to smear positive MDR infection, both in the hospital and the HIV clinic [64].

The prison outbreak was related to inmates who had been inpatients in several outbreak hospitals and then moved to different prisons while ill with active drug-resistant infection. DNA fingerprinting data from isolates indicated that the outbreaks in New York State were epidemiologically related. Specifically, a seven drug-resistant tubercle bacillus strain with a consistent pattern on DNA fingerprinting was the predominant organism in four hospital outbreaks as well as the prison system where this strain was isolated from 33 prisoners in 18 different prisons [33,62,63,78,79,126,127]. Furthermore, clusters of tuberculin skin test conversions after exposure to MDR TB have been reported from a residential substance abuse treatment facility and a medical examiner's office [128,129].

A contributing factor in these outbreaks was the convergence of highly susceptible immunocompromised HIV-positive patients with patients with active MDR TB. Many large urban hospitals have opened dedicated HIV wards. Seven of the hospital outbreaks investigated by the CDC were centered on wards or outpatient clinics dedicated to caring for HIV-infected patients and over 90% of active TB cases in these outbreaks have occurred in persons infected with HIV (Table 3.4) [33,62,63,78,79, CDC, unpublished data].

## (b) Contributing factors

Common features contributing to the nosocomial outbreaks were delays in diagnosis, significant lapses in infection control procedures and delays in the ordering and completion of susceptibility testing. In these outbreaks, the majority of cases in HIV-infected persons were associated with severe immunosuppression (CD4 count 100/µl) [33,62–64] often not exhibiting the characteristic clinical signs and symptoms of TB. In three outbreaks investigated by the CDC, 41 (75%) of 55 patients who had sputum AFB smears submitted were positive [62]. A fourth outbreak hospital did not routinely perform smears. Contributing factors to the delay in diagnoses included failure to order or report smears in a timely manner, failure to treat or isolate patients with AFB seen on a smear assuming that the organisms were *Mycobacterium avium* complex, and discontinuing evaluation for respiratory pathogens after one pathogen, such as *Pneumocystis carinii*, was identified. Some patients had concurrent TB and *Pneumocystis carinii* pneumonia (CDC, unpublished data).

These problems led to long delays, up to 6 months in some cases, in initiating appropriate treatment and isolation [62]. Because the presence of resistant organisms was not recognized quickly, patients remained on inadequate regimens and therefore remained infectious for prolonged periods. Persons were removed from isolation on these inadequate treatments and were returned to the general hospital population under the incorrect assumption that they were not infectious. The use of rapid susceptibility testing using radiometric methods is recommended to remedy this situation, since susceptibility results can usually be completed within 15–30 days of specimen collection [130].

Inadequate isolation of patients known to be infectious also contributed to the outbreaks. Many of the isolation rooms did not have negative air pressure relative to the hall outside the room. In addition, the doors to the rooms were sometimes left open and infectious patients at times left their rooms without a properly worn mask. HIV-infected patients with known TB as well as those with pulmonary symptoms of unknown etiology were hospitalized in HIV-dedicated wards [62]. In one hospital, patients with known TB were placed in isolation rooms sharing an adjoining bathroom with a person with HIV but not TB [CDC, unpublished data].

### (c) Health care workers with drug-resistant tuberculosis

Hospital staff have been affected by this infection as well. In the hospital outbreaks investigated by the CDC, 17 health care workers developed MDR TB [131, CDC, unpublished data]. Of these 17, eight were HIV seropositive. Six are known to have died, four of the HIV-positive group and two of the HIV-negative group that were not TB related. Two health care workers were infected without direct patient contact, one a laboratory worker and the other a pathologist. In three outbreak hospitals, tuberculin skin test conversions were identified after direct exposure to infectious MDR TB patients in 13 (33%) of 39, 6 (50%) of 12, and 24 (22%) of 108 health care workers, respectively [62,131, CDC, unpublished data].

### (d) Prisoners with drug-resistant tuberculosis

Transmission of drug-susceptible TB within prisons has been reported in the past [75,132]. In 1991, transmission of MDR TB occurred in the New York State prison system [78,133]. The increases in cases of MDR TB in the USA are occurring in the same subgroups contributing disproportionately to prison and jail populations. Therefore this difficult-to-treat infection can be easily introduced into the prison system. It is important for prison systems to have protocols and procedures to isolate prisoners with proven or suspected TB properly and to screen inmates and staff with tuberculin skin tests. This screening will help detect transmission and guide prophylaxis or treatment [134]. Protocols should be developed by state prison systems to prevent transfers of ill inmates between facilities until TB is ruled out.

## 3.6 EPIDEMIOLOGY OF TUBERCULOSIS OUTSIDE THE USA

### 3.6.1 Data collection

Worldwide, morbidity information has been collected since 1974 by the World Health Organization (WHO) Expanded Programme on Immunization (EPI), and was reviewed recently [135]. Other reports of the global TB situation include disease burden and cost [136], trends in Western Europe [137], the impact of the HIV epidemic [138,139], and a WHO control strategy [140].

A critical evaluation of global TB surveillance activities must begin by recognizing factors that limit international comparisons. Morbidity data are influenced by access to health care, availability of diagnostic procedures, and completeness of notification or reporting systems. Most developing countries report TB cases among persons who can obtain medical attention and who have evidence of AFB in the sputum smear. In these countries, smear-negative TB patients are not consistently reported. It is estimated that in some developing countries there are 1.22 cases of AFB smear-negative and extrapulmonary cases for every case of AFB smear-positive TB [136].

Other methods used to estimate the number of persons with *M. tuberculosis* infection in a given population include the probability for an un-infected individual to become infected in a one year period [141]. This measure is known as the annual rate of infection, and is calculated from tuberculin skin test surveys. It has been correlated with the number of persons with AFB smear-positive infection and used to predict the number of new cases of active pulmonary TB [142].

### 3.6.2 Developed countries

TB trends have varied between industrialized and developing countries. In Europe and most industrialized countries, TB cases consistently decreased from 1970 through 1989. In these countries, TB among the indigenous population occurred largely in the elderly. More recently, some of these countries have reported an increasing number of TB cases among foreign born persons from developing countries with a high prevalence of this infection [137]. For example, in 1990, foreign born persons accounted for 38% of all TB cases in Denmark, 41% in The Netherlands and 51% in Sweden. Also, a growing proportion of European AIDS patients have been diagnosed with TB. Approximately 10–11% of AIDS patients in France, Germany and Italy have been reported to have TB. In Portugal and Spain, that proportion was 25% and 35%, respectively. Relatively few AIDS patients in Denmark, Switzerland and the United Kingdom have been reported to have TB [137].

### 3.6.3 Developing countries

In contrast to Europe and other industrialized countries, TB cases in the developing countries of Africa and Southeast Asia increased from 1970 through 1989. In Africa, the average rate of TB cases decreased from 60 to 47 cases per 100 000 in non-HIV epidemic countries, while it increased from 51 to 64 per 100 000 in 13 HIV epidemic countries (Burundi, Congo, Cote d'Ivoire, Ethiopia, Kenya, Malawi, Mozambique, Rwanda, Tanzania, Uganda, Zaire, Zambia and Zimbabwe) [135]. In these countries, TB has been reported in 20–44% of AIDS patients, thus becoming one of the most common opportunistic diseases associated with AIDS [139].

### 3.6.4 Worldwide tuberculosis

Most (95%) of the 194 countries participating in the WHO EPI reported TB cases from 1974 through 1979 [135]. The proportion of countries reporting decreased to 85% from 1985 through 1989. Worldwide, an average of 2.5 million TB cases have been reported each year in the past decade [135].

Recently, worldwide TB cases for 1990 were calculated, based on the observed mean and highest number of TB cases reported to WHO by the 194 member countries between 1974 and 1989 [135,136,140]. The range of 1990 calculated TB cases by region, according to the WHO regional classification, is shown in Table 3.5. An estimated 8 million persons had TB worldwide. More than 75% of these occurred in Southeast Asia, the Western Pacific and Africa. An estimated 70% of all cases occur in persons younger than 44 years of age [136]. Additionally, an estimated total of 2.9 million deaths occurred in 1990 due to TB. Given the above calculations, TB deaths appear to be significantly involving the most productive segments of the population in the developing world.

A mechanism has been developed by the International Union Against Tuberculosis and Lung Diseases (IUATLD) in the form of mutual assistance programs to ensure the delivery of diagnosis and treatment of TB

**Table 3.5** Range of estimated tuberculosis cases by world region, 1990[a]

| Region | Range of tuberculosis cases (thousands) | |
|---|---|---|
| Africa | 1160 – | 1400 |
| Americas | 534 – | 560 |
| Eastern Mediterranean | 594 | |
| Southeast Asia | 2470 – | 2480 |
| Western Pacific | 2547 – | 2560 |
| Europe and others | 392 – | 410 |
| HIV-related | 305 | |
| Total | 8002 – | 7410 |

[a] Based on World Health Organization-defined regions [134, 139].

even under the difficult conditions of high prevalence, low resources and sociopolitical instability. Cure rates reportedly approximate 85% in new cases and 80% in retreatment cases in those countries where such programs have been successfully implemented [143]. The elements for effective IUATLD-assisted national TB prevention and control programs include: political commitment; secure supply of drugs and materials; laboratory network for microscopy; proper reporting of cases; adequate supervision of drug therapy; proper training of staff; and stepwise introduction of the program throughout the country. WHO and the United Nations Development Plan have endorsed such programs as an integral part of the global effort to prevent and control TB.

Using TB notification data and HIV seroprevalence information with estimates of future trends, the WHO has projected the morbidity and mortality of TB worldwide and the relationship to HIV infection [144]. An overall increase in total TB cases from 7.54 million in 1990 to 8.77 million, 10.22 million and 11.87 million in 1995, 2000 and 2005, respectively, is predicted. This represents an increase of 57.6% over 15 years. As illustrated in Figure 3.6, a much higher relative increase is predicted in Africa compared with Western Europe and other developed areas. Of the total number of increased cases in 2005 over 1990, 42.8% are predicted to occur in Africa and 31.0% in Southeast Asia. These two areas represent 73.8% of the increase and 61.5% of the total number of cases estimated for 2005.

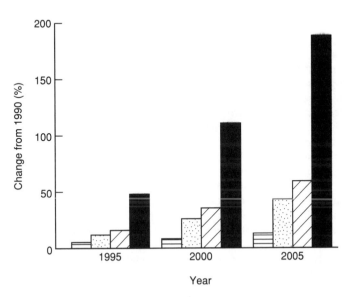

**Figure 3.6** WHO projected percentage increases in TB cases compared with 1990 [144]. Africa (solid shading); Southeast Asia (stippled shading); Western Europe, USA, Canada, Japan, Australia and New Zealand (horizontal line shading); and worldwide (diagonal line shading).

WHO also estimated that total TB deaths will increase by 38.7% from 1990 to 2000 but those TB deaths related to HIV will rise by 331% [144]. The percentage of HIV attributable TB deaths was estimated to increase from 4.6% in 1990 to 14.2% in 2000.

## 3.7 CONCLUSION

TB remains a major public health problem, both in industrialized countries and in the developing world. Since 1985, morbidity from the infection in the USA has increased markedly. Multiple factors, acting independently and in combination, contribute to the increase: the concurrent epidemic of HIV infection and AIDS, increased immigration from countries where TB is endemic and primary transmission among some populations, such as children, ethnic minorities and the homeless. The epidemic of TB and multi-drug-resistant TB is the result of the failure of public health and social programs to effect prompt treatment of active cases, prophylaxis of contacts and screening of high risk populations [109]. The goal of eliminating TB in the USA will be attained only by improving prevention programs and by addressing the problem of endemic TB in the developing world [145].

## REFERENCES

1. Frost, W.F. (1937) How much control of tuberculosis? *Am J Public Health*, **27**, 759–66.
2. Communicable Disease Center (1961) *The Arden House Conference on Tuberculosis*. U.S. Department of Health, Education, and Welfare. Public Health Service publication no. 784 (reprint). Washington, DC.
3. Centers for Disease Control (1989) A strategic plan for the elimination of tuberculosis in the United States. *MMWR*, **38 (S-3)**, 1–25.
4. U.S. Public Health Service (1951) Recommendations of the Committee on Tuberculosis Morbidity Reporting. Public Health Reports, **66**, 1291–2.
5. Centers for Disease Control (1990) Case definitions for public health surveillance. *MMWR*, **39 (RR-13)**, 39–40.
6. Gostin, L.O. (1993) Controlling the resurgent tuberculosis epidemic. A 50-state survey of TB statutes and proposals for reform. *JAMA*, **269**, 255–61.
7. Annas, G.J. (1993) Control of tuberculosis – the law and the public's health. *N Engl J Med*, **328**, 585–8.
8. Marier, R. (1977) The reporting of communicable diseases. *Am J Epidemiol*, **105**, 587–90.
9. Campos-Outcalt, D., England, R. and Porter, B. (1991) Reporting of communicable diseases by university physicians. *Public Health Rep*, **106**, 579–83.
10. Glaser, D. and Hammarsten, J.E. (1978) Pharmacy notification for surveillance and drug utilization review in a metropolitan tuberculosis control program in a low-incidence country. *Maryland Pharmacist*, 10 July 1978.

11. Centers for Disease Control (1953) *Reported Tuberculosis Morbidity and Other Data: Calendar Year 1953*. Public Health Service Publication (CDC) No. 442.

12. Centers for Disease Control (1986) *Tuberculosis in the United States: 1985–1986*. Health and Human Services Publication (CDC) No. 88-8322.

13. Centers for Disease Control (1993) Tuberculosis morbidity – United States, 1992. *MMWR*, **42**, 696–7, 703–4.

14. Bloch, A.B., Rieder, H.L., Kelly, G.D. *et al.* (1989) The epidemiology of tuberculosis. *Semin Resp Infect*, **4**, 157–70.

15. Powell, K.E. and Farer, L.S. (1980) The rising age of the tuberculosis patient: A sign of success and failure. *J Infect Dis*, **142**, 946–8.

16. Styblo, K. (1976) Surveillance of tuberculosis. *Int J Epidemiol*, **5**, 63–8.

17. Bleiker, M.A. (1991) The annual tuberculosis infection rate, the tuberculin survey and the tuberculin test. *Bull Int Union Tuberc Lung Dis*, **66**, 53–6.

18. Barnes, P.F., Bloch, A.B., Davidson, P.T. and Snider, D.E. (1991) Tuberculosis in patients with human immunodeficiency virus infection. *N Engl J Med*, **323**, 1644–50.

19. Centers for Disease Control (1990) Tuberculosis among foreign-born persons entering the United States. *MMWR*, **39 (RR-18)**, 1–21.

20. Centers for Disease Control (1987) Tuberculosis among Asians/Pacific Islanders – United States, 1985. *MMWR*, **36**, 331–4.

21. Centers for Disease Control (1987) Tuberculosis in blacks – United States. *MMWR*, **36**, 212–20.

22. Centers for Disease Control (1987) Tuberculosis in minorities – United States. *MMWR*, **36**, 77–80.

23. Centers for Disease Control (1987) Tuberculosis among Hispanics – United States, 1985. *MMWR*, **36**, 568–9.

24. Centers for Disease Control (1987) Tuberculosis among American Indians and Alaskan Natives – United States, 1985. *MMWR*, **36**, 493–5.

25. Kaplan, G.J., Fraser, R.I. and Comstock, G.W. (1972) Tuberculosis in Alaska, 1970. The continued decline of the tuberculosis epidemic. *Am Rev Respir Dis* **105**, 920–6.

26. Centers for Disease Control (1992) *HIV/AIDS Surveillance Report*. U.S. Public Health Service, Atlanta, GA. pp. 1–23.

27. Centers for Disease Control (1990) Tuberculosis among foreign-born persons entering the United States. *MMWR*, **39 (RR-18)**, 1–21.

28. Murray, J.F. (1991) Tuberculosis and human immunodeficiency virus infection during the 1990's. *Bull Int Union Tuberc Lung Dis*, **66**, 21–5.

29. Selwyn, P.A., Hartel, D., Lewis, V.A. *et al.* (1989) A prospective study of the risk of tuberculosis among intravenous drug users with HIV infection. *N Engl J Med*, **320**, 545–50.

30. Selwyn, P.A., Sckell, B.M., Alcabes, P. *et al.* (1992) High risk of active tuberculosis in HIV-infected drug users with cutaneous anergy. *JAMA*, **268**, 504–9.

31. DiPerri, G., Cruciani, M., Danzi, M.C. *et al.* (1989) Nosocomial epidemic of active tuberculosis among HIV-infected patients. *Lancet*, **2**, 1502–4.

32. Daley, C.L., Small, P.M., Schecter, G.F. *et al.* (1992) An outbreak of tuberculosis with accelerated progression among persons infected with the human immunodeficiency virus. *N Engl J Med*, **326**, 231–5.

33. Edlin, B.R., Tokars, J.I., Grieco, M.H. *et al.* (1992) An outbreak of multi-drug

resistant tuberculosis among hospitalized patients with the acquired immuno-deficiency syndrome. *N Engl J Med*, **326**, 1514–21.

34. Dooley, S.W., Villarino, M.E., Lawrence, M. *et al.* (1992) Nosocomial transmission of tuberculosis in a hospital unit for HIV-infected patients. *JAMA*, **267**, 2632–5.
35. Centers for Disease Control (1993) *HIV/AIDS Surveillance Report.* U.S. Public Health Service, Atlanta, GA. pp. 1–23.
36. Cantwell, M.F., Snider, D.E., Cauthen, G.M. and Onorato, I.M. (1994) Epidemiology of tuberculosis in the United States, 1985–1992. JAMA, **272**, 535–9.
37. Burwan, D.R., Bloch, A.B., Griffin, L.D. *et al.* Unpublished data.
38. Centers for Disease Control (1990) *National HIV Serosurveillance Summary.* Vol 2. U.S. Public Health Service, Atlanta, GA.
39. Onorato, I.M., McCray, E. and the Field Services Branch (1992) Prevalence of human immunodeficiency virus infection among patients attending tuberculosis clinics in the United States. *J Infect Dis*, **165**, 87–92.
40. American Thoracic Society (1994) Treatment of tuberculosis and tuberculosis infection in adults and children. *Am J Respir Crit Care Med*, **149**, 1359–74.
41. Boucot, K.R., Dillon, E.S., Cooper, D.A. *et al.* (1952) Tuberculosis among diabetics. *Am Rev Respir Dis*, **65**, 1–50.
42. Snider, D.E. (1978) The relationship between tuberculosis and silicosis. *Am Rev Respir Dis*, **118**, 455–60.
43. Cowie, R.L., Langton, M.E. and Becklake, M.R. (1989) Pulmonary tuberculosis in South African gold miners. *Am Rev Respir Dis*, **139**, 1086–9.
44. Friedman, L.N., Sullivan, G.M., Bevilaqua, R.P. and Loscos, R. (1987) Tuberculosis screening in alcoholics and drug addicts. *Am Rev Respir Dis*, **136**, 1188–92.
45. Centers for Disease Control (1991) Crack cocaine use among persons with tuberculosis – Contra Costa County, California, 1987–1990. *MMWR*, **40**, 485–9.
46. Reichman, L.B., Felton, C.P. and Edsall, J.R. (1979) Drug dependence, a possible new risk factor for tuberculosis disease. *Arch Intern Med*, **139**, 337–9.
47. Centers for Disease Control (1992) Prevention and control of tuberculosis in migrant farm workers. *MMWR*, **41 (RR-10)**, 1–15.
48. Centers for Disease Control (1986) Tuberculosis among migrant farm workers – Virginia. *MMWR*, **35**, 467–9.
49. Hibbs, J., Yeager, S. and Cochran, J. (1989) Tuberculosis among migrant farm workers. *JAMA*, **262**, 1775.
50. Jacobson, M.L., Mercer, M.A., Miller, L.K. and Simpson, T.W. (1987) Tuberculosis risk among migrant farm workers on the Delmarva peninsula. *Am J Public Health*, **77**, 29–32.
51. Ciesielski, S.D., Seed, J.R., Esposito, P.H. and Hunter, N. (1991) The epidemiology of TB among North Carolina migrant farm workers. *JAMA*, **265**, 1715–19.
52. Centers for Disease Control (1992) Prevention and control of tuberculosis among homeless populations. *MMWR*, **41 (RR-5)**, 13–23.
53. McAdam, J.M., Brickner, P.W., Scharer, L.L. *et al.* (1990) The spectrum of tuberculosis in a New York men's shelter clinic. *Chest*, **97**, 798–805.
54. Nolan, C.M., Elarth, A.M., Barr, H. *et al.* (1991) An outbreak of tuberculosis in a shelter for homeless men. *Am Rev Respir Dis*, **143**, 257–61.
55. Centers for Disease Control (1991) Tuberculosis among residents of shelters for the homeless – Ohio, 1990. *MMWR*, **40**, 869–77.

56. Torres, R.A., Mani, S., Altholz, J. and Brickner, P.W. (1990) Human immuno-deficiency virus infection among homeless men in a New York City shelter. *Arch Intern Med*, **150**, 2030–6.

57. Schieffelbein, C.W. and Snider, D.E. (1988) Tuberculosis control among home-less populations. *Arch Intern Med*, **148**, 1843–6.

58. Brudney, K. and Dobkin, J. (1991) Resurgent tuberculosis in New York City. *Am Rev Respir Dis*, **144**, 745–9.

59. Hutton, M.D., Cauthen, G.M. and Bloch, A.B. (1993) Results of a 29-state survey of tuberculosis in nursing homes and correctional facilities. *Public Health Rep*, **108**, 305–14.

60. Stead, W.W. (1981) Tuberculosis among elderly persons: an outbreak in a nursing home. *Ann Intern Med*, **94**, 606–10.

61. Stead, W.W., Lofgren, J.P., Warren, E. and Thomas, C. (1985) Tuberculosis as an endemic and nosocomial infection among the elderly in nursing homes. *N Engl J Med*, **312**, 1483–7.

62. Centers for Disease Control (1991) Nosocomial transmission of multidrug-resistant tuberculosis among HIV-infected persons – Florida and New York, 1988–91. *MMWR*, **40**, 585–91.

63. Pearson, M.L., Jereb, J.A., Frieden, T.R. *et al.* (1992) Nosocomial transmission of multidrug-resistant *Mycobacterium tuberculosis*: a risk to patients and health care workers. *Ann Intern Med*, **117**, 191–6.

64. Beck-Sague, C., Dooley, S.W., Hutton, M.D. *et al.* (1992) Hospital outbreak of multidrug-resistant *Mycobacterium tuberculosis* infections: factors in trans-mission to staff and HIV-infected patients. *JAMA*, **268**, 1280–6.

65. Ehrenkranz, N.J. and Kicklighter, J.L. (1972) Tuberculosis outbreak in a general hospital: evidence for airborne spread of infection. *Ann Intern Med*, **77**, 377–82.

66. Catanzaro, A. (1982) Nosocomial tuberculosis. *Am Rev Respir Dis*, **125**, 559–62.

67. Hutton, M.D., Stead, W.W., Cauthen, G.M. *et al.* (1990) Nosocomial trans-mission of tuberculosis associated with a draining abscess. *J Infect Dis*, **161**, 286–95.

68. Riley, R. (1967) The hazard is relative. *Am Rev Respir Dis*, **96**, 623–5.

69. Vogeler, D. and Burke, J. (1978) Tuberculosis screening for hospital employees: a five-year experience in a large community hospital. *Am Rev Respir Dis*, **187**, 227–32.

70. Atuk, N. and Hunt, E. (1971) Serial tuberculin testing and isoniazid therapy in general hospital employees. *JAMA*, **208**, 1795–8.

71. Aitken, M.L., Anderson, K.M. and Albert, R.K. (1987) Is the tuberculosis screening program of hospital employees still required? *Am Rev Respir Dis*, **136**, 805–7.

72. Malasky, C., Jordan, T., Potulski, F. and Reichman, L.B. (1990) Occupational tuberculous infections among pulmonary physicians in training. *Am Rev Respir Dis*, **142**, 505–7.

73. Snider, D.E. and Hutton, M.D. (1989) Tuberculosis in correctional institutions. *JAMA*, **261**, 436–7.

74. American College of Physicians, National Commission on Correctional Health Care, and American Correctional Health Services Association (1992) The crisis in correctional health care: the impact of the national drug control strategy on correctional health services. *Ann Intern Med*, **117**, 71–7.

75. Braun, M.M., Truman, B.I., Maguire, B. *et al.* (1989) Increasing incidence of tuberculosis in a prison inmate population: association with HIV infection. *JAMA*, **161**, 393–7.

76. Gobles, M., Iseman, M.D. and Madsen, L.A. (1993) Treatment of 171 patients with pulmonary tuberculosis resistant to isoniazid and rifampin. *N Engl J Med*, **328**, 527–32.

77. Mahmoudi, A. and Iseman, M.D. (1993) Pitfalls in the care of patients with tuberculosis. *JAMA*, **270**, 65–8.

78. Centers for Disease Control (1992) Transmission of multidrug-resistant tuberculosis among immunocompromised persons in a correctional system – New York, 1992. *MMWR*, **41**, 507–9.

79. Alfalla, C., Hewlett, D., Horn, D. *et al.* (1992) *An outbreak of multidrug resistant tuberculosis among 28 patients at a New York City hospital.* Interscience Conference on Antimicrobial Agents and Chemotherapy, Anaheim, CA, American Society for Microbiology.

80. Canetti, G. (1965) Present aspects of bacterial resistance in tuberculosis. *Am Rev Respir Dis*, **92**, 687–703.

81. Iseman, M. and Madsen, L.A. (1989) Drug-resistant tuberculosis. *Clin Chest Med*, **10**, 341–53.

82. Advisory Committee for the Elimination of Tuberculosis (1993) Initial therapy for tuberculosis in the era of multidrug resistance: Recommendations of the Advisory Council for the Elimination of Tuberculosis. *MMWR*, **42 (RR-7)**, 1–13.

83. Des Prez, R.M. and Heim, C.R. (1990) *Mycobacterium tuberculosis*, in *Principles and Practice of Infectious Diseases* (eds G.L. Mandel, R.G. Douglas and J.E. Bennett), Churchill Livingstone, New York, pp. 1877–906.

84. Kent, P.T. and Kubica, G.P. (1985) *Public Health Mycobacteriology: A Guide for the Level III Laboratory.* US Department of Health and Human Services, Public Health Service, Centres for Disease Control, Atlanta, GA, p. 163.

85. Iseman, M.D. and Sbarbaro, J.A. (1992) The increasing prevalence of resistance to antituberculosis chemotherapeutic agents: implications for global tuberculosis control. *Curr Clin Top Infect Dis*, **12**, 188–207.

86. Cohn, M.L. and David, C.L. (1970) Infectivity and pathogenicity of drug-resistant strains of tubercle bacilli studied by aerogenic infection of guinea pigs. *Am Rev Respir Dis*, **102**, 97–104.

87. Mitchison, D.A. (1954) Tubercle bacilli resistant to isoniazid. *Brit Med J*, **1**, 128–30.

88. Snider, D.E., Kelly, G.D., Cauthen, G.M. *et al.* (1985) Infection and disease among contacts of tuberculosis cases with drug-resistant and drug-susceptible bacilli. *Am Rev Respir Dis*, **132**, 125–32.

89. Bloch, A.B., Cauthen, G.M., Onorato, I.M. *et al.* (1994) Nationwide survey of drug-resistant tuberculosis in the United States. *JAMA*, **271**, 665–71.

90. Frieden, T.R., Sterling, T., Pablo-Mendez, A. *et al.* (1993) The emergence of drug-resistant tuberculosis in New York City. *N Engl J Med*, **328**, 521–6.

91. Barnes, P.F. (1987) The influence of epidemiologic factors on drug resistance rates in tuberculosis. *Am Rev Respir Dis*, **136**, 325–8.

92. Riley, L.W., Arathoon, E. and Loverde, V.D. (1989) The epidemiologic patterns of drug-resistant *Mycobacterium tuberculosis* infections. *Am Rev Respir Dis*, **139**, 1282–5.

93. Ben-Dov, I. and Mason, G.R. (1987) Drug-resistant tuberculosis in a Southern California hospital: trends from 1969 to 1984. *Am Rev Respir Dis*, **135**, 1307–10.

94. Pablos-Mendez, A., Raviglione, M.C., Battan, R. *et al.* (1990) Drug resistant tuberculosis among the homeless in New York City. *New York State J Med*, **90**, 351–5.

95. Addington, W.D. (1979) Patient compliance: the most serious remaining problem in the control of tuberculosis in the United States. *Chest*, **76**, 741–3.

96. Byrd, R.B., Horn, B. and Solomon, D.A. (1977) Treatment of tuberculosis by the nonpulmonary physician. *Ann Intern Med*, **86**, 799–802.

97. American Thoracic Society (1992) Control of tuberculosis in the United States. *Am Rev Respir Dis*, **146**, 1623–33.

98. Berning, S.E., Huitt, G.A. and Iseman, M.D. (1992) Malabsorption of anti-tuberculosis medications by a patient with AIDS. *N Engl J Med*, **327**, 1817–8.

99. Kleeberg, H.H. and Olivier, M.S. (1984) *A World Atlas of Initial Drug Resistance*. Tuberculosis Research Institute of the South African Medical Research Council, Pretoria, South Africa.

100. Centers for Disease Control (1981) Drug resistance among Indochinese refugees with tuberculosis. *MMWR*, **30**, 273–5.

101. Nolan, C.M. and Elarth, A.M. (1988) Tuberculosis in a cohort of Southeast Asian refugees. *Am Rev Respir Dis*, **137**, 805–9.

102. Pitchenik, A.E., Russell, B.W., Cleary, T. *et al.* (1982) The prevalence of tuberculosis and drug resistance among Haitians. *N Engl J Med*, **307**, 162–5.

103. Scalcini, M., Carre, G. and Jean-Baptiste, M. (1990) Antituberculous drug resistance in central Haiti. *Am Rev Respir Dis*, **142**, 508–11.

104. Howard, W.L., Maresh, F., Mueller, E.E. *et al.* (1949) The role of pulmonary cavitation in the development of bacterial resistance of streptomycin. *Am Rev Tuberc*, **59**, 391–401.

105. Reichman, L.B. (1986) Tuberculosis as a manifestation of the acquired immunodeficiency syndrome. *JAMA*, **256**, 3093.

106. Hopewell, C.P. (1992) Impact of human immunodeficiency virus infection on the epidemiology, clinical features, management, and control of tuberculosis. *Clin Infect Dis*, **15**, 540–7.

107. Depalo, V.A., Salomon, N., Kolokathis, A. *et al.* (1991) *A rise in drug-resistant Mycobacterium tuberculosis in patients with HIV infection, substance abuse, and homelessness*. Eighth International Conference on AIDS, Florence, Italy, World Health Organization.

108. Centers for Disease Control (1985) Drug-resistant tuberculosis among the homeless – Boston. *MMWR*, **34**, 429–31.

109. Reichman, L.B. (1991) The U-shaped curve of concern. *Am Rev Respir Dis*, **144**, 741–2.

110. Centers for Disease Control (1983) Primary resistance to antituberculosis drugs – United States. *MMWR*, **32**, 521–2.

111. Centers for Disease Control (1980) Primary resistance to anti-tuberculous drugs – United States. *MMWR*, **29**, 345–6.

112. Rudnick, J., Kroc, K., Managan, L. *et al.* (1992) *How prepared are U.S. hospitals to control nosocomial transmission of tuberculosis?* World Congress of Tuberculosis, Bethesda, MD.

113. Doster, B., Caras, G.J. and Snider, D.E. (1976) A continuing survey of primary drug resistance in tuberculosis, 1961 to 1968. *Am Rev Respir Dis*, **113**, 419–25.

114. Schiffman, P.L., Ashkar, B., Bishop, M. *et al.* (1977) Drug-resistant tuberculosis in a large southern California hospital. *Am Rev Respir Dis*, **116**, 821–5.
115. Snider, D.E., Cauthen, G.M., Farer, L.S. *et al.* (1991) Drug resistant tuberculosis. *Am Rev Respir Dis*, **144**, 732.
116. Steiner, M., Steiner, P. and Schmidt, H. (1970) Primary drug-resistant tuberculosis in children: a continuing study of the incidence of disease caused by primarily drug-resistant organisms in children observed between the years 1965 and 1968 at the Kings County Medical Center of Brooklyn. *Am Rev Respir Dis*, **102**, 75–82.
117. Steiner, P., Rao, M., Victoria, M.S. *et al.* (1983) A continuing study of primary drug-resistant tuberculosis among children observed at the Kings County Hospital Medical Center between the years 1961 and 1980. *Am Rev Respir Dis*, **128**, 425–8.
118. Steiner, P., Rao, M., Mitchell, M. *et al.* (1986) Primary drug-resistant tuberculosis in children: emergence of primary drug-resistant strains of *M. tuberculosis* to rifampin. *Am Rev Respir Dis*, **134**, 446–8.
119. Stottmeier, K.D. (1976) Emergence of rifampin-resistant *Mycobacterium tuberculosis* in Massachusetts. *J Infect Dis*, **133**, 88–90.
120. Chaves, A.D., Dangler, F., Abeles, H. *et al.* (1961) Prevalence of drug resistance among strains of *M. tuberculosis* isolated from ambulatory patients in New York City. *Am Rev Respir Dis*, **84**, 744.
121. Chawla, P.K., Klapper, P.J., Kamholz, S.L. *et al.* (1992) Drug-resistant tuberculosis in an urban population including patients at risk for human immunodeficiency virus infection. *Am Rev Respir Dis*, **146**, 280–4.
122. Centers for Disease Control (1987) Multi-drug-resistant tuberculosis – North Carolina. *MMWR*, **35**, 785–7.
123. Centers for Disease Control (1990) Outbreak of multidrug-resistant tuberculosis – Texas, California, and Pennsylvania. *MMWR*, **39**, 369–72.
124. Steiner, M., Chaves, A.D., Lyons, J.A. *et al.* (1970) Primary drug-resistant tuberculosis: report of an outbreak. *N Engl J Med*, **283**, 1353–8.
125. Reves, R., Durward, B., Snider, D.E. *et al.* (1981) Transmission of multiple drug-resistant tuberculosis: report of a school and community outbreak. *Am J Epidemiol*, **113**, 423–5.
126. Kent, J.H., Valway, S.E. and Onorato, I.M. (1992) *Epidemiologically linked outbreaks of multidrug-resistant tuberculosis, New York State, 1990–1992.* World Congress on Tuberculosis, Bethesda, MD.
127. Valway, S. (1992) *Transmission of multidrug-resistant tuberculosis in a New York State Prison, 1991.* World Congress on Tuberculosis, Bethesda, MD.
128. Centers for Disease Control (1991) Transmission of multidrug-resistant tuberculosis from an HIV-positive client in a residential substance abuse treatment facility – Michigan. *MMWR*, **40**, 129–31.
129. Ussery, X.T., Bierman, J.A., Valway, S.E. *et al.* (1992) *Transmission of multidrug resistant Mycobacterium tuberculosis among persons exposed at a medical examiner's office.* Interscience Conference on Antimicrobial Agents and Chemotherapy, Anaheim, CA, American Society for Microbiology.
130. Tenover, F.C., Crawford, J.T., Huebner, R.E. *et al.* (1993) The resurgence of tuberculosis: is your laboratory ready? *J Clin Microbiol*, **31**, 767–70.
131. Valway, S., Pearson, M., Ikeda, R. and Edlin, B. (1993) *HIV infected health care workers with multidrug resistant tuberculosis, 1990–1992.* Interscience

Conference on Antimicrobial Agents and Chemotherapy, New Orleans, LA.

132. Stead, W.W. (1978) Undetected tuberculosis in prison: source of infection for community at large. *JAMA*, **240**, 2544–7.

133. Centers for Disease Control (1992) Transmission of multi-drug resistant tuberculosis among immunocompromised persons in a correctional system. *MMWR*, **41**, 507–9.

134. Centers for Disease Control (1989) Prevention and control of tuberculosis in correctional institutions: Recommendations of the Advisory Committee for the Elimination of Tuberculosis. *MMWR*, **38**, 313–25.

135. Sudre, P., ten Dam, G. and Kochi, A. (1992) Tuberculosis: a global overview of the situation today. *Bull WHO*, **70**, 149–59.

136. Murray, C.J.L., Styblo, K. and Rouillon, A. (1990) Tuberculosis in developing countries: burden, intervention, and cost. *Bull Int Union Tuberc Lung Dis*, **65**, 6–24.

137. Centers for Disease Control (1993) Tuberculosis – Western Europe. *MMWR*, **42**, 628–31.

138. Styblo, K. (1991) The impact of HIV infection on the global epidemiology of tuberculosis. *Bull Int Union Tuberc Lung Dis*, **66**, 27–32.

139. Narain, J.P., Raviglione, M.C. and Kochi, A. (1992) *HIV-Associated Tuberculosis in Developing Countries: Epidemiology and Strategies for Prevention.* WHO document, WHO/TB/92.166.

140. Kochi, A. (1991) The global tuberculosis situation and the new control strategy of the World Health Organization. *Tubercle*, **72**, 1–6.

141. Styblo, K. (1991) Transmission of tubercle bacilli. *Select Pap Roy Neth Tuberc Assoc*, **24**, 40–54.

142. Styblo, K. (1985) The relationship between the risk of tuberculous infection and the risk of developing infectious tuberculosis. *Bull Int Union Tuberc Lung Dis*, **60**, 117–19.

143. Rouillon, A. (1991) The Mutual Assistance Programme of the IUATLD. Development, contribution, and significance. *Bull Int Union Tuberc Lung Dis*, **66**, 159–72.

144. Centers for Disease Control and Prevention (1993) Estimates of future global tuberculosis morbidity and mortality. *MMWR*, **42**, 961–4.

145. Enarson, D.A. (1991) Principles of IUATLD collaborative tuberculosis programmes. *Bull Int Union Tuberc Lung Dis*, **66**, 195–200.

# 4

# Tuberculosis in the adult

Elfatih I.M. Abter, Orlando Schaening, Ronald L. Barbour
Larry I. Lutwick

## 4.1 TUBERCULOSIS OF THE LUNG

### 4.1.1 Pathophysiology

The lung, primary entry site of the tuberculosis (TB) bacillus into the body, is the organ most commonly affected by clinical TB. The initial infection occurs by the inhalation of droplet nuclei which, because of their size, bypass the bronchial mucociliary protective barrier. Settling in an alveolus, a single acid-fast bacillus (AFB) carrying droplet nucleus is adequate to initiate a primary focus of infection [1].

The organisms, initially facing no immune response, multiply with a doubling time of 24 hours [2]. The host's neutrophils and macrophages ingest and destroy the multiplying bacilli, but some remain viable and even replicate within macrophages. This growth and the attraction of cellular elements results in the formation of a primary focus. The organisms spread via lymphatics to the hilar and mediastinal lymph nodes and reach the blood stream, seeding the lung and other organs. The virulence of strains of *Mycobacterium tuberculosis* can be measured by their ability to grow progressively in the lungs of mice [2a]. Avirulent strains were found to have slower doubling times, which could be shortened *in vivo* by cortico-steroid administration with the strains becoming more pathogenic [2a].

Although any tissue can be involved, the upper lung fields, kidney, lymph node, brain and bone seem to provide an environment where foci with viable bacilli are likely to persist. Further spread is limited by the development of cell-mediated immunity, demonstrable by a positive tuber-culin skin test within 4–10 weeks [3]. The infection is not well contained in 2–5% of recently infected individuals, resulting in overt disease within a year. In the remainder of individuals, the granulomatous foci may heal or continue to harbor viable bacilli awaiting reactivation. The risk of re-activation is life long, but the rate declines over the years, with 10% of untreated infected individuals eventually developing active TB [3].

The site of primary infection is often the lower lung fields [2], where the ventilation is best. The primary complex consists of a lung focus with hilar or mediastinal lymph node enlargement. Pleural effusion or atelectasis may occur. These processes can occur alone or in combination and, in many cases, no primary lesions are detected on X-ray [3–5]. The hilar or medi-astinal adenopathy persists longer than the parenchymal lesions and is usually a manifestation of primary TB, while parenchymal and pleural lesions develop both in primary and reactivation TB. In individuals with intact immunity, the primary lesions usually heal, some calcify and symptoms are minimal or absent. In others, the lesions may progress to overt pulmonary or extrapulmonary TB.

Post-primary TB is caused by reactivation of an old focus. Reinfection with a new strain is unusual but may occur in persons exposed to a large infective dose [6] or who have cellular immunosuppression. The latter circumstance has been reported using restriction fragment length poly-morphism demonstrating exogenous reinfection with multi-drug-resistant *M. tuberculosis* [6a]. In cases of reactivation, immunosuppression, mal-nutrition, alcoholism or aging may contribute to the failure of containment. The upper lobe apical and posterior segments are the usual sites for reactivation. This is thought to be due to zonal variation in the ventilation–perfusion relationship with resultant higher oxygen tension in the upper lobes. A second factor may be a relative lack of lymphatic drainage from the upper fields. Both conditions provide a more favorable environment for sustaining the viability and growth of TB [4].

The inflammatory process occurring early in reactivation pulmonary TB is not different from the primary focus. As the lesions progress relatively unchecked, they enlarge and may cavitate and/or rupture into the bronchial or pleural space. An important mode of spread within the lung is bronchogenic or bronchial embolization [4,5]. The parenchymal lesions, as they caseate, spill necrotic contents into the bronchial tree, resulting in extension to areas beyond the lobar boundary. The bronchial wall may become involved, resulting in endobronchial TB characterized by mucosal ulceration, mass lesions or bronchial stenosis [7]. A cavitary lesion can communicate with the pleural space, producing empyema, broncho-pleural fistula or pneumothorax [8].

Miliary TB may be associated with primary or reactivation disease. It usually follows hematogenous dissemination from erosion of a blood vessel by a parenchymal lesion or caseating lymph node. The course is often subacute, but fatal fulminant disease can occur even before the onset of radiographic mottling [4]. Another condition with a high mortality is whole lung TB in which all five lobes are involved [9]. It may occur as a result of diffuse bronchogenic spread and/or hematogenous dissemination.

### 4.1.2 Clinical presentation

The patient with overt pulmonary TB may initially be relatively asymptomatic, reporting mild and nonspecific complaints. More prominent symptoms and signs develop which reflect the progression and extent of disease. Concurrent medical illness can predispose to TB, as well as altering its manifestations, making the diagnosis difficult.

The symptoms and signs of pulmonary TB are categorized as constitutional, pulmonary and other [3,10]. Some manifestations may be suggestive of primary disease and others of reactivation. The findings are not specific and asymptomatic cases may occur.

### (a) Constitutional symptoms

Common symptoms include fatigue, anorexia, irritability and weight loss. Fever is initially low grade, persisting for weeks to months, being more marked with disease progression. The absence of fever, however, should not discount a diagnosis of TB. The fever often develops in the afternoon, subsiding during sleep with the characteristic night sweat [10]. A fever of unknown origin can receive an extensive diagnostic evaluation despite the presence of significant clinical clues for TB. This may result in the use of unneeded diagnostic tests and delay the institution of specific therapy [11]. It should be noted that persistent fever during TB therapy does not necessarily suggest treatment failure, particularly if the patient's sense of well being is improving.

### (b) Pulmonary manifestations

A mild initial cough will progress over weeks to become more frequent, producing mucoid or mucopurulent sputum. Hemoptysis occurs in 8% of adults with active disease and may be significant in those with cavitary lesions [12]. Chest pain can be localized or generalized, may be pleuritic and can indicate more diffuse lung involvement. Dyspnea is uncommon, occurring only with massive lung involvement, large pleural effusion or concomitant cardiac disease.

The physical findings are also nonspecific. Fine rales on deep inspiration may be heard, indicating parenchymal involvement. Pleural signs may or may not be present. The pulmonary physiologic changes are also nonspecific. Arterial $pO_2$ is usually preserved even with extensive lung disease, unless acute respiratory distress syndrome (ARDS) occurs. Pulmonary function tests may reveal a reduction in vital capacity, lung volume and single breath carbon monoxide diffusing capacity in those with extensive disease [3].

Primary TB, previously seen mostly in children, has been noted in adults with increasing frequency, and accounts for up to 30% of adult pulmonary TB in the USA [4]. The infection is, however, commonly asymptomatic and may not be diagnosed until an abnormal X-ray or conversion of the tuberculin test is discovered. In a study of 37 adults with primary TB [13] (assessed using the diagnostic criteria of recent tuberculin conversion and lower lobe disease with hilar node enlargement or lower lobe or anterior segment lung lesions that cleared on specific TB drug treatment) symptoms were absent to mild in 70% of patients and the remainder had moderately symptomatic illness, with the exception of one patient who had miliary TB. Cough and pleuritic chest pain were the most common symptoms and the illness may mimic acute pneumonia [14].

Reactivation TB is more common in the older individual. The symptoms may be nonspecific or masked by other illnesses, reflecting a chronic condition with fever, weight loss and cough. It requires, therefore, a high index of suspicion as the infection is potentially fatal if not treated and, if cavitary disease is present, substantial infectivity exists. In one series, the average delay in diagnosis was 10 days from time of hospital admission and 23.2 days when the diagnosis of TB was not initially included [15].

### (c) Other manifestations

Certain patient populations, especially the elderly and the immunocompromised, are likely to manifest unusual clinical findings that qualify TB as 'the great masquerader' [16]. Hypertrophic osteoarthropathy, which was known to indicate non-TB intrathoracic disease, has been recently reported in patients with pulmonary TB [17]. Erythema nodosum and/ or phlyctenular (vesicular) conjunctivitis may be seen in acute disease, reflecting immunological hyperreactivity [10]. These entities are discussed in Chapter 6. Certain individuals will present with TB in other organs and pulmonary involvement. These are discussed below.

### 4.1.3 Diagnosis

If pulmonary TB is suspected, a chest X-ray should be done, sputum sent for AFB smear and culture and a tuberculin skin test placed. Culture of the tubercle bacillus may take weeks, but it is the most definitive method of diagnosis. A presumptive diagnosis, usually based on X-ray findings with a reactive skin test (Chapter 8) and/or a positive AFB smear (Chapter 7) justifies starting specific therapy (Chapter 12) while awaiting culture results.

Pulmonary TB is now increasingly reported in patients with AIDS, a condition which predisposes to numerous other lung infections, making the diagnosis of TB more difficult (Chapter 5). It is also associated with multi-drug-resistant TB (Chapters 3 and 13). In cities with a high TB incidence, the adoption of specific measures for rapid identification and treatment has been attempted [18,19]. Newer and more rapid diagnostic techniques are now available or being developed (Chapter 7 and below).

*(a) Radiographic findings*

The chest radiograph is usually abnormal in pulmonary TB except in some cases of endobronchial disease [10] or early in miliary disease [4]. The radiographic findings are usually categorized as primary or reactivation, but overlap occurs.

In primary TB the usual radiographic patterns include parenchymal consolidation, hilar or mediastinal lymphadenopathy with or without parenchymal involvement, pleural effusion, lobar atelectasis and miliary disease.

In primary TB the parenchymal infiltrate is located in the lower lobes in more than 50% of patients [5] (Figure 4.1). It may or may not be accompanied by lymphadenopathy or pleural effusion and may also contain cavities. Tuberculous intrathoracic lymphadenopathy is almost always due to primary infection. It may be unilateral or bilateral, hilar, mediastinal or both. The well recognized primary complex of parenchymal pneumonitis with regional adenopathy is more common in children. Isolated mediastinal lymphadenopathy is increasingly described in patients with TB and AIDS (Figure 4.2). The tuberculous pleural effusion is usually seen in

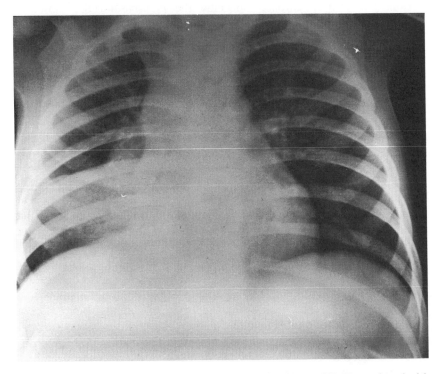

**Figure 4.1** A non-upper lobe consolidation found in primary TB. Reproduced with permission from *Infectious Diseases*, 1st edn, by H.P. Lambert and W.E. Farrar, Gower Medical Publishing, London, UK, 1982.

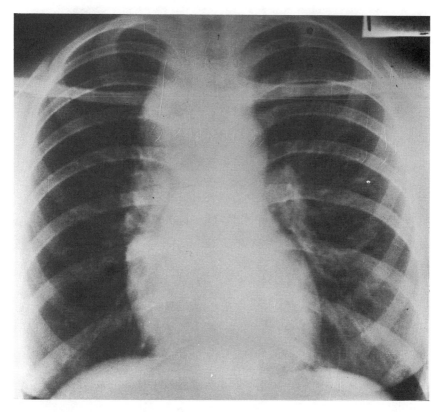

**Figure 4.2** Tuberculous lymphadenopathy with right paratracheal node enlargement. Reproduced with permission from *Infectious Diseases*, 1st edn, by H.P. Lambert and W.E. Farrar, Gower Medical Publishing, London, UK, 1982.

young adults with primary disease, occurring alone or with a parenchymal infiltrate (Figure 4.3). Other radiographic manifestations of primary TB are lobar atelectasis mimicking post-obstructive pneumonia and miliary changes.

Most cases of pulmonary TB are caused by the reactivation of an old focus in the apical or posterior segments of the upper lobe. The radiographic abnormalities usually combine the elements of an acute pneumonic process, seen as patchy ill-defined opacities, and partial healing with nodular or linear fibrosis and calcifications. Cavities occur in 40% of adult patients [5]. They may be thin or thick walled, solitary or numerous and some may show air-fluid levels [20]. When a cavity is solitary, it is almost always surrounded by, or associated with, an inflammatory reaction or infiltration [5]. As the disease extends, mainly by endobronchial spread, multiple lobes and the pleural space become affected, leading to the classical radiographic picture of extensive pulmonary TB (Figure 4.4).

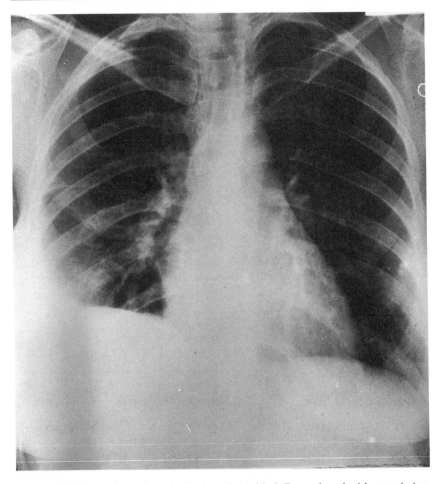

**Figure 4.3** Tuberculous pleural effusion, right sided. Reproduced with permission from *Infectious Diseases*, 1st edn, by H.P. Lambert and W.E. Farrar, Gower Medical Publishing, London, UK, 1982.

Some patients may present with only linear or nodular opacities or pleural thickening. Pneumothorax may also occur. Additionally, tuberculoma, a nodular opacity ranging from less than 1 cm to 3 cm or more which may ultimately calcify, may be seen as a solitary uncalcified nodule and be difficult to distinguish from a neoplastic lesion [4].

Almost any form of pulmonary radiographic abnormality may occur in TB. Terms such as 'old changes' should be used only after reviewing previous radiographs and ascertaining that no changes had occurred during the preceding three to four months [3]. When subtle changes are suspected, further details can be uncovered using computerized tomography (CT) or magnetic resonance imaging (MRI) [3,21]. X-ray abnormalities may be

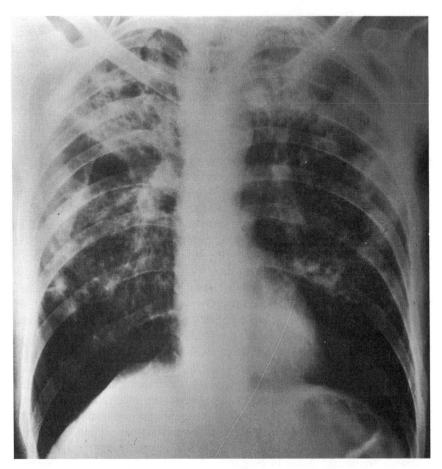

**Figure 4.4** Far advanced TB with extensive nodular shadowing in both lungs, especially in the upper lung fields with contracted upper lobes and probable cavitation on the right. Reproduced with permission from *Infectious Diseases*, 1st edn, by H.P. Lambert and W.E. Farrar, Gower Medical Publishing, London, UK, 1982.

absent or nonspecific in cases of endobronchial TB. A CT scan may be useful in detecting bronchial stenosis in some of these cases [22].

### (b) Microbiological diagnosis

At least three properly obtained sputum specimens containing minimal saliva or nasopharyngeal secretions should be promptly sent to the laboratory. Induction with saline solution (after taking the necessary precautions to prevent nosocomial transmission) may help in persons who are unable to produce sufficient sputum. Likewise, early morning aspiration of gastric secretions may be helpful in hospitalized, debilitated patients and in children [3]. The presence of non-TB mycobacteria limits the value of the smear of gastric aspirates, requiring cultural confirmation of the diagnosis [10]. Gastric smears with large numbers of organisms are likely to represent *M. tuberculosis* [23]. Fiberoptic bronchoscopy with bronchoalveolar lavage (BAL) should be considered when efforts to obtain sputum fail. Post-bronchoscopy sputum should also be collected. Pleural, pericardial, bone marrow or lymph node aspirates may be helpful in certain situations.

The AFB smear has significant clinical and epidemiological importance since the presence of numerous mycobacteria indicates high infectivity. Thus, the experienced microbiologist may be able to estimate the mycobacterial load accurately [3]. Other aspects of the AFB smear are discussed in Chapter 7. A review of sputum AFB smear results obtained from four studies conducted in the USA reported a sensitivity ranging from 22% to 78% with 99% specificity [24]. In a group of 47 patients with pulmonary TB, the sputum smear was positive in 34%, culture was positive in 51%, smear of BAL was positive in 68% and BAL culture positive in 92% [25]. A reported 93% sensitivity was found when cultures of both the sputum and BAL were combined [26]. The sensitivity of the latter combination was not increased significantly by using a biopsy during bronchoscopy [27]. However, trans-bronchial brushing with biopsy and open lung biopsy retain their diagnostic value in the remaining undiagnosed bronchial, parenchymal or lymph node lesions. Bronchoscopy is particularly valuable in endobronchial TB [28].

Sputum culture is still the gold standard for the diagnosis of pulmonary TB. As discussed in Chapter 7, a properly performed sputum AFB culture is the most sensitive and non-invasive procedure available to clinicians. It will identify infected patients with non-diagnostic radiographs and negative smears as demonstrated in an elderly nursing home population [28]. Unlike the smear, which takes a few hours to perform, the culture causes a significant delay in diagnosis. This may subject some patients to inappropriate therapy and/or delay the institution of proper therapy if TB is not appropriately considered and treated while awaiting culture results. For this reason, newer technologies are now being developed to improve on or replace existing techniques. Some of the new tests are currently marketed, while others are limited to reference or research laboratories. They may be performed on sputum, pleural fluid and other clinical specimens and are discussed in some detail in Chapter 7. The tests include radiometric growth systems [29], polymerase chain reaction [30], serum antibody tests [31,32] and adenosine deaminase activity [33].

### 4.1.4 Differential diagnosis

*(a) Primary tuberculosis*

The features of primary TB in adults, including mild to moderate constitutional symptoms and X-ray findings of parenchymal infiltrates, lymphadenopathy and/or pleural effusion are nonspecific. Parenchymal infiltrates with or without effusions can be due to bacterial, atypical or viral pneumonia. Pulmonary TB should be considered in patients with pneumonia, especially in the setting of possible exposure to or risk factors for TB or failure to respond to antibiotics.

Intrathoracic lymphadenopathy with or without parenchymal changes may be due to sarcoidosis. A useful clue is the combination of bilateral mediastinal with unilateral hilar lymphadenopathy, which suggests TB [5]. HIV-infected persons with TB often present with hilar adenopathy [34]. The issue of TB in HIV patients is discussed further in Chapter 5.

### (b) Reactivation tuberculosis

This form of TB is often encountered in the elderly or in patients with diabetes, alcoholism, HIV infection, lung cancer, sarcoidosis, silicosis, post-gastrectomy and organ transplant and those who are receiving corticosteroids or other immunosuppressive therapy [35–37]. Malignancy, sarcoidosis and silicosis may induce inflammatory or destructive pulmonary lesions which can be indistinguishable from TB or may exist with it. AIDS, immunosuppression and organ transplantation predispose to opportunistic infections involving the lung, resembling any of the forms of pulmonary TB. Table 4.1 lists some conditions which can be confused with TB on chest X-ray. Patients with diabetes or HIV and the elderly may exhibit atypical clinical or radiological findings. Lower lobe infiltrates were reported to occur in 20% of diabetic patients with reactivation TB [36]. Most diabetics will, therefore, have typical upper lobe disease with or without cavitation.

**Table 4.1** Conditions that can simulate tuberculosis on chest X-ray

---

**Non-tuberculosis mycobacteria**
In particular *M. kansasii* and *M. avium-intracellulare*

**Fungi**
Including *Histoplasma, Coccidiodes, Blastomyces, Sporothrix, Cryptococcus* and *Aspergillus*

**Bacteria**
Including *Nocardia, Actinomyces* and *Rhodococcus (Corynebacterium) equi*
Purulent lung abscess

**Parasitic diseases**
*Paragonimus westermani, Echinococcus* sp. (cystic or cavitary lesions)
*Pneumocystis carinii, Strongyloides stercorales* (miliary type lesion)

**Viral disease**
Herpes simplex, Varicella-zoster, Cytomegalovirus (miliary type lesions)

**Non-infectious causes**
Including carcinoma, lymphoma, sarcoidosis, silicosis and other pneumoconioses

---

The relationship of lung cancer and TB is significant [38]. Bronchogenic carcinoma is 20 times more common in TB patients than in a population with a similar history of smoking tobacco. TB may be associated with a 'scar carcinoma' in which the malignancy develops in an old inflammatory area. Cancer should be suspected in a TB patient who has progression of one area with regression of others, hilar nodes in adult reactivation disease (Figure 4.5) or atelectasis [39].

### 4.1.5 Pulmonary tuberculosis in the elderly

The incidence of pulmonary TB in the elderly (those aged 65 or over) is usually higher than in younger populations. In the USA in 1987, the incidence was 20.6 cases per 100 000 in the elderly and 4.6 in younger adults [40]. A higher rate in younger people has occurred in recent years in areas of increased TB as detailed in Chapter 3. A rate of 234 per 100 000 has been found in the elderly residing in nursing homes [41]. These data indicate that while older adults often develop TB living in the community, moving into the closed setting of a nursing home places them at an even higher risk.

One report found a rate of purified protein derivative of tuberculin (PPD) reactivity of 25% in persons newly admitted to nursing homes compared with 45% in those residing there for some time [41]. The difference could not be attributed solely to the booster phenomenon (Chapter 8) and was felt to indicate that new infection occurred in some. This finding indicates that TB can be endemic in nursing homes and that institutional transmission occurs [41]. Whether advancing age itself produces an increased TB susceptibility is not clear but this appears not to be the case in a murine model [42].

The magnitude of the problem of pulmonary TB in the elderly is further expanded by the absence of typical clinical manifestations in many cases, making the diagnosis difficult and easy to miss [43]. The combination of fever, cough, night sweats and hemoptysis may not be present. In one study, the time from onset of symptoms to diagnosis was 8 weeks in the elderly compared with 3.5 weeks in a younger group [44]. Weakness was the most frequent complaint and anorexia and weight loss were common. Some elderly persons may present with cough and no other clinical findings [28]. Diseases which are more common in the elderly, such as lung cancer, mimic TB [45]. Several authors reported atypical X-ray findings as well [43]. In a prospective study [46], pure apical lesions were seen in only 7% while 48% had middle field or basal lesions and 46% had a mixed pattern. Atypical radiographic presentations are not necessarily encountered only in the elderly and have been found equally in the elderly and younger adults [47].

Guidelines exist for the prevention and surveillance of TB in chronic care facilities [48]. All persons newly admitted to a nursing home or a chronic care facility should be tuberculin tested, with chest X-rays performed on

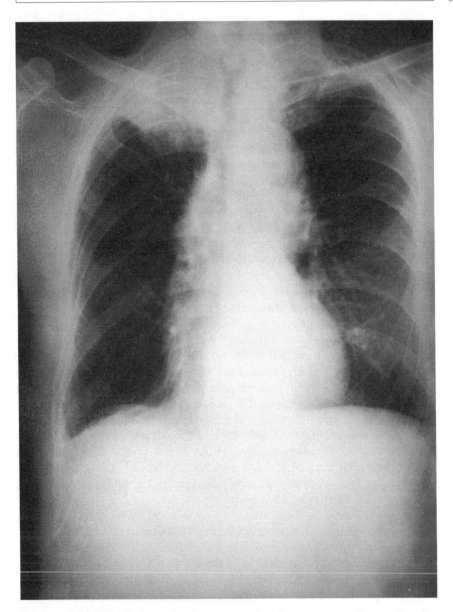

**Figure 4.5** Right upper lobe reactivation TB with right hilar adenopathy sub-sequently found to be a lung carcinoma. Radiograph courtesy of Maimonides Medical Center Radiology Department.

those with a positive test. Those with cough, bronchitis or other symptoms of respiratory infection should have an AFB smear and sputum culture even if the skin test is negative. Those who are tuberculin negative require a repeat PPD whenever a case of active TB is identified in the facility.

Isoniazid (INH) prophylaxis and close follow-up are indicated for all persons with a recent skin test conversion (Chapter 12). A second tuberculin test is often administered 1 week after an initially negative test to evaluate for a booster phenomenon (Chapter 8).

### 4.1.6 Outcome

With the availability of effective therapy, continuous hospitalization for patients with active TB is not required. With clinical improvement, management can be continued at home. In fact, patients who are otherwise well with good home situations may be treated without hospitalization. Clinical indices signifying a good response include improved appetite, reduction in intensity and frequency of cough and disappearance of or decrease in the sputum count of AFB. Fever may persist for two or more months even with effective therapy owing to the infection or may be drug induced [49]. If the sputum culture is still positive after 3 months of treatment, drug resistance should be suspected [1]. The sputum AFB stain, however, may continue to be positive intermittently for up to 6 months on adequate therapy. Such organisms may not be viable by the end of the third week of therapy and often cannot be grown in culture [49].

In 1976, a 5 year follow-up study of 543 patients with TB who were treated successfully revealed a relapse rate of 11.6% [50]. This rate was lowest during the first 2 years and not influenced by the initial pattern of resistance. Patients with radiographic clearing by the end of therapy had the lowest rate of relapse. This study also concluded that there is no indication for yearly follow-up if the individuals return when appropriate symptoms occur. Of interest, only 25% of the relapse cases were detected during routine annual check ups. More recent prospective trials from 1990 found relapse rates of 1.6% and 3.5% [50a,50b]. These rates, from short course therapy protocols, may reflect the risk of relapse with current treatment regimens more accurately.

Primary TB may be associated with endobronchial complications, such as fibrostenosis or ulcerative granulomas. These occur more frequently in patients with parenchymal consolidation or local atelectasis than in those with lymphadenopathy or pleurisy. Patients with lower lobe consolidation or atelectasis should be followed closely for signs of endobronchial disease, which may have serious consequences, including permanent anatomical lung deformity and respiratory failure if not found at an early stage [51,52].

The complications of chronic pulmonary TB are related to the degree of tissue destruction and fibrosis. Fistulae to the pleural space or esophagus may develop [53]. Additionally, residual cavities can serve as a potential space for fungal colonization [54]. Respiratory failure occurred in 0.02% of TB patients in the 'pre-AIDS' era. There was a 30% mortality in those who developed this complication and most of the survivors suffered permanent restrictive lung disability [55]. ARDS and disseminated intravascular coagulation (DIC) rarely occurred and were usually complications of miliary disease [56,57].

Pulmonary TB is almost always a treatable disease. Mortality remains relatively high, however, in persons with AIDS, the elderly and immuno-compromised patients. Atypical clinical and X-ray findings, poor compliance with therapy and a high incidence of concurrent disease contribute to this high mortality. Multi-drug-resistant disease in AIDS patients can result in death rates as high as 93% [18]. In the USA between 1979 and 1989, 60% of deaths due to TB occurred in persons 65 years of age or older. This rate is 10 times higher than in patients 25–44 years old [1]. In cases of TB diagnosed at death, the proportion of cases increased with age from 0.7% in children less than 5 years of age to 18.6% among adults over 85 [58]. There was also a higher representation of extrapulmonary cases diagnosed at death. These observations demonstrate that difficulties in diagnosis contribute significantly to TB mortality in the elderly.

## 4.2 PLEURAL TUBERCULOSIS

### 4.2.1 Organ involvement

Pleural TB has largely been considered a consequence of primary infection [59] but may also complicate reactivation disease. The overall rate was 4.9% in a study of 1738 patients with proven TB [60]. The pathogenesis of the pleural reaction involves a delayed hypersensitivity reaction to AFB, which enter the pleural space from a ruptured caseous focus. Autopsy studies have confirmed direct continuity between the lung parenchyma and pleural space in most cases [59]. A pleural granulomatous reaction occurs with the effusion, but AFB are only found in small numbers, if at all [4]. In the classic case complicating primary TB, the effusion appears 1–4 months after exposure [15].

In industrialized countries, tuberculous pleuritis is more common in middle-aged and older individuals. In a large survey, the median age was 47 years [60]. One report [61] found that 81% of the effusions were associated with primary disease and 19% with reactivation. Most of the patients had a co-existing debilitating condition, such as chronic alcoholism, malignancy or previous gastrectomy. The epidemiology is strikingly different in undeveloped countries where TB and HIV infections are endemic. In this setting, TB is the most common cause of pleural effusion [62], with as many as 86% of pleural effusions caused by TB and 83% of patients with tuberculous pleuritis being HIV seropositive.

### 4.2.2 Presentation and diagnosis

Symptom onset is acute or insidious. Cough, fever, weight loss, dyspnea and chest pain are common, with chills and night sweats less frequent. In a study of 71 patients with TB pleuritis [63], pneumonia was the initial diagnosis in most cases and cough, usually nonproductive, characteristically preceded the chest pain. Purulent sputum was uncommon. Another study revealed a longer duration of cough in those with reactivation rather than primary disease [64].

Examination reveals the signs of pleural fluid with bilateral involvement in less than 10% of cases [64]. Chest X-ray confirms the effusion. Diagnosis requires the direct evaluation of the fluid, even in the presence of a reactive tuberculin test [4,63]. If TB is suspected clinically, thoracentesis should be performed with pleural biopsy [14]. The fluid is typically clear or green tinged, but cloudy or serosanguinous fluid may be obtained [63].

Polymorphonuclear leukocytes (PMNs) may predominate in those with brief illnesses, but a lymphocytic pleocytosis is the rule [59]. Some consider all exudative lymphocytic effusions in PPD-reactive persons to be tuberculous until proved otherwise [60]. Some recommend empiric TB therapy to such patients [4]. The diagnostic value of the phenotypic analysis of fluid lymphocytes has not been proved [65], but the absence of mesothelial cells in the pleural fluid is said to be highly suggestive of TB [59], and pleural fluid eosinophilia is not generally reminiscent of infection with the tubercle bacillus [66].

Tuberculous effusions are exudative; defined as a fluid to serum protein ratio of more than 0.5, a lactate dehydrogenase (LDH) ratio of more than 0.6 and/or a pleural LDH concentration of more than 200 U/l [67]. One study found the LDH concentration was higher than 550 U/l in all cases [64]. The mean pleural fluid protein is about 5 g/dl in most series. In another study [64], pleural fluid glucose was 57 mg/dl in reactivation and 89 mg/dl in primary TB effusion. The use of fluid cholesterol [68] and alkaline phosphatase [67] assists in distinguishing exudative effusions but not in making a diagnosis of TB. Other markers such as tuberculostearic acid [69], adenosine deaminase and interferon gamma have had success diagnostically. One study [70] reported pleural adenosine deaminase levels of more than 47 U/l in all TB effusions with sensitivity of 100% and specificity of 95% while interferon gamma had a sensitivity of 94% and specificity of 92% using a 140 pg/ml threshold. Additionally, the lack of contamination and low bacillary count suggest that pleural fluid may be ideal for testing with polymerase chain reaction for the detection of mycobacterial DNA. In appropriate hands, this technology can be extremely sensitive and specific [30].

As with other forms of TB, a definitive diagnosis of pleural infection requires identification of tubercle bacilli. Pleural fluid, pleural tissue and sputum should be sent for smear and culture. The pleural fluid AFB smear was positive in 27% in reactivation infection and only 7% in those with primary disease [64] and culture was positive in 91% and 66%, respectively. Pleural biopsy [70] revealed granulomata in 25% of those with reactivation and 72% of those with primary disease, with AFB seen in 17% in both groups and culture positivity ranging between 40% and 58%. The sputum

AFB smear and culture were positive in more than 50% of those with reactivation and 0% and 23%, respectively, in primary disease. Pleural biopsy is particularly useful whenever primary pleural TB is suspected [64]. Bedside cultures of pleural fluid, repeated cultures (two or more) and/or culturing 200 ml or more have been felt to increase the diagnostic yield [71]. Imaging techniques, such as chest radiography, CT scan and MRI are useful for the detection of pleural effusion, fluid loculation and complications such as pleural thickening, calcifications and broncho-pleural fistulae. Recently, ultrasound has been evaluated for diagnosing TB pleuritis; the finding of small pleural nodularity is highly specific for pleural TB [72].

### 4.2.3 Outcome

Primary tuberculous pleuritis resolves spontaneously in most patients, including those with massive effusions, without specific chemotherapy [4,59]. As many as 50% of patients, however, will develop pleural thickening with no clinical or laboratory means of predicting the risk of development. Neither pleural fluid characteristics, nor the type of TB therapy or surgical drainage influenced the development of pleural thickening [73]. Further studies are needed to define this risk, however, since in another study none of the 22 patients who were treated, traced and reassessed 2 years later had significant pleural thickening or impairment of lung function [74]. Patients who do not receive chemotherapy are reported to have a 65% chance of developing pulmonary TB within 5 years [59].

When TB pleuritis accompanies reactivation disease, a protracted course with long-term morbidity may ensue. Some complications such as bronchopleural fistula, fibrosis and calcification commonly require surgical management. Treatment with specific chemotherapy and drainage will be required during the acute stage and may be followed by a definitive surgical procedure such as staged thoracoplasty and decortication. These patients will also require long term TB chemotherapy [75].

## 4.3 EXTRAPLEUROPULMONARY TUBERCULOSIS

Although classically a disease of the lung, *M. tuberculosis* infection may involve any organ. Infection of the skin, middle ear, aorta, eye and breast, among others, are well described but will not be considered further. The most common sites outside the lung and its lining are shown in Figure 4.6.

## 4.4 LARYNGEAL TUBERCULOSIS

### 4.4.1 Organ involvement

In the pretherapy era, involvement of the larynx was found in 34–83% of patients with far advanced pulmonary TB [77]. The larynx was felt to be directly infected from contact with infectious sputum. Currently, upper

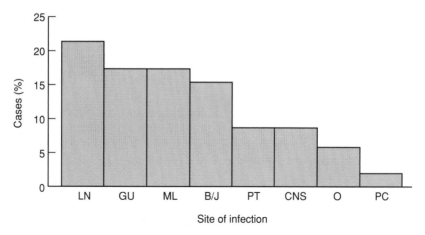

**Figure 4.6** Site of involvement of 207 cases of extrapulmonary TB [76]. LN, lymph node; GU, genitourinary; ML, miliary; B/J, bone/joint; PT, peritoneal; CNS, meningitis; O, other; PC, pericardial.

respiratory tract infection is reported in 1.8% of TB patients [78]. Although most patients have co-existing pulmonary infection, reports of isolated laryngeal infection suggest infection may be an isolated reactivation event [79,80]. Beginning as an erythematous, exudative laryngitis, the infection progresses from discrete nodularity to ulceration with edema and exuberant granulation tissue [81]. Any area of the larynx may be involved but most commonly it affects the true vocal cords (47%), epiglottis (39%) and false cords (29%) [77]. Progression can involve the pharynx, the tonsils and soft palate but unlike malignant or non-TB inflammatory conditions usually does not extend to the hypopharynx or subglottic areas [77].

### 4.4.2 Presentation and diagnosis

Local symptoms of laryngeal TB include cough (94%), sore throat (75%), odynophagia (69%), hoarseness (50%) and otalgia (31%) [78]. Cough is not commonly conspicuous, often being of long standing duration and disregarded as a smoker's cough [82]. Symptoms averaged 4.6 months in duration and were associated with weight loss [78]. The diagnosis is made by demonstrating a granulomatous reaction and the visualization of AFB on stain and/or growth in culture. Because many cases are associated with pulmonary infection, finding AFB in the sputum with a granulomatous laryngeal reaction is adequate for a diagnosis.

The differential diagnosis is laryngeal carcinoma, though other inflammatory conditions such as sarcoidosis, Wegener's granulomatosis, syphilis and fungal infections may merit consideration. The finding of a productive cough, rales on pulmonary auscultation and the absence of cervical lymphadenopathy is supportive of TB and less of malignancy [78].

It has been generally accepted that laryngeal TB is highly infectious but since most cases are associated with far advanced cavitary pulmonary disease, the infectivity of the laryngeal process alone is not clearly proven. In two patients with laryngeal TB without pulmonary disease, no evidence of intrafamilial spread was found, suggesting that laryngeal disease in itself may not be so infectious [80].

### 4.4.3 Outcome

Appropriate drug treatment is adequate to treat this infection. In one report [78], two of 16 patients were left with mild, permanent hoarseness. Persistent symptoms are related to adhesions or fibrosis of the cord [81]. Progressive infection which is not recognized and treated may cause enough damage to need tracheostomy, partial laryngectomy or laryngo-tracheoplasty for respiratory insufficiency [83].

### 4.5 MILIARY TUBERCULOSIS

The term miliary relates to similarities between the 1–2 mm millet seed (Figure 4.7) and the nodular pulmonary infiltrates that often occur during the infection. The chest X-ray in miliary disease may be normal, have nodular shadows which are barely visible or have nodular densities several

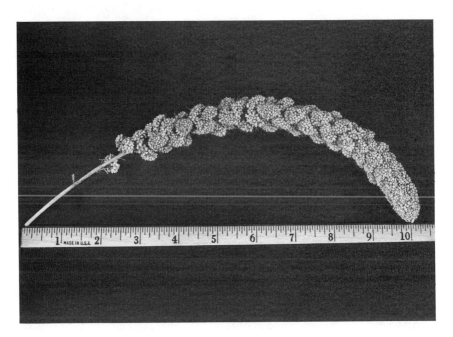

**Figure 4.7** A millet seed sprig.

times or more the size of the millet seed [84]. Classically a disease of the young, over the past few years there has been a progressive increase in the age distribution of miliary TB. In Belfast, for example, of 39 autopsies of individuals dying of this entity before 1949, over half were under 20 years of age; between 1966 and 1969, none was under 30 [85].

### 4.5.1 Organ involvement

Miliary TB results from the acute hematogenous dissemination of tubercle bacilli. The dissemination may be associated with progressive spread following primary infection or a reactivated focus such as a lymph node. The disease process tends to be more severe and more acute in children. Sometimes, especially in the elderly, the seeding is chronic and the symptom complex more difficult to diagnose. This protracted, cryptic form is called chronic hematogenous or late generalized TB [86]. A form of miliary TB known as generalized non-reactive TB or typhobacillosis of Landouzy involves areas of necrosis surrounded by normal tissue with little or no cellular reaction and large numbers of AFB [87]. In rare cases, unusual sources of tubercle bacilli occur, as exemplified by recurrent miliary TB related to a ventriculo–atrial shunt in a patient with TB meningitis [88].

The organs that are well perfused and have reticulo-endothelial function are those with the most involvement in miliary TB. These include lungs, bone marrow, liver, kidneys, adrenals and spleen. In a South African series [89], 63% of endobronchial, 82% of bone marrow and 100% of liver biopsies revealed granulomata, with 50–60% revealing caseation and AFB seen in more than half. Bone marrow is a good source of granulomata but is a poor source of AFB on stain and culture. Slavin's review [86] from 1980 found the frequency of various commonly involved organs as follows: spleen (100%), liver (97%), lungs (86%), bone marrow (77%), kidneys (64%), adrenals (53%) and ocular choroidal lesions (50%). An autopsy survey from 1946 revealed a similar distribution [90].

### 4.5.2 Presentation and diagnosis

The clinical picture of miliary disease is that of a nonspecific systemic illness with weakness, anorexia, fatigue and weight loss [91]. Focal symptoms can vary depending on system involvement and include cough, headache and abdominal pain [85,92]. Physical signs on initial evaluation include fever, pulmonary rales, hepatomegaly, localized lymphadenopathy, splenomegaly and choroidal tubercles [89,91]. Choroidal tubercles have been reported in as many as 95% of miliary cases [92] and are described as gray–white oblong patches seldom greater than 1 mm. The incidence may be related to the diligence with which they are searched for.

Although the disseminated nature of this disease can produce a non-reactive tuberculin skin test, 52% had 9 mm or more induration to 5 TU and 79% reacted if higher strengths were used [91]. Of Munt's 11 patients who were initially negative, all but one developed positivity in the course of illness [91]. The classic diagnostic finding is the miliary pattern on chest X-ray (Figure 4.8). Although it is taught that miliary lesions take up to 6 weeks to develop, one study found that of 12 chest X-rays initially reported to be normal in miliary TB, 10 had subtle lesions on review [93]. Close inspection of the intercostal and retrocardiac spaces is recommended to aid the diagnosis [84]. Most individuals with miliary disease have normal total

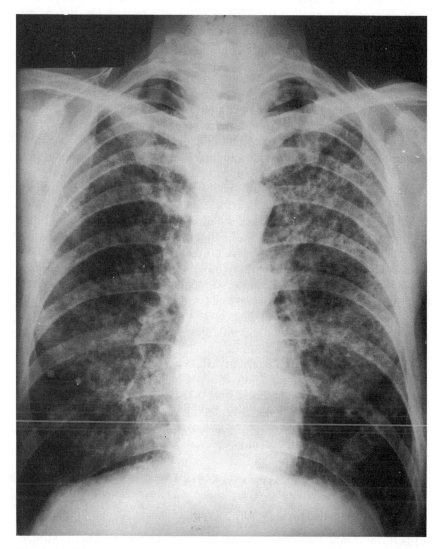

**Figure 4.8** Miliary tuberculosis. Radiograph courtesy of Maimonides Medical Center Radiology Department.

white blood counts but an elevated band count and lymphopenia are both common [89,91]. Hepatic function tests often show cholestatic indices with elevated alkaline phosphatase [90].

The yield of AFB in pulmonary secretions is usually lower than in standard pulmonary TB. One large review found positive sputum AFB smears in 39% and positive cultures in 54% without lung consolidation or cavity formation [91]. Tissue examination may be of value diagnostically, including transbronchial, bone marrow and liver biopsies [89]. Both Maartens, Willcox and Benatar and Munt [89, 91] found a low yield of bone marrow examination for AFB. A diagnostic trial of TB therapy can be attempted and may be used to help diagnose TB while awaiting micro-biological or histological confirmation of the disease.

### 4.5.3 Outcome

The return to an afebrile state in response to specific TB therapy is often slow. In Munt's review, only 14% were afebrile within 1 week and 35% within 2 weeks, with 8% requiring more than 60 days to return to a normal temperature [91]. There was often an increased sense of well being, despite persistent fever, indicating a therapeutic response. Munt did not correlate prolonged fevers with decreased survival. In a more recent series reflect-ing, in part, treatment regimens containing INH and rifampin, Maartens, Willcox and Benatar [89] reported the median duration of fever was 7 days after treatment began, with 76% of patients being afebrile within 2 weeks.

With appropriate therapy, chest X-ray clearing occurs substantially more rapidly than in classical pulmonary TB [94]. The resolution is generally complete without residual changes. Residual miliary calcifications on chest X-ray are most likely related to varicella or histoplasmosis. In Biehl's series [95], most cases had normal findings by 16 weeks with the time to complete resolution generally correlating with the extent of initial involvement, being slower in older patients.

Complications of miliary TB include ARDS (6%), adrenal insufficiency (less than 1%), pancytopenia and death [89]. DIC may also occur [96]. Mortality rates were 21.7% in Munt's series from 1971 [91], and 24% in the series by Maartens, Willcox and Benatar from 1990 [89]. The latter report found six predictors of death: age over 60 years, lymphopenia, thrombocytopenia, hypoalbuminemia, elevated aminotransferase levels and treatment delay.

## 4.6 TUBERCULOUS LYMPHADENITIS

### 4.6.1 Organ involvement

Superficial lymph node involvement is the most common form of extrapul-monary TB. It is often referred to as scrofula, from a latin word for brood sow, or king's evil from the practice of attempting cure by a royal touch.

Since it is often unaccompanied by disease elsewhere, scrofula has been addressed less rigorously than other forms of TB [97]. Lymph node disease is most commonly found in the cervical group (60–90%) but any lymph node group may be involved (Table 4.2) [98–100]. Multiple node groups occur in 10–20% and generalized adenopathy in less than 5% [98,99].

**Table 4.2** Distribution of lymph node involvement in tuberculosis [98, 99, 103]

| Site | Percentage (%) |
|------|----------------|
| Cervical | |
|   Total | 61 |
|   Anterior | 23 |
|   Posterior | 16 |
|   Supraclavicular | 14 |
|   Submandibular | 8 |
| Axillary | 17 |
| Abdominal | 7 |
| Inguinal | 5 |
| Mediastinal | 5 |
| Hilar | 3 |
| Generalized | 2 |

### 4.6.2 Presentation and diagnosis

The affected node begins as an enlarged, firm, mobile, slightly painful or non-tender mass with progression in size and the development of caseation. Node enlargement is generally slow but can be acute with accompanying pain, fever and surrounding inflammation. As the necrosis progresses, abscesses may develop with sinus formation.

The diagnosis is histologic in nature. Caseous granulomatous necrosis on biopsy was seen in 91% of cases [101], with 22% having positive AFB stains and 56% positive cultures. Others report a higher yield with AFB culture [102]. The differential diagnosis of these histologic changes [97] includes diseases with granulomatous changes and AFB (non-TB myco-bacteria, lepromatous leprosy), with necrotizing granulomas without AFB (cat scratch disease, lymphogranuloma venereum, syphilis, tularemia and fungi) and with noncaseating granulomata (sarcoidosis, brucellosis and Hodgkin's disease). A clinical response to TB treatment in a patient with localized adenopathy (particularly cervical) and a reactive tuberculin test are reasonably adequate diagnostic criteria.

### 4.6.3 Outcome

The relapse rate following surgical treatment without TB therapy varies depending on the procedure performed. An 86% recurrence rate occurred after node aspiration, 40% after incision and drainage, 14% after primary excision with abscess present and 3% with excision without abscess [102]. Recurrences following appropriate chemotherapy occur in less than 5% of cases [97].

The major complication of scrofula is a sinus tract which can develop either postsurgically or in unrecognized disease. These sinuses may not heal readily with treatment and surgical excision may be necessary [97]. Damage to the cervical branch of the facial or the posterior auricular nerve may occur, most likely related to surgical intervention.

## 4.7 NEUROTUBERCULOSIS

### 4.7.1 Organ involvement

Tuberculous meningitis generally develops from the breakdown of a 'Rich' focus in a subependymal location. This focus has been found, in almost all autopsies with this form of TB, communicating with and discharging caseous material into the cerebrospinal fluid (CSF) [104]. It may destabilize after many years of quiescence related to advanced age, immunosuppression, debilitation or physical factors such as head trauma. Alternatively, TB meningitis can develop during miliary disease.

The reaction to AFB and necrotic debris produces a thick exudate, most marked in the basilar area of the meninges, and may involve the exiting cranial nerves particularly III, IV and VI. A vasculitis may develop from the direct invasion by *M. tuberculosis* or from extension from the surrounding arachnoiditis. The vessels most commonly involved are branches of the middle cerebral artery, especially the perforating vessels to the basal ganglia [105] and can result in cerebral infarctions.

Similar processes can occur in the spinal subarachnoid space from a 'Rich' focus or TB vertebral osteomyelitis. The epidural space may be involved without meningeal involvement [106].

The tuberculoma, usually intracranial but occasionally in the spinal parenchyma, develops as one or multiple slowly expanding lesions. They may be associated with meningitis and can be silent. The lesions have been observed to appear and disappear on brain imaging studies during medical therapy for meningitis or miliary disease. In areas of the developing world, tuberculomas represent a significant minority of intracranial tumors [106].

### 4.7.2 Presentation and diagnosis

TB meningitis is a subacute disease beginning with vague complaints of weakness, low grade fever, headache and personality changes. Within several weeks, however, a more defined meningoencephalitis syndrome develops with protracted headache, meningeal signs, fever, vomiting and confusion [105,107]. Seizures, focal neurologic signs, particularly related to cranial nerves and long tract signs may develop [108]. The presentation may be more acute and not clinically distinguishable from a pyogenic meningeal process or more chronic with dementia. Physical findings vary based on the extent of the infection. Meningeal irritation signs are present in 80–90% of cases with altered mental status in 40–60% [109]. Other neurologic signs on presentation include papilledema, extensor Babinski sign, hemiparesis and choroidal tubercles [109].

The CSF cell count is 100–400 cells/mm$^3$ in about 50% of cases, with 20% less than 100 and 30% more than 400 [107,109]. Although the typical CSF reveals a prominent lymphocytic predominance, early in the disease a minimal pleocytosis or a PMN cell response can be noted [106]. These can be initial pitfalls in diagnosing this potentially fatal infection. Serial lumbar punctures should show the trend towards the expected lymphocytic pleocytosis. Serial analysis during therapy, however, can show the opposite response, an initial lymphocytic response fluctuating intermittently to granulocytes. This 'therapeutic paradox' has been said to be very suggestive of tuberculous disease [110]. The CSF protein is elevated, most often at 100–500 mg/dl. In 25% of patients it will initially be less than 100 mg/dl and may be less than 40 mg/dl. In 10–20%, the CSF protein may be over 500 mg/dl, sometimes in the range 2–5 g/dl [105,109]. Marked elevation of the CSF protein is associated with a subarachnoid block. CSF glucose is less than 45 mg/dl in 80% or more of cases [105,109].

An increased yield of the AFB stain and culture is produced by the use of multiple CSF examinations. A yield on stain of 37% and culture of 56% could be increased to 87% and 83%, respectively, when up to four CSF specimens were examined [109]. In 30% of the cases, the diagnosis could still be made up to 3 days after therapy was begun so that beginning therapy does not need to be delayed. In the setting of a negative CSF AFB stain, AFB culture results will not be available for weeks. Empiric therapy is clearly indicated while awaiting culture results. A number of newer approaches to diagnosis in the CSF have been evaluated, including indirect tests, such as adenosine deaminase activity [111], and direct ones, such as *M. tuberculosis* antigen detection [112]. Reproducible data on such tests are needed, showing a high degree of sensitivity and specificity before they should be uniformly adopted.

The differential diagnosis of a subacute or chronic lymphocytic meningeal process includes infections such as cryptococcosis, coccidioidomycosis, histoplasmosis, brucellosis, syphilis, Lyme borreliosis and focal parameningeal foci. Non-infectious causes such as lymphomatous or carcinomatous meningitis, sarcoidosis and CNS angiitis may also be considered. In particularly difficult cases, meningeal biopsy has been performed but generally is not helpful, except in malignant meningitis [113].

### 4.7.3 Outcome

In untreated cases, death usually occurs within one or two months [105] but much more prolonged courses are well described. Complications, often related to delayed diagnosis or treatment, include seizures, hemiplegia, cranial nerve palsies, gait disturbances, blindness, deafness, dementia, hydrocephalus and a variety of hypothalamic or pituitary syndromes. The incidence of complications is greatly influenced by the stage of the disease at the onset of treatment. One study [109] found early stage disease had a mortality rate of less than 10% and minimal sequelae, but 46% with late disease died.

Hydrocephalus develops in as many as 80% of cases [104], usually related to poor CSF reabsorption by the arachnoid villi. Noncommunicating hydrocephalus may also occur from obstruction of the ventricular passages. Serial brain imaging studies [114] can be useful in alerting to the need for decompression by external or internal shunting. Adjuvant corticosteroid use can decrease cerebral edema and the risk of spinal fluid block [105]. New focal neurological signs that develop during specific TB treatment may be due to infarction from vasculitis or complications of cerebral hypertension. Tuberculomas can develop paradoxically during therapy and can require surgical decompression if medical measures to diminish intracranial pressure are not successful [115].

## 4.8 GASTROINTESTINAL TUBERCULOSIS

### 4.8.1 Ileocecal tuberculosis

*(a) Organ involvement*

The ileocecal area is the most common portion of the intestinal tract involved by TB. In a report of 67 cases [116], all but six (91%) involved this area. Lesions may be hypertrophic, ulcerative or mixed. After involvement of the mucosa and submucosa, intense inflammation with necrosis occurs in the bowel wall and lymphatic channels encircling it. Caseation necrosis is often found, distinguishing gastrointestinal TB from Crohn's disease. The lymphangitis and endarteritis cause circular transverse mucosal ulceration. Since longitudinal ulcers generally do not develop, the cobblestone appearance seen in Crohn's disease involving both transverse and longitudinal ulcers is rare [117].

TB in the intestinal tract can be related to swallowing sputum tubercle bacilli or the disease reactivation in periintestinal lymphatic tissue. Acquisition of bovine TB is now less common owing to tuberculin programs in cattle and milk pasteurization [118].

*(b) Presentation and diagnosis*

Abdominal pain is the most common symptom, occurring in 77–85% of patients [116,119]. The pain is often located in the right lower quadrant but can be generalized or located elsewhere. It is often a chronic ache which has existed for months or years. In one series, 12% of patients had had pain for more than 5 years [116]. However, 32% of patients presented with acute abdominal pain as a surgical emergency [116]. Other symptoms include weight loss, fever, vomiting, malaise, diarrhea and constipation [116]. A palpable tumor in the right iliac fossa was found in 49 of 67 patients with intestinal TB [119]. The inflammatory mass, due to a thickened cecum, is usually firm, slightly tender and fixed to the posterior abdominal wall. Intestinal obstruction and/or ascites may occur.

The highest culture yield is from a biopsy of the intestinal wall or regional lymph node. The finding of a positive Mantoux test and/or proven pulmonary TB with compatible intestinal disease can support the diagnosis. Most series do not report stool examinations for AFB but a digested, 24 hour specimen after flotation has been used to yield the organism on stain [120]. Since 30% of patients with pulmonary TB without enteritis can yield tubercle bacilli on stool culture [121], such isolation may not be helpful diagnostically in the presence of pulmonary disease.

The diagnosis of gastrointestinal TB may be made endoscopically. Stenoses, ulcerations and ileocecal valve deformities are found and valve destruction strongly favors the diagnosis [122]. Although the X-ray picture can be indistinguishable from a malignant process or Crohn's disease, failure to fill the cecum with barium, cecal retraction and a gaping, rigid ileocecal valve with loss of the normal ileocecal angle are typical of TB enteritis [117].

*(c) Outcome*

Obstruction of the small or large bowel occurs in 12–60% of cases and is the most common complication requiring surgical intervention [121]. Entero-enteral and enterocutaneous fistulae may develop. Intestinal perforation is uncommon, occurring in only 10 of 734 cases in one series [123]. The low incidence of perforation is related to the marked fibrosis and thickening of the bowel wall with adherent mesentery. Overt intestinal bleeding is also uncommon.

**4.8.2 Peritoneal tuberculosis**

*(a) Organ involvement*

TB of the peritoneal surface can develop as a local reactivation or be related to active disease in the adjacent gastrointestinal or gynecological systems. The disease is manifest from the seeding of tubercles throughout the peritoneal surface. It has been described as occurring in either ascitic (exudative) or plastic (adhesive or dry) forms. The former is more common and is characterized by obvious free fluid and the latter by fibrous adhesions and discomfort rather than overt abdominal swelling [124].

*(b) Presentation and diagnosis*

The most common symptoms are abdominal pain and swelling [125–127]. Other symptoms include fever and chills, anorexia, weight loss, night sweats and constipation or diarrhea. At presentation, abdominal swelling may have existed for several months with pain for a longer period [125]. Frank rigors can occur, especially with rapidly increasing ascites [128].

Physical findings include fever in 60–100% of patients, ascites in 60–90% and a palpable abdominal mass in 25–50% [125–128]. The mass is often tender and may be multiple. One of the classical findings, the 'doughy' abdomen, is relatively rare and nonspecific. There is often concomitant pulmonary infection and pleural involvement occurs in at least 30–40% [129]. Pericardial involvement may also occur.

Ascitic fluid analysis reveals a lymphocytic exudate. The cell count ranges from 150 to 1500 per $mm^3$ with more than 80% lymphocytes. The total protein is often greater than 3.5 g/dl. Direct AFB smear is positive in about 10% of patients and cultures positive in about 50% [124,126,127]. A higher yield (83%) with culture of 1 liter of ascitic fluid is reported [129]. The diagnostic test of choice is laparoscopy, finding the peritoneum studded with nodules (Figure 4.9) which on biopsy reveal granulomas with caseation. With the availability of laparoscopy, blind Cope needle biopsy of the peritoneum or laparotomy is rarely needed for diagnosis.

This form of TB is easily confused with other diseases. It should be considered in the differential diagnosis of inflammatory bowel disease and abdominal or pelvic malignancies. Care must be taken not to overlook TB in evaluating the patient with alcoholic cirrhosis and ascites. Significant overlap in the ascitic fluid parameters occurs [126,130].

*(c) Outcome*

Palpable abdominal masses and ascites disappear within several months of adequate treatment [125,126]. Intestinal obstruction owing to adhesions may be a late complication. Such fibrotic complications can occur in 5–15% of cases [125,129]. Corticosteroids may diminish this risk [129].

### 4.8.3 Miscellaneous gastrointestinal tuberculosis

*(a) Esophageal tuberculosis*

Esophageal TB is rare. It was found in 3 of 117 cases of gastrointestinal disease from South Africa and felt to be primarily due to spread from adjacent tuberculous lymph nodes [131]. Dysphagia was found in 60% of

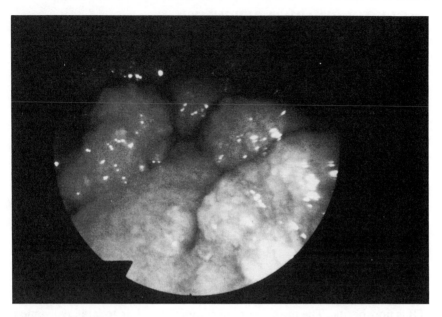

**Figure 4.9** Laparoscopic view of peritoneal tuberculosis. Photograph courtesy of Dr Eliot Zimbalist, Maimonides Medical Center.

patients, weight loss in 22% and retrosternal pain in 20% [132]. It is very difficult to distinguish clinically from carcinoma without histologic confirmation. Tracheoesophageal fistulae occur.

### (b) Gastroduodenal tuberculosis

Gastric ulcers may be tuberculous in origin. Infiltration of the stomach wall produces an X-ray appearance indistinguishable from linitis plastica [131]. Pyloric obstruction occurs related to ulcerative or infiltrative disease or large sub-pyloric lymphadenopathy. Isolated duodenal TB may occur, appearing similar to peptic ulcer disease with gastric outlet obstruction; it can cause duodeno-renal or duodeno-aortic fistulae [132].

### (c) Pancreatic tuberculosis

Isolated pancreatic TB presents as abdominal pain, obstructive jaundice, chronic pancreatitis or splenic vein thrombosis. The biopsy of a suspected pancreatic carcinoma is needed to evaluate for the possibility of TB in the appropriate setting [133].

## 4.9 GENITOURINARY TUBERCULOSIS

### 4.9.1 Urinary tuberculosis

*(a) Organ involvement*

Reactivation of a renal focus may be unilateral or bilateral and begins in the cortex spreading towards the papillae and medulla [134]. As the infection progresses, the kidney lesion may caseate, cavitating to discharge material containing viable AFB into the renal pelvis and ureter. Infection produces edema and eventual fibrosis at the calyceal neck, ureteropelvic junction and ureterovesicular junction. The process can spread to the bladder producing a small capacity, thick walled, fibrotic structure.

*(b) Presentation and diagnosis*

Generally a disease of young adulthood, Narayana [135] reported that 75% of 66 patients were below 50 years of age. Two other reports found an average age of 30 [136] and 47 [137] years. The symptomatology of urinary TB is nonspecific. The most common complaints relate to late involvement of the bladder and include frequency (60%), dysuria (34%) and hematuria (28%) [135]. This study found that 21% of patients presented with symptoms unrelated to the urinary tract. In fact, 72% of Lattimer's cases [138] of advanced cavitary renal TB had minimal renal symptoms. Constitutional complaints are the exception rather than the rule. Other symptoms related to urinary TB include renal colic due to clots and/or debris from open cavitary kidney lesions and a cold abscess presenting as a non-tender flank mass.

The urinalysis typically shows an acid pH, pyuria, proteinuria and hematuria and a negative routine urine culture. An abnormal urinalysis is found in 93% of cases [139]. Routine urine cultures may be positive for enteric bacilli, especially if structural abnormalities are present. Although a direct urine AFB stain can be positive [135], saprophytic AFB are visualized as well. The microbiological benchmark is isolation of *M. tuberculosis* from culture, with first voided morning urine having replaced 24 hour urine for culture. Comparing over 3600 clinical specimens, the yield of tubercle bacilli from the morning void was equal to the 24 hour urine, more convenient and less prone to contamination [140]. Urine cultures are positive in 80–90% [136,139] with the additional cases diagnosed on reactive skin tests, characteristic X-rays and/or isolation of TB from other sites. The initial urine culture was found positive in 77% and at least one of the first two cultures in 91% [141]. Positive urine cultures may also occur with normal urinalyses. These individuals usually have obvious disease elsewhere with subclinical renal seeding.

Radiographically, the intravenous pyelogram (IVP) can reveal calyceal dilation, stricture, cavitary papillary disease and calcification. Multiple ureteral strictures causing a beaded appearance and a small scarred bladder may also be seen. A typical IVP is shown in Figure 4.10. Early in disease,

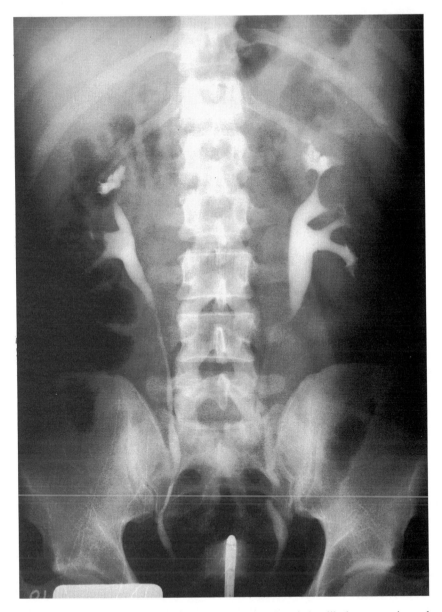

**Figure 4.10** Renal tuberculosis. Pyelogram showing infundibular stenosis and calyceal scarring. There is a stricture at the left ureteropelvic junction. Radiograph courtesy of Maimonides Medical Center Radiology Department.

the pyelogram can be normal. Cystoscopy may be helpful in revealing edema, hyperemia and shallow bladder ulcers. A variety of urinary tract disorders may produce similar X-ray changes. Among systemic infections, urinary brucellosis may closely mimic TB [142].

### (c) Outcome

Based on a higher than expected tuberculin reaction rate in children of individuals with urinary TB without pulmonary disease, it was suggested that transmission may have occurred via the urine [143]. No direct data exist to support this and no evidence to support this route of transmission was found in 1720 relatives of 290 urogenital TB patients [144].

Although therapy is quite effective, significant diminution in renal function is caused by this infection. Diminished creatinine clearance in 58% of 117 patients has been noted with 5% considered to be severe [145]. Azotemia may affect the dosing of antitubercular drugs. The renal disease is usually caused by granulomatous destruction but can be caused by tuberculous interstitial nephritis [146].

Although nephrectomy has been advocated for the non-functioning TB kidney, it now appears unnecessary if urine culture conversion is obtained and the drug treatment completed [139,141]. Surgical intervention is used for strictures and nephrolithiasis, which can cause obstruction and predispose to recurrent infection. Hypertension as a complication is rare [139].

### 4.9.2 Male genital tuberculosis

### (a) Organ involvement

Involvement of multiple sites in the male genital tract is often seen. Christensen [136] reported clinical involvement of prostate in 37%, epididymis 31%, testes 23% and seminal vesicles 9%. Similar comparative rates are reported [147] in an autopsy series. Penile TB is quite rare. This form of skin TB can be acquired from sexual contact. It was a complication in ritual circumcisions in the pretherapeutic age. It can also be a manifestation of either local or hematogenous spread [148]. Because concomitant or previous renal TB occurs in many cases (44–80%) [149], genital involvement is thought to follow a descending infection from the kidney. Renal involvement, however, may be difficult to document because intravenous pyelograms can appear normal in the setting of microscopic renal disease. Clinical studies, therefore, underestimate kidney involvement. Genital TB may also occur through: hematogenous spread with late reactivation; direct extension from adjacent foci; or lymphatic spread. Female to male venereal transmission is extremely rare [150].

## (b) Presentation and diagnosis

Most cases occur between the ages of 20 and 40 with few before puberty. The onset of symptoms is often insidious and constitutional symptoms are often absent. Prostatic involvement manifests as urinary frequency, urgency, hematuria or hematospermia. Digital rectal examination is often not remarkable until disease progression, when an enlarged, nodular prostate is detected [151]. If caseation occurs, soft areas that depress on digital examination may be noted. Such necrosis can perforate through the prostate capsule into the rectum or produce perineal sinuses [149]. Biopsy reveals granulomatous inflammation with AFB. Noncaseating granulomas may be seen and do not rule out *M. tuberculosis* [151]. In TB prostatitis, semen cultures are often positive [152].

Epididymitis rarely presents acutely with the rapid onset of a focal, painful scrotal swelling [153]. More commonly, it manifests as scrotal swelling, with or without pain, developing over several months. As many as 40–50% of advanced cases have scrotal fistulae [149,153]. Examination of TB epididymitis at an early stage reveals irregular nodularity. With progression, the epididymis enlarges to four or five times its usual size. Involvement of the testes, usually combined with epididymal disease, presents as progressive swelling.

As with all forms of genitourinary TB, a combination of typical signs and symptoms, a reactive Mantoux tuberculin test, AFB cultures of urine and seminal fluids and, when available, histopathologic findings and cultures of appropriate biopsy material are needed to produce an accurate diagnosis. Fine needle aspiration of mass lesions may be helpful [150]. Sonographic studies may help in distinguishing solid from cystic structures and localizing intrascrotal pathology [154].

The differential diagnosis of genital TB includes acute epididymitis due to pyogenic Gram-negative bacilli, *Neisseria gonorrheae* or *Chlamydia*. Chronic processes such as brucellosis, blastomycosis, malignancy, non-TB AFB, and sarcoidosis also need to be considered.

## (c) Outcome

Early therapy may prevent fibrosis during healing, but fibrotic lesions already present will not resolve with treatment. Surgery is rarely needed but should be considered if there is no response after several months of therapy, a large caseating mass is present or there is significant obstruction. Surgery may be used diagnostically in those in whom a concern about malignancy exists [153]. Abnormal semen analysis is the rule [152], with a marked decrease in fertility and a high incidence of sterility. Among the findings are decreased volume of seminal fluid, blockage of the lumen of the epididymitis or vas deferens and decreased sperm counts.

### 4.9.3 Female genital tuberculosis

*(a) Organ involvement*

Pathologically, the fallopian tube is the most common site of involvement; it is affected in 80–100% of cases, usually bilaterally [155,156]. The tube is likely seeded during the primary infection with subsequent reactivation. The endometrium is also commonly (70–90%) involved, probably related to spread from the fallopian tubes [157]. The myometrium and myosalpinx are involved by direct spread. Conversely, involvement of the serosal uterine surface is related to local TB peritonitis from contamination of the pelvic peritoneal surface from the ends of the fallopian tubes.

Less commonly, the uterine cervix and vagina may be involved. Both of these areas are infected from endometrial involvement. Direct ovarian infection has been reported in 20–43% of cases in which the disease was severe enough to require surgery [156,157]. Female genital TB due to venereal transmission causes vulvar ulcers and inguinal adenopathy resembling lymphogranuloma venereum [158].

*(b) Presentation and diagnosis*

The average age at diagnosis has increased and the disease now involves more postmenopausal women [157]. Presenting symptomatology includes lower abdominal pain (often bilateral) and menstruation abnormalities, such as postmenopausal bleeding and oligo- or amenorrhea [155]. The latter is more likely to be related to general debility than any pelvic pathology. Between 7% and 13% [155,157] of women present with infertility. Many have a history of failure to respond to standard antimicrobial therapy for pelvic inflammatory disease.

Physical examination reveals lower abdominal and pelvic tenderness. On bimanual pelvic examination, unilateral or bilateral adnexal masses are often found. Pelvic pain is less than that of pyogenic pelvic inflammatory disease [155]. The patient is often afebrile with no leukocytosis, which can help to distinguish this disease from pyogenic processes.

A diagnosis can be made by endometrial curettage with AFB stain and culture. The optimal time to perform the curettage is late in the menstrual cycle [155]. Cervical biopsy and culdoscopy is also useful. TB isolation is successful in 30–65% of cases [156,157]. In as many as 65% of cases [156], no diagnosis is made until histopathologic examination of surgically removed tissue is performed. The use of endoscopy (laparoscopy and hysteroscopy) has been found to be useful diagnostically [159] with tubercles seen on the surface of the organs, nodular, thickened tubes and fibrous adhesions.

*(c) Outcome*

Chemotherapy is usually effective. A 97% cure rate is reported in patients followed for an average of 2.5 years [156]. Surgical intervention should be used only if therapy is not successful from persistent large adnexal masses, recurrent endometrial infection or continued uterine bleeding. In a series of 709 cases, the need for follow-up surgical intervention dropped from 11% to 0% using modern TB regimens [156].

The chances of reversing infertility are slim because of blockage of the fallopian tubes. In an Indian study of 101 cases of pelvic TB [159], 11 (15%) subsequent intrauterine pregnancies occurred. Three patients developed ectopic pregnancies (27% of total conceptions). Another report [160] found no pregnancies in 47 cases followed for 169 patient-years in the pretherapeutic era and a 11.7% pregnancy rate after antitubercular therapy. Of these 18 pregnancies, only seven viable babies (39%) were produced with a 33% ectopic pregnancy rate. Clearly, any pregnancy in a patient who has had genital TB should be considered to be high risk.

## 4.10 BONE AND JOINT TUBERCULOSIS

### 4.10.1 Organ involvement

Bone and joint involvement with *M. tuberculosis* occurs in 1% of TB patients and 5% or more with extrapulmonary disease [161]. It is usually a late manifestation of hematogenous spread to bone from the primary pulmonary infection. Less commonly, spread from a contiguous area of activity such as pleura, kidney or periaortic lymph node occurs. Predisposing factors include trauma, race (higher incidence in Blacks), debilitating systemic diseases, intra-articular injection of steroids and intravenous drug use.

The site most frequently involved is the vertebral body, representing 36–50% of the total of bone and joint TB [161,162]. Spinal TB is known as Pott's disease after Sir Percival Pott, an 18th century physician who described the disease and its neurologic complications. Involvement of the spine occurs most commonly (48–67%) in the lower thoracic and upper lumbar areas. Weight bearing joints are involved most frequently such as the knee (12–15%) and hip (9–15%) [161,163]. Any bone or joint, however, can be involved. Rib TB is not frequent, but is the most common inflammatory lesion of the rib [164].

Invasion of the joint is direct via the blood stream to the synovium or indirect from lesions in epiphyseal bone eroding into the joint space. Initially, the synovium develops a granulomatous reaction with effusion. Fibrin debris precipitates in the effusion, forming so-called rice bodies. The pannus of inflammatory tissue begins to erode and destroy cartilage and bone ultimately leading to progressive demineralization with caseation necrosis. Cartilage is destroyed peripherally first, preserving the joint space for a considerable length of time. In far advanced disease, para-osseous abscesses develop involving tissue surrounding the bone or joint.

### 4.10.2 Presentation and diagnosis

The incidence of bone and joint TB has fallen dramatically during the past 30 years in developed countries such as the USA and the UK. This decline has not been shared, however, by underdeveloped nations. Today, spinal TB is a disease of children in developing nations and of the elderly in the USA and Europe. The disease most commonly involves a single joint, though it may be multifocal [165]. A recent report of four cases of multicentric TB bone disease from Canada emphasizes the difficulty of distinguishing this entity from a malignant process [166].

The commonest early evidence of illness is the insidious onset of local pain and swelling. TB should always be considered when evaluating skeletal pain. Limitation of motion can also be found along with constitutional symptoms such as fever, night sweats, anorexia and weight loss. Buttock pain occurs with sacroiliac TB which can cause gluteal abscesses [167]. Chronically swollen, infected joints may be associated with draining sinuses. Very often, patients tolerate the symptoms for many months and even years before seeking medical attention. In vertebral disease, back pain can progress to focal neurological symptoms and signs [162].

X-rays of affected joints typically show some decrease in the articular space with destruction of adjacent cartilage and bone. In Pott's disease, classical involvement is of two vertebrae with destruction of the intervening intervertebral disc (Figure 4.11). Normal radiographs, however, do not exclude the condition, particularly if the disease is of recent onset (less than 3 months). Thirteen cases of atypical spinal TB were reported [168] including: neural arch involvement only; intraspinal cold abscesses; and infection of a single vertebra with collapse. CT and MRI are important in defining spine and cauda equina involvement. Intraspinal cold abscesses as well as paravertebral (psoas) abscesses can easily be found by these means. Psoas abscess is seen in a significant number of patients with advanced Pott's disease.

The diagnosis is best made by biopsy with culture and histology. For practical purposes, a histologic appearance of granulomatous synovitis in an individual with a reactive tuberculin test is sufficient to start a patient on chemotherapy, even in the absence of positive cultures. The yield of AFB stain for joint fluid is 25%, with higher yields using synovial tissue [169]. An individual with a positive tuberculin test and a compatible spinal X-ray must be treated for Pott's disease, even in the absence of a tissue diagnosis. AFB stains on material obtained from vertebrae or disc tissue are positive in 27% and culture in 53–59% [163,170].

### 4.10.3 Outcome

A microbiologic cure is possible with therapy, even in far advanced disease. Failure to diagnose a bone or joint problem as tuberculous will delay

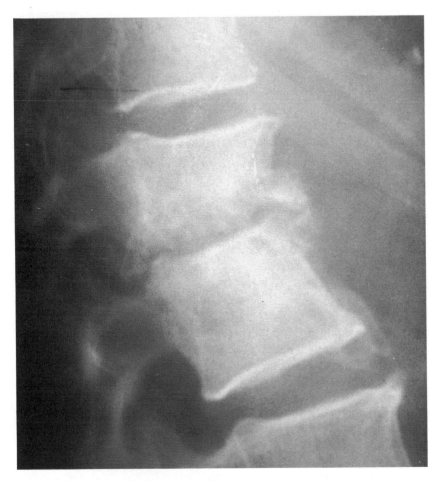

**Figure 4.11** Tuberculous lumbar spondylitis. X-ray showing involvement of two adjacent vertebrae with some collapse. Radiograph courtesy of Maimonides Medical Center Radiography Department.

treatment and allow further destruction. Prompt recognition and treatment can prevent destructive arthritis or vertebral collapse with kyphosis and scoliosis (gibbus formation).

Outcome of joint TB, in general, is fair. The results of the treatment of 10 patients with wrist TB [170] were microbiologically satisfactory in that the activity of the disease was controlled throughout the period of observation. Six of these patients, however, needed arthrodesis. Eleven patients with sacroiliac TB all returned to full activity and none had significant functional impairment despite marked radiographic changes [167].

The outcome in Pott's disease changes if the infection penetrates through the dura [171]. Spinal cord or root compression are possible complications of vertebral TB. The degree of neurologic involvement observed on the physical examination can serve as a prognostic measure. Those with complete loss of motor function have a poor prognosis while those with preservation of some voluntary muscle control, sphincter control and sensory function have a better prognosis. Surgical decompression is useful in more severe cases if carried out expeditiously. In most cases of TB of the spine, however, immobilization and/or surgery is unnecessary. Chemotherapy should provide appropriate treatment [162,169].

## 4.11 PERICARDIAL TUBERCULOSIS

### 4.11.1 Organ involvement

In countries where TB is highly endemic, tuberculous involvement is the most common form of pericardial disease. In industrialized countries, this entity may attract increased interest because of the current TB resurgence and its propensity to produce life-threatening cardiac tamponade or disabling constrictive pericarditis. In the USA, TB has been reported to cause 4% of acute pericardial disease, 5% of cardiac tamponade and 6% of constrictive pericarditis [172]. The pericardium is involved in 1–2% of cases of pulmonary TB and 5% of extrapulmonary TB [172].

Generally, the infection reaches the pericardial space directly following reactivation of TB in latent mediastinal lymph node rupturing into the pericardial space. The lymph nodes at the tracheal bifurcation are the most common source of infection. Rarely, direct extension from contiguous pulmonary, pleural or bony structures or hematogenous spread from a nearby or distant organ occurs [172,173]. In one autopsy series of 10 patients, all had concomitant mediastinal TB adenitis, nine had pulmonary and five had pleural involvement [174].

The process begins as a hypersensitivity reaction to mycobacterial proteins with the attraction of cellular elements and the deposition of fibrin. PMNs predominate at the onset but lymphocytes rapidly replace them. With the development of a granulomatous reaction, an effusive phase occurs with the collection of fluid in the pericardial sac. The amount is usually several hundred milliliters, but up to 3.5 liters has been reported [173]. The fluid is hemorrhagic in as many as 80% [172]. Despite a prominent granulomatous reaction, few AFB are noted histologically. Later, the fluid is slowly absorbed with the development of pericardial thickening, adhesions and fibrosis. The thickening is considered the hallmark of the disease as it progresses to a constrictive phase. Microscopically, the lymphohistiocytic infiltration, fibrosis and necrosis may not be limited to the pericardium, but may involve the myocardium as well [175]. The calcifications, when they occur, are patchy or form a diffuse sheet surrounding the heart.

## 4.11.2 Presentation and diagnosis

Affected persons are usually in their third to fifth decade with a male preponderance [174]. The disease is more common in Blacks compared with other races and the higher ratio persisted even after adjustment for the high prevalence of TB in Black populations [174]. In HIV-infected persons, the disease may be encountered as the initial manifestation of AIDS [176]. The clinical manifestations of TB pericarditis can be caused by the infective process *per se*, or reflect disability due to organ involvement with the heart and lung most commonly affected. Cough, dyspnea and weight loss are by far the most common complaints, occurring in 80% or more of the cases, followed by shortness of breath, chest pain, fever, night sweats, ankle edema and hemoptysis [172–174].

Physical examination reveals some degree of cardiomegaly in up to 95% of patients. Fever and tachycardia are also common. Other findings are pulsus paradoxus, pleural effusion, friction rub, distant heart sounds, neck vein distension and hepatomegaly [172–174]. The signs and symptoms of cardiac tamponade and constrictive pericarditis caused by TB are not different from those occurring in pericarditis from other etiologies.

The chest X-ray usually shows cardiomegaly. Concomitant evidence of pulmonary TB has been found in 72% [172]. In another report, pleural effusion was seen in about 70% and more than a third of these effusions were confirmed as TB [174].

Electrocardiographic, echocardiographic and angiographic findings are largely nonspecific. Their usefulness is retained for confirmation of the presence, size and hemodynamic significance of the effusion, but cannot establish the etiology. The electrocardiogram may show ST depression, low voltage and rarely ST elevation. Real time echocardiography offers a readily available sensitive bedside means of evaluating cardiac tamponade. Thickening of the pericardium with stranding and adhesions occurs commonly in TB pericarditis [172]. Right heart catheterization, although invasive, is also useful for evaluation of constrictive pericarditis and cardiac tamponade.

For the non-invasive diagnosis of constrictive pericarditis, CT may be the test of choice. In a study of 212 patients with impaired diastolic filling, it could clearly differentiate between constrictive TB pericarditis and restrictive cardiomyopathy. Magnetic resonance imaging is also capable of detecting pericardial thickening, but is inferior to CT because of its inability to detect pericardial calcifications [177].

The pericardial fluid is usually exudative and either serosanguinous or grossly hemorrhagic. The cells in the fluid are predominantly lymphocytes, but a significant number of PMNs is not unusual initially. The diagnosis is often based on the identification of AFB in the sputum or pleural fluid because of the common coexistence of pulmonary and/or pleural TB. In a large study of 189 proven cases of TB pericarditis, the pericardial fluid culture was positive in 59% of the patients and pericardial biopsy was diagnostic in 70% of the patients [178]. In the same series, 11% of the patients had a positive sputum culture. DNA amplification by polymerase chain reaction is suitable for use with uncontaminated fluids, such as pericardial fluid, and can confirm a diagnosis rapidly [179].

The list of differential diagnoses includes many infectious and non-infectious conditions. Viral infections, malignancy, uremia, autoimmune disease and hypothyroidism are common causes of pericardial effusions. Some authors favor early pericardial biopsy to establish the diagnosis [173]. TB may also complicate a pre-existing pericardial disease [173].

### 4.11.3 Outcome

Without chemotherapy, the mortality of TB pericarditis is 90% or more [180]. With the advent of specific therapy, it has been reduced to less than 40% [174]. Major causes of death relate to the cardiac complications of tamponade, constriction and myocarditis. The patient will usually require hospitalization and observation for the initiation of diagnostic testing. It is justified to treat those with a positive tuberculin test and rapidly progressive pericardial disease empirically for 4–6 weeks while following the response if bacteriological diagnosis cannot be confirmed [172]. Emergent pericardiocentesis may be required for cardiac tamponade and pericardiectomy may be indicated if this complication recurs during therapy. A pericardial window may be tried in some cases, but if pericardial thickening is present, pericardiectomy should be performed. The surgical mortality of pericardiectomy is high if it is done at a late stage, particularly after onset of calcification.

Early surgical intervention with pericardiectomy was advocated in some older studies [181] claiming a better outcome, but recent studies reported a good clinical response to medical therapy if started in the acute phase, obviating the need for pericardiectomy in such patients [182]. Medical management is not different from other forms of extrapulmonary TB. However, corticosteroids are considered an integral part of the therapy of TB pericarditis. Adding corticosteroids to the regimen, usually 40–60 mg/day of prednisone, is reported to improve the clinical outcome [178].

### REFERENCES

1. Yoshikawa, T.T. (1992) Tuberculosis in aging adults. *J Am Geriatr Soc,* **40**, 178–86.
2. Sbarbaro, J.A. (1980) Tuberculosis. *Med Clin N Am*, **64**, 417–31.
2a. North, R.J. and Izzo, A.A. (1993) Mycobacterial virulence. Virulent strains of *Mycobacterium tuberculosis* have faster, in vivo doubling time and are better equipped to resist growth-inhibited function of macrophages in the presence and absence of specific immunity. *J Exp Med*, **177**, 1723–33.

3.  Bass, J.B., Farer, L.S., Hopewell, P.C. *et al.* (1990) Diagnostic standards and classification of tuberculosis. *Am Rev Respir Dis*, **142**, 725–35.
4.  Buckner, C.B. and Walker, C.W. (1990) Radiologic manifestations of adult tuberculosis. *J Thorac Imag*, **5**, 28–37.
5.  Miller, W.T. and Miller, W.T. (1993) Tuberculosis in the normal host: radiographic findings. *Semin Roentgenol*, **28**, 109–18.
6.  Nardell, E., McInnis, B., Thomas, B. *et al.* (1986) Exogenous reinfection with tuberculosis in a shelter for the homeless. *N Engl J Med*, **315**, 1570–5.
6a. Small, P.M., Shafer, R.W., Hopewell, P.C. *et al.* (1993) Exogenous reinfection with multi-drug-resistant *Mycobacterium tuberculosis* in patients with advanced HIV infection. *N Engl J Med*, **328**, 1137–44.
7.  Van den Brande, P.M., Van de Mierop, F., Verbeken, E.K. *et al.* (1990) Clinical spectrum of endobronchial tuberculosis in elderly patients. *Arch Intern Med*, **150**, 2105–8.
8.  Johnson, T.M., McCann, W. and Davey, W.N. (1975) Tuberculous bronchopleural fistula. *Am Rev Respir Dis*, **107**, 30–41.
9.  Tsao, T.C.Y., Juang, Y., Tsai, Y. *et al.* (1992) Whole lung tuberculosis: A disease with high mortality which is frequently misdiagnosed. *Chest*, **101**, 1309–11.
10. Mayock, R.L. and MacGregor, R.R. (1976) Diagnosis, prevention and early therapy of tuberculosis. *DM*, **22**, 24–59.
11. Larson, E.B., Featherstone, H.J. and Petersdorf, R.G. (1982) Fever of undetermined origin: Diagnosis and follow-up of 105 cases, 1970–1980. *Medicine*, **61**, 269–92.
12. Johnston, R.N., Lockhart, W. and Smith, D.H. (1960) Haemoptysis. *Brit Med J*, **1**, 592–5.
13. Stead, W.W., Kerby, G.R., Schlueter, D.P. and Jordahl, C.W. (1968) The clinical spectrum of primary tuberculosis in adults. *Ann Intern Med*, **68**, 731–44.
14. Bailey, W.C. (1980) Diagnosis of tuberculosis. *Clin Chest Med*, **1**, 209–17.
15. Nagiami, P.H. and Yoshikawa, T.T. (1983) Tuberculosis in the geriatric patient. *J Am Geriatr Soc*, **31**, 356–63.
16. Hanania, H. and Hoffstein, V. (1993) Tuberculosis presenting with generalized lymphadenopathy, pulmonary infiltrates and bone destruction in a young man. *Arch Intern Med*, **153**, 1265–7.
17. Kelly, P., Manning, P., Corcoran, P. and Clancy, L. (1991) Hypertrophic osteoarthropathy in association with pulmonary tuberculosis. *Chest*, **99**, 769–70.
18. Centers for Disease Control (1993) Outbreak of multi-drug-resistant tuberculosis in a hospital – New York City, 1991. *MMWR*, **42**, 427, 433.
19. Lutwick, S.M., Abter, E.I.M., Chapnick, E.K. *et al.* (1992) Tuberculosis in patients infected with human immunodeficiency virus: A problem-solving approach. *Am J Infect Control*, **20**, 156–8.
20. Cohen, J.R., Amorosa, J.K. and Smith, P.R. (1978) The air–fluid level in cavitary pulmonary tuberculosis. *Radiology*, **127**, 315–6.
21. Im, J., Webb, W.R., Han, M.C. and Park, J.H. (1991) Apical opacity associated with pulmonary tuberculosis: High-resolution CT findings. *Radiology*, **178**, 727–31.
22. Choe, K.O., Jeong, H.J. and Sohn, H.Y. (1990) Tuberculous bronchial stenosis: CT findings in 28 cases. *Am J Roentgenol*, **155**, 971–6.

23. Strumph, I.J., Tsang, A.Y., Schork, M.A. *et al.* (1976) The reliability of gastric smears by auramine-rhodamine staining technique for the diagnosis of tuberculosis. *Am Rev Respir Dis*, **114**, 971–6.

24. Daniel, T.M. (1990) The rapid diagnosis of tuberculosis: A selective review. *J Lab Clin Med*, **116**, 277–82.

25. Baughman, R.P., Dohn, M.N., Loudon, R.G. and Frame, P.T. (1991) Bronchoscopy and bronchoalveolar lavage in tuberculosis and fungal infections. *Chest*, **99**, 92–7.

26. Chan, H.S., Sun, A.J.M. and Hoheisel, G.B. (1990) Bronchoscopic aspiration and bronchoalveolar lavage in the diagnosis of sputum smear negative pulmonary tuberculosis. *Lung*, **168**, 2125–30.

27. Miro, A.M., Gibilara, E., Powell, S. and Kamholtz, S.L. (1992) The role of fiberoptic bronchoscopy for diagnosis of pulmonary tuberculosis in patients at risk for AIDS. *Chest*, **101**, 1211–14.

28. Morris, C.D.W. (1991) Sputum examination in the screening and diagnosis of pulmonary tuberculosis in the elderly. *Quart J Med*, **81**, 999–1004.

29. Woodhead, M. (1992) New approaches to the rapid diagnosis of tuberculosis. *Thorax*, **47**, 264.

30. de Lassence, A., Lecossier, D., Pierre, C. *et al.* (1991) Detection of mycobacterial DNA in pleural fluid from patients with tuberculous pleurisy by means of the polymerase chain reaction: comparison of two protocols. *Thorax*, **47**, 265–9.

31. Bothamley, G.H., Rudd, R., Restenstein, F. and Ivanyi, J. (1992) Clinical value of the measurement of *Mycobacterium tuberculosis* specific antibody in pulmonary tuberculosis. *Thorax*, **47**, 270–5.

32. Fadda, G., Grillo, R., Santori, L. *et al.* (1992) Serodiagnosis and follow-up of patients with pulmonary tuberculosis by enzyme-linked immunosorbent assay. *Eur J Epidemiol*, **8**, 81–7.

33. Banales, J.I., Pineda, P.R., Fitzgerald, J.M. *et al.* (1991) Adenosine deaminase in the diagnosis of tuberculous pleural effusions. A report of 218 patients and review of the literature. *Chest*, **99**, 355–7.

34. Long, R., Maycher, B., Scalcini, M. and Manfreda, J. (1991) The chest roentgenogram in pulmonary tuberculosis patients seropositive for human immunodeficiency virus type 1. *Chest*, **99**, 123–7.

35. Stead, W.W. and Dutt, A.K. (1981) What's new in tuberculosis? *Am J Med*, **71**, 1–4.

36. Weaver, R.A. (1974) Unusual radiographic presentation of pulmonary tuberculosis in diabetic patients. *Am Rev Respir Dis*, **69**, 162–3.

37. Qunibi, W.Y., Al-Sibai, G.A., Taher, S. *et al.* (1990) Mycobacterial infection after renal transplantation. Report of 14 cases and review of literature. *Quart J Med*, **77**, 1039–60.

38. Straus, S.E., Pizzo, P.A. and Lutwick, L.I. (1982) Infectious complications of lung cancer, in *Lung Cancer: Clinical Diagnosis and Treatment*, 1st edn (ed. M.J. Straus), Grune & Stratton, New York, pp. 293–314.

39. Mok, C.K., Nandi, P. and Ong, G.B. (1978) Co-existent bronchogenic carcinoma and active pulmonary tuberculosis. *J Thorac Cardiovasc Surg*, **76**, 469–72.

40. Dutt, A.K. and Stead, W.W. (1992) Tuberculosis. *Clin Geriatr Med*, **8**, 761–36.

41. Stead, W.W. (1989) Special problems in tuberculosis. Tuberculosis in the

elderly and residents of nursing homes, correctional facilities, long-term care hospitals, mental hospitals, shelters for the homeless and jails. *Clin Chest Med*, **10**, 397–405.

42. North, R.J. (1993) Minimal effect of advanced aging on susceptibility of mice to infection with *Mycobacterium tuberculosis. J Infect Dis*, **168**, 1059–62.

43. Stewart, R.B. (1991) Tuberculosis in the elderly: incidence, manifestation, PPD skin tests, and preventive therapy. *Ann Pharmacother*, **25**, 650–5.

44. Van Dijk, J.M. and Rosin, A.J. (1993) A comparison of clinical features of mycobacterial infection in the young and elderly patients. *Neth J Med*, **42**, 12–15.

45. Van Den Brande, P., Lambrechts, M., Tack, J. and Demedts, M. (1991) Endobronchial tuberculosis mimicking lung cancer in elderly patients. *Respir Med*, **85**, 107–9.

46. Morris, C.D.W. (1989) The radiography, hematology and biochemistry of pulmonary tuberculosis in the aged. *Quart J Med*, **71**, 529–36.

47. Van Den Brande, P. and Palemous, W. (1989) Radiographic features of pulmonary tuberculosis in elderly patients. *Age Aging*, **18**, 205–7.

48. Centers for Disease Control (1990) Prevention and control of tuberculosis in facilities providing long term care to the elderly. Recommendation of the Advisory Committee for Elimination of Tuberculosis. *MMWR*, **39 (RR-10)**, 7–13.

49. Harris, A.A. and Karakusis, P. (1979) Diagnosis and management of tuberculosis. *Primary Care*, **6**, 43–62.

50. Pamra, S.P., Prasad, G. and Mathur, G.P. (1976) Relapse in pulmonary tuberculosis. *Am Rev Respir Dis*, **113**, 67–72.

50a. Cohn, D.L., Catlin, B.J., Peterson, K.L. *et al.* (1990) A 62-dose, 6-month therapy for pulmonary and extrapulmonary tuberculosis. A twice-weekly directly observed, and cost effective regimen. *Ann Intern Med*, **112**, 407–15.

50b. Combs, D.L., O'Brien, R.J. and Geiter, L.J. (1990) USPHS tuberculosis short-course chemotherapy trial 21 – effectiveness, toxicity, and acceptibility. *Ann Intern Med*, **112**, 397–406.

51. Chang, S., Lee, P. and Perng, R. (1991) The value of roentgenographic and fiberbronchoscopic findings in predicting outcome of adults with lower lung field tuberculosis. *Arch Intern Med*, **151**, 1581–3.

52. Tse, C.Y. and Natkunam, R. (1988) Serious sequelae of delayed diagnosis of endobronchial tuberculosis. *Tubercle*, **69**, 213–6.

53. Raghu, G. and Dillard, D. (1990) Esophagobronchial fistula and mediastinal tuberculosis. *Ann Thorac Surg*, **50**, 647–9.

54. Varkey, B. and Rose, H.D. (1976) Pulmonary aspergilloma. A rational approach to treatment. *Am J Med*, **61**, 626–31.

55. Agarwal, M.K., Muthuswany, P.P., Banner, A.S. *et al.* (1977) Respiratory failure in pulmonary tuberculosis. *Chest*, **72**, 605–9.

56. Murray, H.W., Tuazon, C.U., Kirmani, N. and Sheagren, J.N. (1978) The adult respiratory distress syndrome associated with miliary tuberculosis. *Chest*, **73**, 37–43.

57. Stein, D.S. and Libertin, C.R. (1990) Disseminated intravascular coagulation in association with cavitary tuberculosis. *South Med J*, **83**, 60–2.

58. Rieder, H.L., Kelly, G.D., Block, A.B. *et al.* (1991) Tuberculosis diagnosed at death in the United States. *Chest*, **100**, 678–81.

59. Herbert, A. (1986) Pathogenesis of pleurisy, pleural fibrosis, and mesothelial proliferation. *Thorax*, **41**, 176–89.

60. Seibert, A.F., Haynes, J., Middleton, R. and Bass, J.B. (1991) Tuberculous pleural effusion. Twenty-year experience. *Chest*, **99**, 883–6.

61. Epstein, D.M., Kline, L.R., Albelda, S.M. and Miller, W.T. (1991) Tuberculous pleural effusions. *Chest*, **91**, 106–9.

62. Batunguanayo, J., Taelman, H., Allen, S. *et al.* (1993) Pleural effusion, tuberculosis and HIV-1 infection in Kigali, Rwanda. *AIDS*, **7**, 73–9.

63. Levine, H., Szanto, P.B. and Chagell, D.W. (1968) Tuberculous pleurisy. *Arch Intern Med*, **122**, 329–32.

64. Antoniskis, D., Amin, K. and Barnes, P.F. (1990) Pleuritis as a manifestation of reactivation tuberculosis. *Am J Med*, **89**, 447–50.

65. Guzman, J., Bross, K.J., Wurtemberger, G. *et al.* (1989) Tuberculous pleural effusions: Lymphocyte phenotypes in comparison with other lymphocyte-rich effusions. *Diagnost Cytopathol*, **5**, 139–44.

66. Bower, G. (1967) Eosinophilic pleural effusion. *Am Rev Respir Dis*, **95**, 746–51.

67. Syabbalo, N.C. (1991) Use of alkaline phosphatase content to diagnose tuberculous effusions. *Chest*, **99**, 522–3.

68. Valdes, L., Pose, A., Suarez, J. *et al.* (1991) Cholesterol: a useful parameter for distinguishing between pleural exudates and transudates. *Chest*, **99**, 1097–102.

69. Yew, W.W., Kwan, S.Y., Cheung, S.W. *et al.* (1991) Diagnosis of tuberculous pleural effusion by the detection of tuberculostearic acid in pleural aspirates. *Chest*, **100**, 1261–3.

70. Valdes, L., San Jose, E., Alvarez, D. *et al.* (1993) Diagnosis of tuberculous pleurisy using the biologic parameters adenosine deaminase, lysozyme and interferon-gamma. *Chest*, **103**, 458–65.

71. Maartens, G. and Bateman, E.D. (1991) Tuberculous pleural effusions: increased culture yield with bedside inoculation of pleural fluid and poor diagnostic value of adenosine deaminase. *Thorax*, **46**, 96–9.

72. Akhan, O., Demirkazik, F.B., Ozen, M.N. *et al.* (1992) Tuberculous pleural effusions. Ultrasonic diagnosis. *J Clin Ultrasound*, **20**, 461–5.

73. Barbas, C.S., Cukier, A., de Varvacho, C.R. *et al.* (1991) The relationship between pleural fluid findings and the development of pleural thickening in patients with pleural tuberculosis. *Chest*, **100**, 1264–7.

74. Chan, C.H., Arnold, M., Chan, C.Y. *et al.* (1991) Clinical and pathologic features of pleural effusion and its long-term consequences. *Respiration*, **58**, 171–5.

75. Johnson, T.M., McCann, W. and Winthrop, N.D. (1975) Tuberculous bronchopleural fistula. *Am Rev Respir Dis*, **107**, 30–41.

76. Alvarez, S. and McCabe, W.R. (1984) Extrapulmonary tuberculosis revisited: a review of experience at Boston City and other hospitals. *Medicine*, **63**, 25–55.

77. Lindell, M.M., Jing, G.S. and Wallace, S. (1977) Laryngeal tuberculosis. *Am J Roentgenol*, **129**, 677–80.

78. Rohwedder, J.J. (1974) Upper respiratory tract tuberculosis. Sixteen cases in a general hospital. *Ann Intern Med*, **80**, 708–12.

79. Kilgore, T.L. and Jenkins, D.W. (1983) Laryngeal tuberculosis. *Chest*, **83**, 139–41.

80. Horowitz, G., Kaslow, R. and Friedland, G. (1976) Infectiousness of laryngeal tuberculosis. *Am Rev Respir Dis*, **114**, 241–4.

81. Getson, W.R. and Park, Y.W. (1992) Laryngeal tuberculosis. *Arch Otolaryngol Head Neck Surg*, **118**, 878–81.
82. Bull, T.R. (1966) Tuberculosis of the larynx. *Brit Med J*, **2**, 991–2.
83. Soda, A., Rubis, H., Salazar, M. *et al.* (1989) Tuberculosis of the larynx: clinical aspects in 19 patients. *Laryngoscope*, **99**, 1147–50.
84. Sahn, S.A. and Neff, T.A. (1974) Miliary tuberculosis. *Am J Med*, **56**, 495–505.
85. Jacques, J. and Sloan, J.M. (1970) The changing pattern of miliary tuberculosis. *Thorax*, **25**, 237–40.
86. Slavin, R.E., Walsh, T.J. and Pollack, A.D. (1980) Late generalized tuberculosis: a clinical-pathologic analysis and comparison of 100 cases in the pre-antibiotic and antibiotic eras. *Medicine*, **59**, 352–66.
87. Singh, R., Joshi, R.C. and Christie, J. (1989) Generalized non-reactive tuberculosis: a clinicopathological study of four patients. *Thorax*, **44**, 952–5.
88. Shibolet, S., Dan, M., Jedwab, M. *et al.* (1979) Recurrent miliary tuberculosis secondary to infected ventriculo-atrial shunt. *Chest*, **76**, 328–30.
89. Maartens, G., Willcox, P.A. and Benatar, S.R. (1990) Miliary tuberculosis: rapid diagnosis, hematologic abnormalities, and outcome in 109 treated adults. *Am J Med*, **89**, 291–6.
90. Chapman, C.B. and Wharton, C.M. (1946) Acute generalized miliary tuberculosis in adults. *N Engl J Med*, **235**, 239–48.
91. Munt, P.W. (1971) Miliary tuberculosis in the chemotherapy era: with a clinical review in 69 American adults. *Medicine*, **51**, 139–55.
92. Debre, R. (1952) Miliary tuberculosis in children. *Lancet*, **2**, 545–9.
93. Berger, H.W. and Samartin, T.G. (1970) Miliary tuberculosis: diagnostic methods with emphasis on the chest roentgenogram. *Chest*, **58**, 586–9.
94. Massaro, D. and Katz, S. (1964) Rapid clearing in hematogenous pulmonary tuberculosis. *Arch Intern Med*, **113**, 573–7.
95. Biehl, J.P. (1958) Miliary tuberculosis. A review of 68 adult patients admitted to a municipal general hospital. *Am Rev Tuberc Pulm Dis*, **77**, 605–22.
96. Goldfine, I.D., Schachter, H., Barclay, W.R. and Kingdon, H.S. (1969) Consumption coagulopathy in miliary tuberculosis. *Ann Intern Med*, **71**, 775–7.
97. Hooper, A.A. (1972) Tuberculous peripheral lymphadenitis. *Brit J Surg*, **59**, 353–9.
98. Kent, D.C. (1967) Tuberculous lymphadenitis: not a localized disease process. *Am J Med Sci*, **254**, 866–73.
99. Priel, I. and Doley, E. (1982) Tuberculous lymphadenitis: a survey of 94 cases. *J Infect Dis*, **146**, 710.
100. Newcombe, J.F. (1971) Tuberculous cervical lymphadenopathy. *Postgrad Med J*, **47**, 713–17.
101. Des Prez, R.M. and Heim, C.R. (1991) *Mycobacterium tuberculosis*, in *Principles and Practice of Infectious Diseases*, 3rd edn (eds G.L. Mandell, R.G. Douglas and J.E. Bennett), Churchill Livingstone, New York, pp. 1877–906.
102. Mason Browne, J.J. (1957) Discussion on tuberculous cervical adenitis: incidence of disease. *Proc R Soc Med*, **50**, 1060–3.
103. Cantrell, R.W., Jenson, J.H. and Reid, D. (1975) Diagnosis and management of tuberculous cervical adenitis. *Arch Otolaryngol*, **101**, 53–7.
104. Rich, A.R. and McCordock, H.A. (1933) Pathogenesis of tuberculous meningitis. *Bull Johns Hopkins Hosp*, **52**, 5–37.

105. Leonard, J.M. and Des Prez, R.M. (1990) Tuberculous meningitis. *Infect Dis Clin N Am*, **4**, 769–87.
106. Kocen, R.S. and Parsons, M. (1970) Neurological complications of tuberculosis. *Quart J Med*, **39**, 17–30.
107. Ogawa, S.K., Smith, M.A., Brennessel, D.J. and Lowy, F.D. (1987) Tuberculous meningitis in an urban medical center. *Medicine*, **66**, 317–26.
108. Gordon, A. and Parsons, M. (1972) The place of corticosteroids in the management of tuberculous meningitis. *Br J Hosp Med*, **7**, 651–5.
109. Kennedy, D.H. and Fallon, R.J. (1979) Tuberculous meningitis. *JAMA*, **241**, 264–8.
110. Smith, H.V. (1964) Tuberculous meningitis. *Int J Neurol*, **4**, 134–57.
111. Ribera, E., Martinez-Vazquez, J.M., Ocaña, I. *et al.* (1987) Activity of adenosine deaminase for the diagnosis and follow-up of tuberculous meningitis in adults. *J Infect Dis*, **155**, 603–7.
112. Kadival, G.V., Samuel, A.M., Mazarelo, T.B.M.S. and Chapras, S.D. (1987) Radioimmunoassay for detecting *Mycobacterium tuberculosis* antigen in cerebrospinal fluids of patients with tuberculous meningitis. *J Infect Dis*, **155**, 608–11.
113. Anderson, N.E. and Willoughby, E.W. (1987) Chronic meningitis without predisposing illness – a review of 83 cases. *Quart J Med*, **63**, 283–95.
114. Kingsley, D.P.E., Hendrickse, W.A., Kendall, B.E. *et al.* (1987) Tuberculous meningitis: role of CT in management and prognosis. *J Neurol Neurosurg Psych*, **50**, 30–6.
115. Teoh, R., Humphries, M.J. and O'Mahony, G. (1987) Symptomatic intracranial tuberculomas developing during treatment of tuberculosis: a report of 10 patients and review of the literature. *Quart J Med*, **63**, 449–60.
116. Klimach, O.E. and Ormerod, L.P. (1985) Gastrointestinal tuberculosis: a retrospective review of 109 cases in a district general hospital. *Quart J Med*, **56**, 569–78.
117. Tabrisky, J., Lindstrom, R.R., Peters, R. and Lachnan, R.S. (1975) Tuberculous enteritis – review of a protean disease. *Am J Gastroenterol*, **63**, 49–57.
118. Dankner, W.M., Waecker, N.J., Essey, M.A. *et al.* (1993) *Mycobacterium bovis* infection in San Diego: a clinico-epidemiologic study of 73 patients and a historical review of a forgotten pathogen. *Medicine*, **72**, 11–37.
119. Wig, K.L., Chitkara, N.L., Gupta, S.P. *et al.* (1961) Ileocecal tuberculosis with particular reference to isolation of *Mycobacterium tuberculosis*. *Am Rev Respir Dis*, **84**, 169–78.
120. Foster, G.S. and Galdabini, J.J. (1980) Case records of the Massachusetts General Hospital – Case 33 – 1980. *N Engl J Med*, **303**, 445–51.
121. Thoeni, R.F. and Margulis, A.R. (1979) Gastrointestinal tuberculosis. *Surg Roent*, **14**, 283–94.
122. Bretholz, A., Strasser, H. and Knoblauch, M. (1978) Endoscopic diagnosis of ileocecal tuberculosis. *Gastrointest Endoscopy*, **24**, 250–1.
123. Jordan, G.L. and DeBakey, M.E. (1954) Complications of tuberculous enteritis during antimicrobial therapy. *Arch Surg*, **69**, 688–93.
124. Johnston, F.F. and Sanford, J.P. (1961) Tuberculous peritonitis. *Ann Intern Med*, **54**, 1125–33.
125. Borhanmanesh, F., Hekmat, K., Vaezzadeh, K. and Rezai, H.R. (1972) Tuberculous peritonitis. Prospective study of 32 cases in Iran. *Ann Intern Med*, **76**, 567–72.

126. Karney, W.W., O'Donoghue, J.M., Ostrow, J.H. *et al.* (1977) The spectrum of tuberculous peritonitis. *Chest*, **72**, 310–15.
127. Bastani, B., Shariatzadeh, M.R. and Dehdashti, F. (1985) Tuberculous peritonitis – report of 30 cases and review of the literature. *Quart J Med*, **56**, 549–57.
128. Hyman, S., Villa, F., Alvarez, S. and Steigmann, F. (1962) The enigma of tuberculous peritonitis. *Gastroenterology*, **42**, 1–6.
129. Singh, M.M., Bhargawa, A.N. and Jain, K.P. (1969) Tuberculous peritonitis – an evaluation of pathogenic mechanisms, diagnostic procedures and therapeutic measures. *N Engl J Med*, **281**, 1091–4.
130. Burack, W.R. and Hollister, R.M. (1960) Tuberculous peritonitis. A study of 47 proven cases encountered by a general medical unit in 25 years. *Am J Med*, **28**, 510–23.
131. Werbeloff, L., Novis, B.H., Bank, S. and Marks, I.N. (1973) The radiology of tuberculosis of the gastro-intestinal tract. *Brit J Radiol*, **46**, 329–36.
132. Eng, J. and Sabanathan, S. (1991) Tuberculosis of the esophagus. *Digest Dis Sci*, **36**, 536–40.
133. Desai, D.C., Swaroop, V.S., Mohandas, K.M. *et al.* (1991) Tuberculosis of the pancreas: report of three cases. *Am J Gastroenterol*, **86**, 761–3.
134. Horne, N. and Tulloch, W.S. (1975) Conservative management of renal tuberculosis. *Brit J Urol*, **47**, 481–7.
135. Narayana, A.S. (1982) Overview of renal tuberculosis. *Urology*, **19**, 231–7.
136. Christensen, W.I. (1974) Genitourinary tuberculosis: review of 102 cases. *Medicine*, **53**, 377–90.
137. O'Boyle, P. and Gon, J.G. (1976) Genitourinary tuberculosis: study of 20 patients. *Brit Med J*, **1**, 141–3.
138. Lattimer, J.K. (1975) Renal tuberculosis. *N Engl J Med*, **273**, 208–11.
139. Simon, H.B., Weinstein, A.J., Pasternak, M.D. *et al.* (1977) Genitourinary tuberculosis. Clinical features in a general hospital population. *Am J Med*, **63**, 410–20.
140. Kenney, M., Loechel, A.B. and Lovelock, F.J. (1960) Urine cultures in tuberculosis. *Am Rev Respir Dis*, **82**, 564–7.
141. Teklu, B. and Ostrow, J.H. (1976) Urinary tuberculosis: a review of 44 cases treated since 1963. *J Urol*, **115**, 507–9.
142. Kelalis, P.P., Greene, L.F. and Weed, L.A. (1962) Brucellosis of the urogenital tract: a mimic of tuberculosis. *J Urol*, **88**, 347–53.
143. Vasquez, G. and Lattimer, J.K. (1959) Danger to children of infection from exposure to urine containing tubercle bacilli. *JAMA*, **171**, 115–19.
144. Obrant, K.O. (1966) Infection risk for relatives of patients with urogenital tuberculosis. *Am Rev Respir Dis*, **94**, 108–11.
145. Wisnia, L.G., Kukolj, J.S., DeSanta Maria, J.L. and Camuzzi, F. (1978) Renal function damage in 131 cases of urogenital tuberculosis. *Urology*, **11**, 457–61.
146. Morgan, S.H., Eastwood, J.B. and Baker, L.R.I. (1990) Tuberculous interstitial nephritis – the tip of an iceberg? *Tubercle*, **71**, 5–6.
147. Rosenberg, S. (1963) Has chemotherapy reduced the incidence of genitourinary tuberculosis? *J Urol*, **90**, 317–23.
148. Lewis, E.L. (1946) Tuberculosis of the penis: a report of 5 new cases and a complete review of the literature. *J Urol*, **56**, 737–45.
149. Gorse, G.J. and Belshe, R.B. (1985) Male genital tuberculosis: a review of the literature with instructive case reports. *Rev Infect Dis*, **7**, 511–24.

150. Wolf, J.S. and McAninch, J.W. (1991) Tuberculous epididymo-orchitis: diagnosis by fine needle aspiration. *J Urol*, **145**, 836–8.

151. O'Dea, M.J., Moore, S.B. and Greene, L.F. (1978) Tuberculous prostatitis. *Urology*, **11**, 483–5.

152. Veenema, R.J. and Lattimer, J.K. (1957) Genital tuberculosis in the male: clinical pathology and effect on fertility. *J Urol*, **78**, 65–77.

153. Ross, J.C., Gow, J.G. and St. Hill, C.A. (1961) Tuberculous epidydimitis. A review of 170 patients. *Brit J Surg*, **48**, 663–6.

154. Das, K.M., Indudhara, R. and Vaidyanathan, S. (1992) Sonographic features of genitourinary tuberculosis. *Am J Roentgenol*, **158**, 327–9.

155. Brown, A.B., Gilbert, C.R.A. and TeLinde, R.W. (1953) Pelvic tuberculosis. *Obstet Gynecol*, **2**, 476–83.

156. Sutherland, A.M. (1985) Tuberculosis of the female genital tract. *Tubercle*, **66**, 79–83.

157. Falk, V., Ludviksson, K. and Agren, G. (1980) Genital tuberculosis in women. *Am J Obstet Gynecol*, **138**, 974–7.

158. Lattimer, J.K., Colmore, H.P., Sanger, G. *et al.* (1954) Transmission of genital tuberculosis from husband to wife via the semen. *Am Rev Tuberc*, **69**, 618–24.

159. Merchant, R. (1989) Endoscopy in the diagnosis of genital tuberculosis. *J Reprod Med*, **34**, 468–74.

160. Snaith, L.M. and Barns, T. (1962) Fertility in pelvic tuberculosis. *Lancet*, **1**, 712–16.

161. Davidson, P.T. and Horowitz, I. (1970) Skeletal tuberculosis. A review with patient presentations and discussion. *Am J Med*, **48**, 77–84.

162. Davies, P.D.D., Humphries, M.J., Byfield, S.P. *et al.* (1984) Bone and joint tuberculosis. A survey of notifications in England and Wales. *J Bone Joint Surg*, **66B**, 326–9.

163. Gorse, G.J., Pais, M.J., Kusske, J.A. and Cesario, T.C. (1983) Tuberculous spondylitis. A report of six cases and a review of the literature. *Medicine*, **62**, 178–93.

164. Brown, T.S. (1980) Tuberculosis of the ribs. *Clin Radiol*, **31**, 681–4.

165. Newton, P., Sharp, J. and Barnes, K.L. (1982) Bone and joint tuberculosis in Greater Manchester 1969–79. *Ann Rheum Dis*, **41**, 1–6.

166. Muradali, D., Gold, W.L., Vellend, H. and Beeker, E. (1993) Multifocal osteoarticular tuberculosis: report of four cases and review of management. *Clin Infect Rev*, **17**, 204–9.

167. Pouchot, J., Vinceneux, P., Barge, J. *et al.* (1988) Tuberculosis of the sacroiliac joint: clinical features, outcome, and evaluation of closed needle biopsy in 11 consecutive cases. *Am J Med*, **84**, 622–8.

168. Ur-Rahman, N. (1980) Atypical forms of spinal tuberculosis. *J Bone Joint Surg*, **62B**, 162–5.

169. Berney, S., Goldstein, M. and Bishko, F. (1972) Clinical and diagnostic features of tuberculous arthritis. *Am J Med*, **53**, 36–42.

170. Omari, B., Robertson, J.M., Nelson, R. and Chiu, L.C. (1969) Pott's disease. A resurgent challenge to the thoracic surgeon. *Chest*, **95**, 145–50.

171. Brasheur, J.R. and Winfield, H.G. (1975) Tuberculosis of the wrist: a report of ten cases. *South Med J*, **68**, 1345–9.

172. Fowler, N.O. (1991) Tuberculous pericarditis. *JAMA*, **266**, 99–103.

173. Ortbals, D.W. and Avioli, L.V. (1979) Tuberculous pericarditis. *Arch Intern Med*, **139**, 231–4.

174. Rooney, J.J., Crocco, J.A. and Lyons, H.A. (1970) Tuberculous pericarditis. *Ann Intern Med*, **72**, 73–8.

175. Dave, T., Naruca, J.P. and Chopra, P. (1990) Myocardial and endocardial involvement in tuberculous constrictive pericarditis: difficulty in biopsy distinction from endomyocardial fibrosis as a cause of restrictive heart disease. *Internat J Cardiol*, **28**, 245–51.

176. Suchet, I.B. and Horowitz, T.A. (1992) CT in tuberculous constrictive pericarditis. *J Comp Assist Tomograph*, **16**, 391–400.

177. Hammersmith, S.M., Colleti, P.M., Moris, S.L. *et al.* (1991) Cardiac calcifications: difficult MRI diagnosis. *Magnetic Reson Imaging*, **9**, 195–200.

178. Strang, J.I.G., Gibson, D.G., Mitchison, D.A. *et al.* (1988) Controlled clinical trial of complete open surgical drainage and of prednisolone in treatment of tuberculous pericardial effusion in Transkei. *Lancet*, **2**, 759–63.

179. Godfrey–Faussett, P., Wilkins, E.G., Khoo, S. and Stoker, N. (1991) Tuberculous pericarditis confirmed by DNA amplification. *Lancet*, **337**, 176–7.

180. Hageman, J.H., D'Esopo, N.D. and Glenn, W.W.L. (1964) Tuberculosis of the pericardium. A long-term analysis of forty-four proved cases. *N Engl J Med*, **270**, 327–32.

181. Larrieu, A.J., Tyers, F.O., Williams, E.H. and Derrick, J.R.(1980) Recent experience with tuberculous pericarditis. *Ann Thorac Surg*, **29**, 464–8.

182. Long, R., Younes, M., Patton, H. and Hershfield, E. (1989) Tuberculous pericarditis. Long-term outcome in patients who received medical therapy alone. *Am Heart J*, **117**, 1133–9.

# 5 | Tuberculosis in HIV-infected individuals

Douglas V. Sepkowitz

## 5.1 EPIDEMIOLOGY

When the AIDS epidemic began in the early 1980s, the incidence of tuberculosis (TB) in the USA had been falling for more than 30 years. From 1953 to 1984, the number of reported cases of TB decreased by 73.6% (from 84 304 to 22 255) [1]. In 1985, however, the decline in the number of cases stopped, and in 1986, the number of TB cases increased by 3%. There was a further increase of 5% in 1989 and 6% in 1990 [2].

The TB resurgence has closely paralleled the epidemic caused by the human immunodeficiency virus (HIV) and there are epidemiologic data to suggest that the resurgence of TB is closely related to the HIV epidemic. Areas of both the USA and Africa that have experienced the heaviest burden of HIV infection have suffered the greatest increases in the incidence of TB [3,4]. Certain demographic groups highly affected by HIV infection, such as intravenous drug users [5] and Haitians [6], are those groups which have sustained the highest increases in TB.

Poverty, overcrowding and homelessness are socioeconomic factors common to groups and areas most affected by co-infection with TB and HIV. In a New York City retrospective study of patients with both infections, more than two-thirds of these patients earned less than $10 000 a year and 52% had lived in a shelter within the past year [7]. Another similar study of HIV prevalence in TB patients found that in Brooklyn, 15% of patients were admitted to the hospital directly from prison and 8% were homeless at the time of admission [8]. A third study from Harlem of 224 patients with HIV and TB found that 45% were homeless, 23% had unstable housing and 82% were unemployed [9].

In groups of HIV-infected individuals that do not have a high risk of TB exposure, however, such as middle class male homosexuals, there is a lower rate of the infection. Since this group represents a significant majority of HIV-infected patients, it will still account for substantial numbers of co-infection with HIV and TB.

Of the infections associated with the HIV epidemic, TB has a special importance. It is probably the only HIV-related infection that is readily transmissible regardless of whether the exposed person is infected with HIV [10]. If diagnosed promptly, TB is treatable [11]. Additionally, there are studies that suggest that TB chemoprophylaxis can be effective in HIV patients [12].

## 5.2 PATHOGENESIS IN HIV-INFECTED PATIENTS

In immunocompetent individuals, TB infection is usually contained and clinical disease does not develop, although small numbers of dormant bacilli remain. Reactivation disease develops in approximately 10% of infected persons over the course of a lifetime and is thought often to occur through defects in T cell or macrophage function [13]. HIV infection is well known to cause dysfunction and depletion of the T helper cell population. The function of macrophages and monocytes is also disturbed [14]. Because of these effects, HIV impairs the mechanisms whereby newly acquired TB infection is contained and latent TB is suppressed.

### 5.2.1 Rapid development of tuberculosis after primary exposure

There are several studies documenting an accelerated course of TB in HIV-infected patients who have been recently infected with the tubercle bacillus. An outbreak of TB in a residential facility for HIV-infected individuals occurred where 31 residents were exposed to patients with pulmonary TB and 11 developed active disease within a 4 month period [15]. In contrast, among 28 staff members who had been similarly exposed, none developed active infection though six had tuberculin test conversions. Despite similar rates of new infections, the HIV-infected patient was much more likely to develop active disease.

Another outbreak from Italy [16] reported 18 HIV-infected patients who were inadvertently exposed to other patients with pulmonary TB. Within 60 days of the diagnosis of the index cases, seven of the 18 had developed active disease. Although no typing of any of the acid-fast bacilli (AFB) was done, the outbreak was thought to be to new infection rather than re-activation. Hospital staff and volunteers exposed to the index patients were considered control groups and only one of 25 of the hospital staff developed active pulmonary TB. Of nine exposed volunteers, six had previously negative tuberculin skin tests and four of these converted. No cases of active disease occurred. The rate of active TB (39%) was notably higher in HIV-infected patients than in hospital workers or volunteers (3%).

Outbreaks of multi-drug-resistant disease have provided additional data on the progression of recently acquired TB among HIV-infected individuals. In one New York City hospital, nine of 13 patients with newly diagnosed multi-drug-resistant TB had been exposed for 30–105 days before the diagnosis of tubercular disease [17]. Of another eight cases, six were diagnosed with TB after exposures to multi-drug-resistant strains 50–180 days earlier. A cluster of 22 cases of multi-drug-resistant disease was described [18] where contact with the resistant strains occurred in an HIV clinic. In some cases, the interval between exposure and development of active TB was as short as 22 days.

### 5.2.2 Increased risk of reactivation disease

In addition to accelerated progression of recently acquired TB, individuals with HIV infection have an increased incidence of reactivation of latent disease. In a study of intravenous drug users [19], 49 of 217 HIV-seropositive subjects (23%) and 62 of 303 HIV-seronegative subjects (20%) had positive skin tests. Rates of tuberculin test conversion were similar (11% and 13%, respectively) as well. Active TB developed in eight HIV-seropositive subjects, seven of whom had positive tuberculin tests. None of the seronegative subjects developed active disease. Over the 2 year study period, 14% of the HIV-seropositive patients who had prior positive tuberculin tests developed active TB.

Additionally, besides latent reactivation or accelerated progression of new infection, it has been shown that HIV-infected patients already infected with the tubercle bacillus can be clinically reinfected with a new, exogenous strain [20].

### 5.3 PREVALENCE OF HIV INFECTION AMONG TUBERCULOSIS PATIENTS

During 1988 and 1989, a study was conducted concerning HIV seroprevalence among patients attending TB clinics in the USA [21]. Sixty-four clinics in 29 cities were studied with an HIV seroprevalence rate of 3.4%, ranging from 0.3% in Honolulu to 46.3% in New York City. The seroprevalence rates were highest in the 30–39 year old age group and nearly equal for men and women. Seroprevalence rates were not statistically higher in Blacks than in Whites. Of 178 consecutive patients who were hospitalized in Brooklyn for the treatment of newly diagnosed, previously untreated TB, 82 were HIV seropositive, 62% were intravenous drug users, 18% were Haitian and 10% were homosexual [8]. An earlier report from San Francisco reviewed all TB cases reported between 1981 and 1985 [22]. There were 287 cases of disease in non-Asian born males and 35 (12%) had AIDS; most of these (28 of 35) were homosexual.

The epidemiologic differences in these two studies reflect the fact that different populations are infected by HIV, and these vary geographically. There is a preponderance of data suggesting that, in the industrialized world, intravenous drug users and heterosexuals are the groups most affected by TB and HIV co-infection (21,23).

In Africa, approximately half the adult population aged 20–40 years is infected with the tubercle bacillus [24]. Not surprisingly, there are substantially more people co-infected with TB and HIV. The prevalence of HIV infection in patients with TB from sub-Saharan Africa ranges from 20% in Zaire to 67% in Uganda [4]. The degree of HIV incidence in TB patients supports the recommendation of HIV antibody testing in newly diagnosed TB patients [5].

## 5.4 PREVALENCE OF TUBERCULOSIS IN HIV PATIENTS

The incidence of TB in HIV-infected patients is also increased. The rate is less in the USA than in Africa. In the USA in 1984, the incidence of tubercular disease was 9.4 per 100 000 population [1]. Studies of the incidence of the disease among AIDS patients from the same period ranged from 7% to 60% [6,25–27]. Haitians and intravenous drug users were the groups most affected with incidence rates of 60% and 21%, respectively.

In Africa, TB is the most common opportunistic infection seen in HIV-infected patients [4]. In Zimbabwe and Ethiopia, a third of AIDS patients have TB [24]. A rate of 40% has been reported from Zambia [4]. An autopsy study from Abidjan revealed that miliary TB was present in 36% of 265 consecutive HIV-seropositive patients [4]. Another study from Abidjan reported on 473 HIV-positive patients whose predominant cause of death was TB; 40% had disseminated TB at autopsy [28]. A retrospective study of women of child bearing age from Zaire found HIV-seropositive women were more likely to develop TB than seronegative women. Of 249 (7.6%) seropositive subjects, 19 developed TB compared with 1 of 310 seronegative subjects (0.3%) [29], a 25-fold increased rate.

Using TB notification data, the World Health Organization has published estimates of future global TB morbidity and mortality [29a]. The total number of TB deaths in 1990 was estimated at 2.53 million with 4.6% attributable to HIV. Projected mortality for the year 2000 is 3.51 million with 14.2% being attributable to HIV. Most of the increase is related to increases in the Africa region.

## 5.5 CLINICAL ASPECTS OF TUBERCULOSIS IN HIV-INFECTED PATIENTS

### 5.5.1 Clinical presentation

Several trends have emerged concerning the presentation of TB in HIV-

infected individuals (Table 5.1). TB often precedes any other AIDS defining illness. It is more virulent than most other opportunistic infections
and thus may occur earlier [10]. In several reviews of co-infection, 75%
of patients had TB prior to the diagnosis of AIDS (Table 5.2) [22, 25–
27,30].

**Table 5.1** Tuberculosis in AIDS patients

- Tuberculosis often precedes other AIDS defining illnesses
- The incidence of extrapulmonary tuberculosis is increased
- Presentation is dependent on level of immune function
- Symptoms are usually nonspecific
- Chest X-rays may by atypical
- A higher percentage of culture-positive sputa are smear negative

**Table 5.2** Presentation of tuberculosis prior to the diagnosis of AIDS

| Location | Number of patients with co-infection | Patients with TB before AIDS (%) | Reference |
|---|---|---|---|
| San Francisco | 35 | 63 | 22 |
| New York | 24 | 62 | 25 |
| New York | 30 | 60 | 26 |
| Newark, NJ | 29 | 48 | 27 |
| Los Angeles | 39 | 67 | 30 |

It was recognized early in the HIV epidemic that the incidence of extrapulmonary TB (EPTB) was greatly increased in HIV-infected individuals
[22,26,27,30–32]. As many as 60–70% of patients co-infected with the
tubercle bacilli and HIV had EPTB. With recognition of this, in 1987 the
Centers for Disease Control (CDC) classified EPTB as an AIDS defining
illness [33]. By 1993, pulmonary TB was included as well [34]. Much of
the data concerning co-infection emerged from cross-sectional studies
rather than longitudinal studies, and the changing definitions of AIDS
have skewed the data, probably underestimating the number of those co-
infected.

The clinical presentation of TB is dependent on the immune status of the
individual infected. Subjects with higher CD4 counts (250–500/mm$^3$) were
more likely to have pulmonary disease, while those with counts of less than
100/mm$^3$ were more prone to miliary disease (Figure 5.1) [4].

Fever, cough, chest pain and weight loss are seen in most HIV patients
co-infected with TB. Chronic diarrhea and generalized lymphadenopathy are often present. Unfortunately, many of the HIV-related illnesses
produce similar symptoms making an accurate diagnosis difficult [21,30,
31,35].

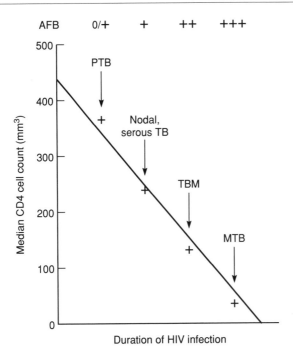

**Figure 5.1** The clinical and immunopathological course of HIV-related tuberculosis. AFB indicates the density of tubercle bacilli in lesions from few (o/+) to many (+++); PTB, pulmonary tuberculosis; TBM, tuberculous meningitis; and MTB, miliary tuberculosis. The data points are derived from studies from Australia, USA and Africa. Reproduced with permission from the *Journal of the American Medical Association*, September 23/30, **268**, 1581–7, copyright 1992, American Medical Association [4].

### 5.5.2 Radiographic studies

Despite the increased frequency of EPTB in HIV-infected patients, pulmonary disease is the most common form of TB [2]. There are a variety of radiographic findings in HIV-infected patients with pulmonary TB. Hilar adenopathy, diffuse infiltrates (which can be confused with pulmonary pneumocystosis), and lower lobe involvement are seen more frequently than is typically expected in pulmonary TB [10,21,30,31]. Pleural effusions are often present [30,31]. Chest X-rays have been reported to be normal in as many as 10% of HIV-infected individuals with pulmonary TB [35a]. The disease, therefore, cannot be entirely excluded on radiographic grounds in the HIV-infected patient.

The degree of immunosuppression caused by HIV infection is probably directly related to how atypical the X-ray appears [2]. In one study [32], where the average CD4 count was 326/mm³, the radiographic findings in the seropositive group were not significantly different from those of a seronegative group. Cavitary disease or focal infiltrates were seen in the majority of cases. Hilar adenopathy, cavitation and pleural effusion are significant X-ray findings because they are rarely found in pneumocystis pneumonia, the most common pulmonary infection in AIDS [2].

### 5.5.3 Sputum studies

Reports vary as to how often sputum AFB smears are positive in HIV-infected patients, with a 31–82% range [2,30]. In one study [36], 45% of the seropositive group had a positive AFB smear whereas 81% of seronegative patients were positive. The initial AFB smear was positive only 29% of the time in seropositive patients, compared with 61% in the seronegative group. Sixty per cent of the HIV-infected patients and 13% of seronegative patients had more than five negative smears. Patients with milder immune dysfunction have similar results to HIV antibody negative individuals regarding AFB smear and culture yields.

Because of the higher incidence of non-diagnostic sputum examinations, bronchoscopy, with or without biopsy, may be required for diagnostic purposes. In one study [31], however, bronchoscopic alveolar lavage (BAL) yielded a positive AFB smear in two of 21 cases and a positive culture in 12. With transbronchial biopsy, three of 21 cases had a positive smear, nine had a positive culture and four had granulomas seen on biopsy. Bronchoscopy or other procedures which can increase coughing should be done in appropriately controlled environments to minimize the potential transmission of the tubercle bacillus from an, as yet, undiagnosed TB patient to others.

### 5.5.4 Extrapulmonary tuberculosis

Extrapulmonary TB occurs in approximately 15% of people with TB who are not infected with HIV, but it is present in about 70% of patients with AIDS and TB. In patients with TB and less advanced HIV disease, EPTB is diagnosed in between 25% and 45% of cases [37]. Intravenous drug users account for almost half of all cases of EPTB and have the highest rate of EPTB among all HIV risk groups [38].

EPTB in HIV-infected patients can involve any organ system. Lymphadenitis and disseminated disease (involvement of blood, bone marrow or more than two noncontiguous extrapulmonary sites) are the most common forms of EPTB in AIDS patients [2,22,25,27,39]. Blood cultures are frequently positive in these patients, ranging in incidence from 26% to 56% [2,31,39,40]. In a review of tubercle bacillus bacteremia [40], the average CD4 count in these HIV-infected patients was 198/mm$^3$. In six of 34 patients, the only positive culture was from the blood.

Genitourinary and meningeal TB are also fairly common in HIV-infected patients. In one study, 37% of co-infected patients had evidence of genitourinary TB [39]. Genitourinary symptoms were rarely present; 40% had an abnormal urinanalysis, and 61 of 73 patients had a positive urine culture. At autopsy, 11 patients had renal involvement, three had testicular disease and one had a rectoprostatic fistula. Of 73 patients, 59 had concomitant pulmonary TB and 33 had TB of at least one other extra-pulmonary site [39]. A review of TB meningitis in HIV-infected patients found that 10% of co-infected patients had meningitis [41]. Eighteen of 26 had abnormal CT scans, including 11 with hydrocephalus, seven with non-enhancing lesions, six with meningeal enhancement and four with enhancing lesions. CSF pleocytosis was usually present but four patients had fewer than 5 WBC/mm$^3$. The CSF protein was normal in 43% of the patients and four of 18 had a positive AFB CSF smear.

Overt TB abscesses may be more common in HIV-infected individuals [42]. Purulent collections have been described in a variety of locations including pancreas [43], spleen [44,45], breast [46], liver [42], abdominal wall [42], psoas muscle [42], pericardium [47] and mediastinum [42]. It is possible that the minimal immune response in such patients makes it more likely for a focal TB abscess to develop.

## 5.6 TUBERCULIN SKIN TESTING IN HIV-INFECTED PATIENTS

It has often been assumed that tuberculin skin tests will be non-reactive in HIV-infected patients with TB. The results are dependent, however, on the degree of immune dysfunction in the patient. In one review [32], 12 of 17 (70%) patients with a median CD4 count of 326/mm$^3$ had induration of 10 mm or more on the Mantoux test. In another report of HIV-seropositive patients with TB [35], only one of nine with a lower CD4 count had a reactive skin test. A review of AIDS patients with TB from Florida found that a patient was more likely to have a positive Mantoux skin test if the TB was diagnosed prior to the diagnosis of AIDS, compared with being diagnosed following another AIDS defining illness [48] when the CD4 count is likely to be lower.

Cell mediated immune function is progressively depressed by HIV infection. In 1989, the CDC recommended that tuberculin skin reactions of 5 mm or more should be considered indicative of TB infection in an HIV-infected person [5]. Studies involving Haitians [49] and intravenous drug users [50] support the need for reducing the definition of a positive reaction. In both studies, the prevalence of tuberculin skin test reactivity at 10 mm was less in seropositive subjects compared with seronegative subjects. However, when the induration size was lowered, to 5 mm or more in the Haitian study and 2 mm or more in the intravenous drug users study, the prevalence rates for tuberculin test positivity equalized in the sero-negative and seropositive groups.

## 5.7 TREATMENT

TB therapy is effective in HIV-infected individuals when therapy is begun promptly. Many reports indicate that seropositive patients with TB respond as well as seronegative patients [4,6,25,27,32,35,39]. In the largest study of the treatment of TB in HIV-infected patients, 125 individuals were studied retrospectively [11]. The median time from the start of therapy to clearance of AFB from the sputum was 10 weeks with three relapses and one case of failure. In those patients with pulmonary TB, the chest X-ray improved or stabilized in two-thirds. When the radiograph worsened, it was found to be caused by a non-TB cause. Some studies, especially from Africa, are not as promising. Perriens et al. [51] documented a relapse rate three times higher in HIV-positive patients compared with HIV-negative patients.

There is an increased incidence of drug toxicity in HIV-infected patients receiving chemotherapy [4,11,24]. In one study [11], 18% of patients needed alterations of therapy due to adverse reactions. Rifampin was the drug most likely to cause adverse reactions. Another study [22] demonstrated an increased incidence of adverse drug reactions in seropositive compared with seronegative patients, 26% versus 3%, respectively. It is not understood why HIV patients have an increased rate of adverse drug reactions but similar increases have been seen with other medications such as trimethoprim/sulfamethoxazole [10,52].

When appropriate anti-TB therapy is delayed, either because of unsuspected drug resistance [53] or the lack of a diagnosis, mortality increases. When treatment was begun within 15 days of presentation in one report [31], four of 27 patients (15%) died of TB but if therapy was delayed (23–119 days after presentation, median 57 days), the mortality rate due to TB more than doubled (36%). In this study, the reasons for the delay in diagnosis were usually due to not considering TB as a diagnosis rather than because of an atypical presentation.

Recent outbreaks of multi-drug-resistant TB have made treatment much more problematic [17,18,29,53–57]. Frieden et al. [54] examined the incidence and characteristics of multi-drug-resistant isolates in New York City for April 1991. Of 518 patients, 33% had isolates resistant to one or more drugs; 26% of the isolates were resistant to isoniazid (INH) and 19% were resistant to both INH and rifampin. The probability of resistance increased if the patient had received prior anti-TB therapy (44%). The incidence of resistance in patients who had never received anti-TB chemotherapy was 10% in 1982–1984 and had increased to 23% in 1991. People who were co-infected with HIV were more likely to have resistant strains than were seronegative patients.

The CDC has recently issued new guidelines for the treatment of TB in the era of multi-drug resistance [58]. For individuals co-infected with TB and HIV, the CDC recommends at least 9 months of therapy or at least six months after sputum conversion. Because of the persistence of the immunologic deficit, consideration of continuing INH suppression following the treatment course may be in order.

Directly observed treatment (DOT) is prominent among the CDC recommendations since patient compliance in taking TB therapy is poor. Studies report a third of patients do not complete therapy [59,60]. In the study by Brudney and Dobkin of 178 TB patients discharged from an inner city hospital, only 19 (11%) were compliant; 99 (56%) did not return for subsequent therapy, 49 (28%) had less than 3 months of therapy, and 11 (6%) were lost to follow-up after 3 months of therapy [9]. The data from Frieden et al.'s study strongly suggest that the recent multi-drug-resistant TB epidemic is directly related to poor compliance [54].

Immunological adjuvant therapy may be of value in HIV-infected individuals with TB. A recent report in mice [60a] showed the utility of interferon-$\gamma$ in animals deficient in this lymphokine. Such therapy may be useful in HIV-infected individuals particularly those with multi-drug-resistant TB who retain some CD4 function.

## 5.8 CHEMOPROPHYLAXIS

It appears that INH prophylaxis is beneficial in HIV-infected individuals, as has been shown to be the case in the normal host (Chapter 12). Selwyn et al. [12] studied intravenous drug users with patients classified according to HIV status and tuberculin skin test results. Twelve months of INH treatment was given to HIV-infected individuals with a skin test of 5 mm induration or more. Active TB did not develop in anyone who received prophylaxis, either during or after 12 months of therapy. Similarly, a study from Zambia demonstrated a nine-fold reduction in the incidence of TB when HIV-infected patients received 6 months of INH prophylaxis [4].

There is debate regarding who should receive chemoprophylaxis, when it should begin, what drugs should be used, and for how long it should continue. Selwyn et al.'s study [12] recommended INH prophylaxis in anergic, as well as tuberculin test reactive, HIV-infected individuals in areas where TB is prevalent. Some believe chemoprophylaxis should begin when the CD4 count falls below 500/mm$^3$, and it should be extended beyond 12 months [61].

## 5.9 BACILLE CALMETTE-GUERIN (BCG)

It is not known if BCG vaccination is helpful or detrimental in HIV-infected people [4,24,62]. There are reports of dissemination following BCG vaccination. Two patients developed BCG-related disease 30 years after vaccination [63,64]. The study by Ong and Mandal, although small, did not show any protective benefit from BCG vaccination [35]. On the other hand, data from the Congo has revealed that infants born to HIV-infected mothers did not suffer from routine BCG vaccination [65]. The current WHO guidelines are to withhold BCG vaccination in cases of symptomatic HIV infection and in cases of HIV infection where the risk of TB is low [66].

Chapter 9 gives a more detailed discussion on BCG. It may be the case that either the current form or a modified form of BCG will be used increasingly in the future. One circumstance where an even partially effective BCG vaccine would be useful is the health care worker involved in high risk procedures (such as bronchoscopy) with HIV-infected patients who may be infected with multi-drug-resistant TB. In this group, the diagnosis may be more difficult to make and INH prophylaxis can be ineffective.

## 5.10 PROGNOSIS

Despite evidence that anti-TB chemotherapy and chemoprophylaxis are effective in HIV-infected individuals, the prognosis for people with both infections is poor. Several reports document a much higher mortality rate in people with both TB and HIV compared with those with TB alone

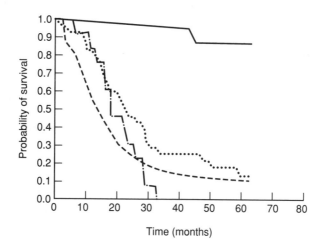

**Figure 5.2** A comparison of the cumulative probability of survival from the diagnosis of TB in patients who were HIV seronegative (solid line), HIV seropositive (dotted line), a subset of seropositive patients with < 200 CD4 cells/mm³ (dot-dash-dot line) and from a diagnosis of pneumocystosis (dashed line) in 1985 and 1986. Reproduced with permission from *Archives of Internal Medicine*, 1992, **152**, 2033–7, copyright 1992, American Medical Association [7].

[24,26,41,51,67]. Much of the increased mortality rate is probably related to other opportunistic infections associated with HIV infection.

The median survival from the time of the diagnosis of TB ranges from 7.4 months [21] to 21 months [67]. Stoneburner *et al.* [7] showed, not surprisingly, that the median survival time varied directly with the CD4 count (Figure 5.2). The prognosis associated with multi-drug-resistant TB infection is worse. Patients with this resistant disease and HIV infection had a median survival time of 2.1 months, compared with 14.6 months for HIV-infected patients with sensitive strains of TB [53].

## REFERENCES

1. Rieder, H., Cauthen, G., Kelly, G. *et al.* (1989) Tuberculosis in the United States. *JAMA*, **262**, 385–9.
2. Barnes, P., Bloch, A., Davidson, P. *et al.* (1991) Tuberculosis in patients with human immunodeficiency virus infection. N Engl J Med, **324**, 1644–50.
3. Centers for Disease Control (1986) Tuberculosis – United States, 1985. The possible impact of human T-lymphotrophic virus type III/lymphadenopathy-associated virus infection. *MMWR*, **35**, 74–6.
4. De Cock, K., Soro, B., Coulibaly, I. *et al.* (1992) Tuberculosis and HIV infection in sub-Saharan Africa. *JAMA*, **268**, 1581–7.
5. Centers for Disease Control (1989) Tuberculosis and human immunodeficiency virus infection: Recommendations of the Advisory Committee for the Elimination of Tuberculosis (ACET). *MMWR*, **38**, 236–8, 243–50.
6. Pitchenik, A., Cole, C., Russell, B. *et al.* (1984) Tuberculosis, atypical mycobacteriosis, and the acquired immunodeficiency syndrome among Haitian and non-Haitian patients in south Florida. *Ann Intern Med*, **101**, 641–5.
7. Stoneburner, R., Laroche, E., Prevots, R. *et al.* (1992) Survival in a cohort of human immunodeficiency virus-infected tuberculosis patients in New York City. *Arch Intern Med*, **152**, 2033–7.
8. Shafer, R., Chirgwin, K., Glatt, A. *et al.* (1991) HIV prevalence, immunosupression, and drug resistance in patients with tuberculosis in an area epidemic for AIDS. *AIDS*, **5**, 399–405.
9. Brudney, K. and Dobkin, J. (1991) Resurgent tuberculosis in New York City. *Am Rev Respir Dis*, **144**, 745–9.
10. Hopewell, P. (1992) Impact of human immunodeficiency virus infection on the epidemology, clinical features, management, and control of tuberculosis. *Clin Infect Dis*, **15**, 540–7.
11. Small, P., Schecter, G., Goodman, P. *et al.* (1991) Treatment of tuberculosis in patients with advanced human immunodeficiency virus infection. *N Engl J Med*, **324**, 289–94.
12. Selwyn, P., Sckell, B., Alcabes, P. *et al.* (1992) High risk of active tuberculosis in HIV-infected drug users with cutaneous anergy. *JAMA*, **268**, 504–9.
13. Edwards, D. and Kirkpatrick, C. (1986) The immunology of mycobacterial diseases. *Am Rev Respir Dis*, **134**, 1062–71.
14. Bender, B., Davidson, B., Kline, R. *et al.* (1988) Role of the mononuclear phagocyte system in the immunopathogenesis of human immunodeficiency

virus infection and the acquired immunodeficiency syndrome. *Rev Infect Dis*, **10**, 1142–54.

15. Daley, C., Small, P., Schecter, G. *et al.* (1992) Tuberculosis in persons infected with HIV. *N Engl J Med*, **326**, 231–5.

16. Di Perri, G., Danzi, M., De Checchi, G. *et al.* (1989) Nosocomial epidemic of active tuberculosis among HIV-infected patients. *Lancet*, **1**, 1502–4.

17. Edlin, B., Tokars, J., Grieco, M. *et al.* (1992) An outbreak of multidrug-resistant tuberculosis among hospitalized patients with the acquired immunodeficiency syndrome. *N Engl J Med*,**326**, 1514–21.

18. Fischl, M., Uttamchandani, R., Daikos, G. *et al.* (1992) An outbreak of tuberculosis caused by multiple-drug-resistant tubercle bacilli among patients with HIV infection. *Ann Intern Med*, **117**, 177–82.

19. Selwyn, P., Hartell, D., Lewis, V. *et al.* (1989) A prospective study of the risk of tuberculosis among intravenous drug users with human immunodeficiency virus infection. *N Engl J Med*, **320**, 545–50.

20. Small, P., Shafer, R., Singh, S. *et al.* (1993) Exogenous reinfection with multidrug-resistant *Mycobacterium tuberculosis* in patients with advanced HIV infection. *N Engl J Med*, **328**, 1137–44.

21. Onorato, I., McCray, E. and the Field Services Branch (1992) Prevalence of human immunodeficiency virus infection among patients attending tuberculosis clinics in the United States. *J Infect Dis*, **165**, 87–92.

22. Chaisson, R., Schecter, G., Theuer, C. *et al.* (1987) Tuberculosis in patients with the acquired immunodeficiency syndrome. *Am Rev Respir Dis*, **136**, 570–4.

23. Centers for Disease Control (1987) Tuberculosis and acquired immunodeficiency syndrome – New York City. *MMWR*, **36**, 785–95.

24. Harries, A.D. (1990) Tuberculosis and human immunodeficiency virus infection in developing countries. *Lancet,* **335**, 387–90.

25. Louie, E., Rice, L. and Holzman, R. (1986) Tuberculosis in non-Haitian patients with acquired immunodeficiency syndrome. *Chest*, **90**, 542–5.

26. Handwerger, S., Mildvan, D., Senie, R. *et al.* (1987) Tuberculosis and the acquired immunodeficiency syndrome at a New York City hospital: 1978–1985. *Chest*, **91**, 176–80.

27. Sunderam, G., McDonald, R., Maniatis, T. *et al.* (1986) Tuberculosis as a manifestation of the acquired immunodeficiency syndrome (AIDS). *JAMA*, **256**, 362–6.

28. Abouya, Y.L., Beaumel, A., Dago-Akribi, A. *et al.* (1992) *Pneumocystis carinii* pneumonia. *Am Rev Respir Dis*, **145**, 617–20.

29. Braun, M.M., Badi, N., Ryder, R. *et al.* (1991) A retrospective cohort study of the risk of tuberculosis among women of childbearing age with HIV infection in Zaire. *Am Rev Respir Dis*, **143**, 501–4.

29a. Centers for Disease Control and Prevention (1993) Estimates of future global tuberculosis morbidity and mortality. *MMWR*, **42**, 961–4.

30. Modilevsky, T., Sattler, F. and Barnes, P. (1989) Mycobacterial disease in patients with human immunodeficiency virus infection. *Arch Intern Med*, **149**, 2201–5.

31. Kramer, F., Modilevsky T., Waliany, A. *et al.* (1990) Delayed diagnosis of tuberculosis in patients with human immunodeficiency virus infection. *Am J Med*, **89**, 451–6.

32. Theuer, C., Hopewell, P., Elias, D. *et al.* (1990) Human immunodeficiency virus infection in tuberculosis patients. *J Infect Dis*, **162**, 8–12.

33. Centers for Disease Control (1987) Revision of the CDC surveillance case definition for acquired immunodeficiency syndrome. *MMWR*, **36**, 1S–6S.

34. Centers for Disease Control (1992) 1993 revised classification system for HIV infection and expanded surveillance case definition for AIDS among adolescents and adults. *MMWR*, **41**, 1–19.

35. Ong, E. and Mandal, B.K. (1991) Tuberculosis in patients infected with the human immunodeficiency virus. *Quart J Med*, **80**, 613–17.

35a. FitzGerald, J.M., Grzybowski, S. and Allen, E.A. (1991) The impact of human immunodeficiency virus infection on tuberculosis and its control. *Chest*, **100**, 191–200.

36. Klein, N., Duncanson, F., Lenox, T. *et al.* (1989) Use of mycobacterial smears in the diagnosis of pulmonary tuberculosis in AIDS/ARC patients. *Chest*, **95**, 1190–2.

37. Slutsker, L., Castro, K., Ward, J. *et al.* (1993) Epidemiology of extrapulmonary tuberculosis among persons with AIDS in the United States. *Clin Infect Dis*, **16**, 513–18.

38. Braun, M., Byers, R., Heyward, W. *et al.* (1990) Acquired immunodeficiency syndrome and extrapulmonary tuberculosis in the United States. *Arch Intern Med*, **150**, 1913–16.

39. Shafer, R., Kim, D., Weiss, J. *et al.* (1991) Extrapulmonary tuberculosis in patients with human immunodeficiency virus infection. *Medicine*, **70**, 384–96.

40. Bouza, E., Diaz–Lopez, M., Moreno, S. *et al.* (1993) *Mycobacterium tuberculosis* bacteremia in patients with and without human immunodeficiency virus infection. *Arch Intern Med*, **153**, 496–9.

41. Berenguer, J., Moreno, S., Laguna, F. *et al.* (1992) Tuberculosis meningitis in patients infected with the human immunodeficiency virus. *N Engl J Med*, **326**, 668–72.

42. Lupatkin, H., Brau, N., Flomenberg, P. *et al.* (1992) Tuberculosis abscesses in patients with AIDS. *Clin Infect Dis*, **14**, 1040–4.

43. Eyer-Silva, W.A., Moraid de Sa, C.A., Pinto, J.F.C. *et al.* (1993) Pancreatic tuberculosis as a manifestation of infection with the human immunodeficiency virus. *Clin Infect Dis,* **16**, 332.

44. Pedro-Botet, J., Maristany, M., Miralles, R. *et al.* (1991) Splenic tuberculosis in patients with AIDS. *Rev Infect Dis*, **13**, 1069–71.

45. Khalil, T., Uzoaru, I., Nadimpalli, V. *et al.* (1992) Splenic tuberculosis abscess in patients positive for human immunodeficiency virus: report of two cases and review. *Clin Infect Dis*, **14**, 1265–6.

46. Hartstein, M. and Leaf, H. (1992) Tuberculosis of the breast as a presenting manifestation of AIDS. *Clin Infect Dis*, **15**, 92–3.

47. Horn, D., Hewlett, D., Alfalla, C. *et al.* (1992) Undiagnosed HIV infections in acute care hospitals. *N Engl J Med*, **327**, 1816–17.

48. Rieder, H., Cauthen, G., Bloch, A. *et al.* (1989) Tuberculosis and acquired immunodeficiency syndrome – Florida. *Arch Intern Med*, **149**, 1268–73.

49. Johnson, M., Coberly, J., Clermont, H. *et al.* (1992) Tuberculin skin test reactivity among adults infected with human immunodeficiency virus. *J Infect Dis*, **166**, 194–8.

50. Graham, N., Nelson, K., Solomon, L. *et al.* (1992) Prevalence of tuberculin

positivity and skin test anergy in HIV-1-seropositive and seronegative intravenous drug users. *JAMA*, **267**, 369–73.

51. Perriens, J., Colebunders, R., Karahunga, C. *et al.* (1991) Increased mortality and tuberculosis treatment failure rate among human immunodeficiency virus (HIV) seropositive compared with HIV seronegative patients with pulmonary tuberculosis treated with 'standard' chemotherapy in Kinshasa, Zaire. *Am Rev Respir Dis*, **144**, 750–5.

52. Gordin, F.M., Simon, G.L., Wofsy, C.B. and Mills, J. (1984) Adverse reations to trimethoprim-sulfamethoxazole in patients with the acquired immunodeficiency syndrome. *Ann Intern Med*, **100**, 95–9.

53. Fischl, M., Daikos, G., Uttamchandani, R. *et al.* (1992) Clinical presentation and outcome of patients with HIV infection and tuberculosis caused by multiple-drug-resistant bacilli. *Ann Intern Med*, **117**, 184–90.

54. Frieden, T., Sterling, T., Pablos-Mendez, A. *et al.* (1993) The emergence of drug-resistant tuberculosis in New York City. *N Engl J Med*, **328**, 521–6.

55. Monno, L., Carbonara, S., Costa, D. *et al.* (1991) Emergence of drug-resistant *Mycobacterium tuberculosis* in HIV-infected patients. *Lancet*, **337**, 852.

56. Pearson, M., Jereb, J., Frieden, T. *et al.* (1992) Nosocomial transmission of multidrug-resistant *Mycobacterium tuberculosis*. *Ann Intern Med*, **117**, 191–96.

57. Pitchenik, A., Burr, J., Laufer, M. *et al.* (1990) Outbreaks of drug-resistant tuberculosis at AIDS centre. *Lancet*, 336, 440–1.

58. Centers for Disease Control (1993) Initial therapy for tuberculosis in the era of multidrug resistance. *MMWR*, **42**, 1–8.

59. Addington, W. (1979) Patient compliance: the most serious remaining problem in the control of tuberculosis in the United States. *Chest*, **76**, 741–3.

60. Iseman, M., Cohn, D. and Sbarbaro, J. (1993) Directly observed treatment of tuberculosis. *N Engl J Med*, **328**, 576–8.

60a. Flynn, J.L., Chan, J., Triebold, K.J. *et al.* (1993) An essential role for interferon-γ in resistance to *Mycobacterium tuberculosis* infection. *J Exp Med*, **178**, 2249–54.

61. Di Perri, G., Vento, S., Cruciani, M. *et al.* (1991) Tuberculosis and HIV infection. *N Engl J Med*, **325**, 1882–4.

62. Subcommittee of the Joint Tuberculosis Committee of the British Thoracic Society (1992) Guidelines on the management of tuberculosis and HIV infection in the United Kingdom. *Brit Med J*, **304**, 1231–3.

63. Reynes, J., Perez, C., Lamaury, I. *et al.* (1989) Bacille Calmette-Guerin adenitis 30 years after immunization in a patient with AIDS. *J Infect Dis*, **160**, 727.

64. Armbruster, C., Junker, W., Vetter, N. *et al.* (1990) Disseminated bacille Calmette-Guerin infection in an AIDS patient 30 years after BCG vaccination. *J Infect Dis*, **162**, 1216.

65. Lallemant-Le Coeur, S., Lallemant, M., Cheynier, D. *et al.* (1991) Bacillus Calmette-Guerin immunization in infants born to HIV-1-seropositive mothers. *AIDS*, **5**, 195–9.

66. World Health Organization (1987) Special programme on AIDS and expanded programme on immunization. Consultation on human immunodeficiency virus (HIV) and routine childhood immunization. *Wkly Epiderm Rec*, **62**, 297–9.

67. Colebunders, R., Ryder, R., Nzilambi, N. *et al.* (1989) HIV infection in patients with tuberculosis in Kinshasa, Zaire. *Am Rev Respir Dis*, **139**, 1082–5.

# Pediatric aspects of tuberculosis | 6

Amin Hakim, Joyce R. Grossman

## 6.1 INTRODUCTION

Pediatric infection with *Mycobacterium tuberculosis* can be different from that in adults. In children, symptomatic disease in many organs may occur earlier in the course of infection, with the full spectrum of tuberculosis (TB) seen more often than in adults. As pointed out by Edith Lincoln [1], a modern pioneer in childhood TB, in children one can easily study what Wallgren [2] called the 'time table of tuberculosis' with the evolution of disease from overt primary infection to classical reactivation pulmonary disease. In the days of pediatric TB wards, every form of the disease was seen. Although the number of reported pediatric patients is only a small percentage of the total annual cases, adults often represent a reservoir that acquired the infection as children. We regard TB as a childhood disease which can affect adults. This is similar to herpes zoster in adults, occurring as a late manifestation of childhood varicella.

## 6.2 EPIDEMIOLOGY

The annual pediatric toll of TB worldwide is estimated to be 1.3 million cases, causing 450 000 deaths in children under 15 years of age [3]. The epidemiology of TB is discussed in detail in Chapter 3. Since 1987, the number of TB cases among children less than 5 years of age has increased 39% in the USA [4]. Recent data reported by the Centers for Disease Control (CDC) revealed an increase in cases of TB in children less than 15 years of age of nearly 50% from 1988 to 1991 [5]. Of the total increase, 76% was attributed to cases in Hispanics, both US and foreign born. The age distribution, which did not change over the study period, found

58% of cases in children less than 5 years old with 19% in 1 year olds, 13% in 2 year olds and 10% in those less than 1 year of age.

Infection in almost all pediatric cases is acquired from adults with cavitary pulmonary disease through the inhalation of aerosolized droplets containing tubercle bacilli. It is not surprising, therefore, that the rising incidence of pediatric TB mirrors that of adult disease. Consequently, the diagnosis of TB in a child generally indicates the presence of an infectious adult, usually in the immediate household and often a parent or grandparent. Adolescents, by virtue of their activity, are more likely than younger children to acquire infection from non-household sources. Prevention of the spread of TB among children (and adults) is best achieved, therefore, by rapid identification and effective treatment of active cases as well as by investigation of their contacts. This is even more relevant in households containing HIV-infected children. Bakshi *et al.* [6] stressed the risk of tubercle bacillus infection in these children often came from a parent with both HIV and TB. Such transmission was recognized in four of 60 families with HIV-infected children.

In certain areas of the USA and in many parts of the world, unpasteurized milk is still available. Therefore, infection with *M. bovis* from ingestion of unpasteurized dairy products still occurs, but usually accounts for only a small number of cases of TB in industrialized countries. In San Diego, however, 13% of cases in children over a 13 year period were found to be due to *M. bovis* [7]. It was manifest primarily in Hispanic patients as lymph node or abdominal disease.

Seven states (California, Florida, Georgia, Illinois, New York, South Carolina, Texas) account for 63% of the reported cases of TB among children less than 5 years of age [5]. The number of cases is highest in cities with populations greater than 250 000, with New York and Miami accounting for a majority of the cases. Socio-economic conditions, the incidence of HIV infection, and the number of immigrants contribute to the prevalence of TB in these communities. The majority of infected children were American born, but the proportion of foreign born children with TB has increased [5].

## 6.3 PEDIATRIC DIAGNOSIS

A key to the diagnosis of pediatric TB is given in Table 6.1.

### 6.3.1 History

The physician should always question the child's parents and other care givers regarding a history of TB exposure. Definitive answers may not be forthcoming unless general questions are asked regarding complaints such as unexplained cough or weight loss. A travel history to or from highly

**Table 6.1** Keys to the diagnosis of pediatric tuberculosis

---

**History (in child and contacts)**
Travel to or from highly endemic areas
Unexplained cough or weight loss
Tuberculin reactivity in family members
Drug sensitivity/treatment compliance in contacts
Previously treated tuberculosis in child or contacts

**Tuberculin reactivity**
5 TU Mantoux intradermal test is standard
Annual tests for high risk children
Nutritional, immunologic and viral factors can cause a false negative test

**Radiology**
Primary pulmonary infection can involve any lung segment
Mediastinal lymphadenopathy is prominent
Changes of primary infection usually resolve slowly regardless of therapy

**Specimen Collection**
Gastric lavage
Overall yields of positive cultures are lower in children

---

endemic areas should also be sought for the child and close contacts. When a child's close contact is identified as an active or treated TB case, it is vital to ascertain the details of treatment, drug sensitivity of the infecting organism, adherence to the regimen and degree of follow-up. Routine review of previous tuberculin tests can aid in uncovering missed cases. Assessment of the family's environment, level of education and comprehension are vital for the success of any treatment plan, as these factors contribute to compliance with treatment.

### 6.3.2 Tuberculin skin testing

The American Academy of Pediatrics recommends TB screening annually for children 1 year of age or older who are known to be at high risk [8]. Children at high risk include those listed in Table 6.2. It is not recommended that children in low risk groups receive routine testing. In such settings, positive skin tests are more likely to be false-positive results [8]. In a high prevalence area, however, only two new tuberculin convertors were found in hospitalized children (0.66%) in one recent study from Texas [9]. The purified protein derivative of tuberculin (5 TU PPD) test is the standard test; it is traditionally applied to the exterior surface of the left forearm. Chapter 8 reviews information on the interpretation of the tuberculin test. Although not specifically mentioned in the current US American Thoracic Society/ CDC guidelines, some authors [10] recommend that children aged 4 years or under should be included in the 10 mm cutoff for positivity. The tine test, a multipuncture technique, has continued to be used for screening children in the USA because of its ease of administration. Positive reactions should always be confirmed by PPD. This test can have a significant false-negative rate which has prompted certain regional health authorities (e.g. New York City) to make the use of the PPD test mandatory, instead of the tine test, for screening children before admission to school [11]. The American Academy of Pediatrics now no longer recommends the use of any multipuncture tests for diagnostic purposes.

**Table 6.2** Children at high risk for tuberculosis

---

- Socio-economically deprived
- Medical risk factors for tuberculosis reactivation[a]
- Households with one or more cases of tuberculosis
- Neighborhoods of higher rates of tuberculosis
- Heritage from high risk areas: Asia, Africa, Middle East, Latin America or Caribbean
- Ethnic background, such as Black, Hispanic, Asian or Native American
- Incarcerated children
- HIV-infected children
- Children frequently exposed to high risk adults[b]

---

[a] Hematologic or lymphoid malignancies, diabetes mellitus, malnutrition, chronic renal failure.
[b] HIV-infected, homeless, drug user, migrant worker, resident of shelter or nursing home.

In children, tuberculin reactivity first appears 3–6 weeks after the start of primary infection. A positive skin test, however, may not develop for up to 3 months [10]. A variety of host related factors including age, nutrition, immunosuppression (including the use of corticosteroids), viral infections, immunization with live viral vaccines and the presence of disseminated TB can alter tuberculin reactivity. The latter factor can explain why certain children who rapidly develop progressive infection after exposure are not skin test reactive. Measles infection and live measles virus vaccination are known to induce immunosuppression, resulting in PPD anergy for several weeks [12]. It is not clear, however, that this nonreactivity translates into an increased incidence of overt TB. Children in the USA are screened for TB before or at the same time as they are given a measles vaccination to avoid a false-negative result. If a child acquires the measles virus by infection or vaccination before screening, a 6–8 week interval should ideally elapse before PPD testing. Whenever a factor that may modify the PPD reaction is recognized in a child, the diagnosis of TB may need to be based on clinical and epidemiologic factors.

The tuberculin test is not useful in newborns since the vast majority do not react. This nonreactivity is not, however, necessarily related to an innate deficiency but rather to the incubation period. Prospective surveillance of infants immunized at birth with BCG shows that tuberculin reactivity develops within 6–9 weeks in 97% of cases [13].

Tuberculin reactivity following infection with *M. tuberculosis* is life long and not altered by anti-TB therapy. PPD reactivity is clinically useful even with a history of BCG vaccination in early childhood. Most Vietnamese refugees under 18 years of age who received BCG were nonreactive to intradermal tuberculin [14]. A Finnish survey found that 24% of previously BCG vaccinated children aged 4–6 years had no reaction to the Mantoux test [15]. The mean size of positive reactions in children younger than 4.5 years was 6.6 mm, and only 34% had strong reactions (10 mm or greater in diameter). The overall prevalence of strong reactions was 14%, and it was 11% in children older than 5.5 years. There is no evidence that severe reactions to tuberculin occur after BCG vaccination. Apparently, certain BCG strains may elicit reactivity of significantly longer duration (up to 12 years) [16], but data clearly differentiating responses to BCG from TB are not available [16–19]. In our opinion, the issue of skin reactivity after BCG vaccination is muddled by the high incidence of TB in countries such as India and Pakistan where tuberculin reactivity in school-aged children had been attributed to BCG, but could be due to TB itself. Unpublished data collected at our hospital, where patients come from diverse regions around the world, indicate that PPD is negative within 2 years of neonatal BCG vaccination in children coming from the former Soviet Union and from China. As a rule, therefore, reactions of 10 mm or greater in normal children who have been inoculated with BCG should be managed as being due to *M. tuberculosis*.

### 6.3.3 Radiological studies

The most common X-ray features of primary TB in children are hilar lymphadenopathy and parenchymal abnormalities, seen in as many as 70–90% of overt cases. The parenchymal densities represent segmental consolidation rather than atelectasis. These changes are more prevalent in children younger than 3 years of age [20]. All segments of the lung can be affected in primary TB [21].

Hilar lymphadenopathy often occurs during primary infection and is best seen on a lateral film of the chest. The presence of hilar and/or mediastinal lymph node enlargement on the chest X-ray is almost synonymous with the diagnosis of primary TB. Based on the location of the primary focus, different lymph nodes will be involved with drainage predominantly from left to right [22]. The right upper tracheal lymph nodes are the most often affected [23]. However, other conditions, notably sarcoidosis, may also cause a similar X-ray appearance. Isolated unilateral hilar lympha-denopathy is more likely seen in TB and with a right sided pulmonary focus. Left sided foci often lead to bilateral hilar adenopathy.

Lymph node size and air space consolidation often progress in the first few months of disease, even if adequate therapy is given. Complete resolu-tion is unusual during the first six treatment months. Parenchymal and lymph node calcification less frequently occur since the advent of effective therapy. Consolidation often disappears within 1 year, but may persist for up to 2 years. Residual parenchymal scarring, appearing as linear opacities, is evident in a small number of patients who have received adequate therapy. Most successfully treated patients will eventually have normal chest X-rays.

### 6.3.4 Specimen collection

In adults, demonstration of acid-fast bacilli (AFB) on a sputum smear is a valuable tool in making a prompt diagnosis. Infants and young children, however, usually quickly swallow their sputum, making it difficult to obtain adequate specimens. Gastric lavage can be an important method of collecting specimens from children who do not expectorate and has been reported to be equivalent or superior to bronchoalveolar lavage (BAL) for the diagnosis of TB in children [24]. The pulmonary procedure is, also, more invasive and may not be suitable for all patients.

To obtain optimal results, gastric lavage should be performed on the child immediately on waking, so that the gastric contents which have accumulated during sleep will be obtained. The patient should fast after dinner on the night before collection. Early morning collection is important to reduce dilution of gastric contents with saliva and tears swallowed after waking, which may additionally initiate peristalsis. Older children may drink 30–60 ml of sterile water before the gastric contents are aspirated via a nasogastric tube. Smaller amounts can be given to younger infants via the tube. The authors prefer to place the nasogastric tube on the night before the procedure, so that the early morning anxieties of the parents and child are lessened. The material should be collected daily for 3 days, and delivered promptly to the laboratory for processing. Although under optimal conditions tubercle bacilli have been recovered in 50–90% of gastric aspirates, the average hospital yield for the technique is 25–33% [25]. Care should be taken in the interpretation of a positive AFB stain of gastric contents since non-TB mycobacteria may be found.

In areas where there is a significant risk of drug resistance, identification and susceptibility testing of *M. tuberculosis* is extremely important in management. In children, if the adult index case can be identified and information is available on the isolate, appropriate treatment for the child [26] can be chosen.

In older children, inhalation of nebulized, superheated saline via a mask or a tent for 15–20 minutes can enhance sputum production [27]. Overall, however, relatively low yields of sputum cultures (30–50%) are reported in children [10]. Care should be taken to protect the health care worker involved in the collection of the specimen from aerosolized infectious material.

Samples from other body sites should be collected as dictated by the clinical situation. If renal involvement is suspected, several first morning urines should be collected and delivered promptly to the laboratory. In immunosuppressed patients and those with suspected miliary TB, stains and cultures of blood and bone marrow aspirate may yield the organism.

## 6.4 TUBERCULOSIS DURING THE PERINATAL PERIOD

### 6.4.1 Tuberculosis during pregnancy

TB may first appear or can relapse during pregnancy. Although a number of diseases may be more severe in pregnancy, including varicella, coccidioidomycosis and hepatitis E, the clinical manifestations of TB in pregnant patients are similar to those in non-pregnant women. Hedvall [28] noted that, since Hippocrates, pregnancy had been thought to be beneficial to the course of TB, but since the mid-1890s a more unfavorable outcome has been suggested. In the chemotherapeutic era, the outcome of TB treatment is unchanged by the pregnant state. One study in 1959 [29] found no differences in X-ray stabilization, sputum conversion and cavity closure in treated pregnant women compared with non-pregnant women. Pregnancy does not seem to alter tuberculin reactivity [30] and is not a contraindication for tuberculin skin testing. TB, also, does not affect the course of pregnancy or the type of delivery required, although any severe disease during pregnancy may increase the incidence of miscarriage. With the use of first line anti-TB agents, routine therapeutic abortion is not medically indicated [31].

Pregnant women with active TB should be treated without delay when the diagnosis is strongly suspected or established. Untreated infection represents a greater hazard to pregnant women and to their fetuses than do the anti-TB drugs. TB screening by Mantoux tuberculin test in high risk women should be incorporated into prenatal care. A history, physical examination and a chest X-ray should be obtained whenever a skin test is interpreted as positive. It is preferable to obtain the X-ray, with proper abdominal shielding, after the twelfth week of gestation [32].

The incidence of congenital defects is not increased in babies of mothers receiving isoniazid (INH) during pregnancy. Although animal studies have shown that ethambutol has potential teratogenic effects, none have been reported in humans [33,34]. Otoxicity caused by streptomycin is clearly a potential risk to the fetus throughout gestation and this antibiotic should be avoided [35]. Para-aminosalicylic acid appears to be safe during pregnancy. Rifampin has shown varying degrees of teratogenicity in animals, including hydrocephalus and skeletal abnormalities, but data supportive of a teratogenic role in man have not been substantiated [36].

Small amounts of most of the anti-TB agents are secreted in breast milk. No contraindications to breast feeding exist after the mother is deemed non-infectious. Mothers who are being treated with TB medication and wish to breast feed their infants should be informed of the baby's exposure to the drug.

### 6.4.2 Management of infants of tuberculous mothers

Infants born to mothers who have completed anti-TB therapy in the past with no evidence of current active disease have no risk of acquiring the infection from the mother. Most frequently, the scenario confronting a physician is a healthy newborn of a mother with a prenatal positive tuberculin test and negative chest X-ray. In this circumstance, the risk to the infant is minimal unless the mother was a convertor during gestation or active infectious pulmonary disease is present in household contacts. Care should be taken by the pediatrician, therefore, to assess whether any other member of the family has symptoms compatible with pulmonary TB. If a tuberculous mother is noncompliant with therapy or is thought to be actively infectious, temporary separation may be used to protect the infant.

BCG vaccination should be considered in infants at high risk of intimate and prolonged exposure to pulmonary TB, especially if the child cannot be separated from the source or be placed on long term preventive treatment because of noncompliance or resistance [37]. None of 30 BCG vaccinated infants of actively infected mothers and 38 of 95 unvaccinated infants developed TB [38]. It was felt that this experience and the known inadequacy of an imperfectly followed regimen of isolation and INH prophylaxis combined to make BCG vaccination the method of choice for prevention of disease in newborns at risk. The increasing incidence of INH resistance further underscores this recommendation.

If a mother has active TB during pregnancy, her baby is at risk for congenital infection and should be treated with INH for 3 months or at least until the mother is known to be smear and culture negative. The mother's compliance with therapy must be monitored. The infant should be tuberculin tested at birth and at 3 month intervals. If, after 3 months of treatment, the mother is felt to be noninfectious and the infant is tuberculin negative with a normal chest X-ray, INH may be discontinued in the infant. If at 3 months the infant has a tuberculin reaction greater than 5 mm of induration, examination for pulmonary and extrapulmonary disease is in order. If any infection is found, the child should be treated with at least two additional drugs.

### 6.4.3 Congenital tuberculous infection

True congenital TB is rare and has a poor prognosis if not diagnosed and treated promptly. Bacteremic disease in the mother may spread to the fetus from an infected placenta. The fetus may also acquire TB *in utero* by swallowing infected amniotic fluid. The major site of involvement in congenital TB is the liver, with the formation of a primary complex similar to the Ghon complex in the lung. This observation supports transmission through either the umbilical vessels or gastrointestinal tract.

The manifestations of congenital TB are nonspecific, consisting of respiratory distress, fever, hepatosplenomegaly, poor feeding, lethargy and irritability. Less frequent findings include lymphadenopathy, abdominal distension and failure to thrive [39]. Skin lesions are unusual but, if present, histologic and cultural examination of biopsy material may aid in the diagnosis [40]. Congenital TB should be considered in the differential diagnosis of any infant with a consistent clinical picture, even if the patient has been separated from the mother since birth [41].

Cantwell *et al.* [42], recently reviewed the first two US cases of congenital TB reported since 1982. Both presented at 3–4 weeks of age with respiratory distress and poor feeding, had smear and culture positive gastric and endotracheal tube aspirates, were treated and survived. Interestingly, the diagnosis of TB was made in the mothers after it was confirmed in the infants. One of these cases [43] was associated with tuberculin skin test conversion in one of 33 health care workers exposed to the intubated infant.

The newborn at risk for congenital TB must be carefully examined and a tuberculin skin test and chest X-ray performed. The X-ray may show a miliary pattern, nonspecific changes, or be unremarkable. Cultures of gastric washings, urine, blood and CSF should be done as well as bone marrow aspiration for microscopic examination and culture. The infant may not develop a positive PPD for approximately 3–5 weeks if infection had been acquired shortly before delivery. Anti-TB therapy should be strongly considered pending the culture results. If TB is isolated, drug sensitivity should be determined. A seriously ill newborn may not have a reactive skin test, and this should not dissuade the pediatrician from starting therapy. Congenital TB is very difficult to distinguish from sepsis due to the usual bacterial pathogens. A high index of suspicion must be maintained and a careful history obtained from the mother in order to arrive at a correct diagnosis.

### 6.4.4 Neonatal infection

Infants may acquire infection from their mothers at or after birth through swallowing or aspirating infected material in the birth canal, inhalation of infectious droplet nuclei or ingestion of breast milk. Physicians should keep in mind that TB may also be transmitted to babies in the nursery from infectious medical personnel. The infant can be infected from non-pulmonary TB foci as well. Schaaf *et al.* [44] reported four cases of TB in the neonatal period in which 2 mothers had genitourinary TB. Primary infection in the neonate is usually not recognized because of lack of specific symptoms. However, patients are at high risk of developing serious morbidity early in life since the infection may rapidly disseminate to the meninges, bone or other organs.

A series of 47 infants less than 12 months of age with neonatal TB [45] was reported of which 45 survived. The diagnoses came from the evaluation of a symptomatic infant in 79%, case contact studies in 19%, and skin testing in 2%. Presenting symptoms were cough, fever and anorexia. A South African series of 38 infants under 3 months of age [46] reported cough in 87% and tachypnea in 82%. Only 18% of the infants had less than 15 mm of induration on the Mantoux test. Chest X-rays in 27 infants showed miliary disease in seven (26%) and hilar adenopathy in 14 (52%) with airway compression in 56%. Diagnostically, 92% of the infants had positive gastric aspirate cultures. Of the 30 mothers evaluated, seven were found to have previously unsuspected pulmonary TB.

## 6.5 PRIMARY TUBERCULOSIS IN CHILDHOOD

The primary pulmonary focus is generally located in the subpleural tissues. Lincoln and Sewell [47] describe Ghon and Kudlich's data derived between 1909 and 1928 which showed that the primary focus was in the lung in 96% of children, with 2.4% undetermined, 1.1% intestinal, 0.14% cutaneous and the rest in the eye, nose and throat. During initial infection, which is typically unrecognized, tubercle bacilli disseminate throughout the body. Immunity and hypersensitivity to tuberculin develop within 3–5 weeks after infection, and the spread of infection abates as the foci are walled off by inflammatory cells. The organism then remains dormant for a variable length of time, depending on several factors such as the host immune system, then can reactivate, causing disease. Children are at a higher risk of developing secondary disease when they acquire TB in the early years of life, often within one year from the onset of infection.

The median age of pediatric patients with primary TB in Houston, Texas was 24 months [48]. Of these children, 56% were asymptomatic and discovered by screening contacts of adult cases. Lincoln [49] describes the onset of primary TB as heralded by a fever rarely over 102°F lasting 3–10 days associated with lassitude and/or anorexia with no other symptoms or signs. It is usually at the onset of fever that tuberculin reactivity develops. Although fatigue and anorexia may be the sole manifestations of primary TB, other common symptoms include cough and weight loss. However, primary TB can have an insidious onset with children asymptomatic at the time of diagnosis to be identified only by skin testing. The patient's healthy appearance may belie the extent of pulmonary involvement (Figure 6.1).

Abnormal pulmonary auscultation signs are not prominent, even with significant parenchymal changes on X-ray. In fact, the absence of rales is so characteristic that the presence of even a few constant moist rales should suggest either local progressive TB disease or a non-TB pulmonary infection [1]. Symptoms and signs related to bronchial encroachment are, however, characteristic, including a harsh cough, which can be brassy in character, and wheezing. At times, the onset may be quite abrupt, simulating the clinical and X-ray picture of lobar pneumococcal pneumonia [1]. The presence of hilar lymphadenopathy and a positive tuberculin test

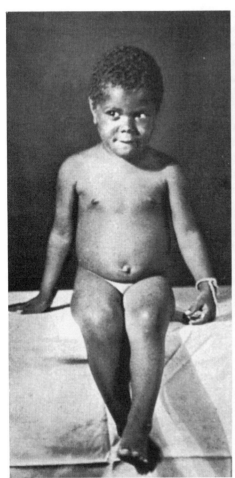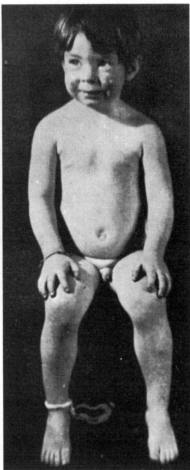

**Figure 6.1** Photographs of the healthy appearance of two young children who had X-ray evidence of extensive primary pulmonary TB. Reproduced from [49] with permission of the publisher.

should suggest the correct diagnosis. Typical findings on chest radiographs may alert the physician to the diagnosis, but the primary complex may not be visible for several weeks after the onset of symptoms. It does not appear that specific chemotherapy speeds the disappearance of the enlarged lymph nodes or parenchymal infiltrates of the primary complex.

Although the infectivity of children with cavitary TB is comparable to that of adults, the risk of transmission in primary TB under ordinary circumstances is generally small. Most young children with primary infection often have little or no cough and produce no sputum. Lincoln and Sewell, in fact, state that Wallgren has repeatedly affirmed the conviction that primary TB in patients in the pediatric age group who are not ill should be assumed to be noninfectious [50]. Wallgren's observations are supported by the observation that children with pulmonary disease of non-TB origin who spent months or years in hospitals for tuberculous children have failed to become tuberculin reactive [50].

In the pretherapeutic age, Lincoln reported a 23.6% mortality rate in children with progressive primary TB [1]. She found that 90% of the deaths were within 1 year of the initial diagnosis and 58% were within 3 months (Figure 6.2). The age of acquisition was also an important factor, with 55% of infants aged under 6 months, 28% of those 1–2 years of age and 15% of children 4–9 years of age succumbing to the infection (Figure 6.3). In this series, 60% of the deaths were caused by TB meningitis, and 95% of the total mortality was related to meningitis, miliary infection or progressive pulmonary infection [1].

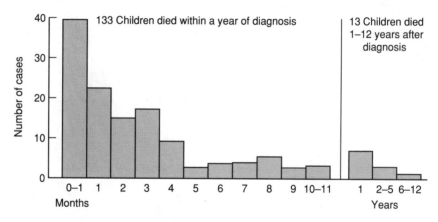

**Figure 6.2** Interval between the diagnosis of TB and death in children, illustrating the relationship between mortality and the duration of primary tuberculosis. Reprinted from the *American Journal of Medicine*, **9**, 623–32 [1].

## 6.6 PROGRESSIVE PULMONARY PRIMARY TUBERCULOSIS

Occasionally, the primary focus continues to enlarge despite the development of hypersensitivity. The area of caseation expands and softens, spilling its contents into a bronchus, resulting in disseminated pulmonary involvement. Rarely, tuberculous cavities rupture into the pleural space, producing a pneumothorax, caseous pyopneumothorax and/or fistulae into the pleura, pericardium or mediastinum. The clues to advancing local disease are progressive weight loss, persistent prominent fever, and persistent cough. Moist rales can be heard over the affected area. X-rays reveal radiolucency within the area of infiltrate, which is referred to as a 'highlight'. It can be quite difficult to distinguish this entity, which in the prechemotherapeutic era had a mortality rate of 25–65%, from a simple

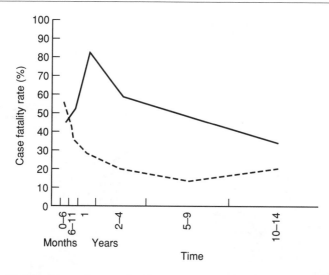

**Figure 6.3** The decreasing case fatality rate of primary tuberculosis with age (dashed line) and the variation in incidence of tubercular meningitis as a cause of death in children (solid line). Reprinted from the *American Journal of Medicine*, **9**, 623–32 [1].

TB focus with a superimposed bacterial pneumonia [23]. In later stages, clinical findings are indistinguishable from advanced chronic pulmonary TB.

## 6.7 ENDOBRONCHIAL TUBERCULOSIS

The most prominent aspect of primary TB is the large size of the involved lymph nodes compared with the parenchymal focus. Obstruction of the bronchus occurs most commonly from pressure on the lumen by the enlarged node [51]. Other mechanisms of obstruction include plugging by caseous material discharged into the bronchial tree and the development of tuberculous endobronchial granulomatous tissue. Bronchial obstruction can rarely cause sudden death [52].

Obstructive hyperaeration (obstructive emphysema) of a lung segment, lobe or an entire lung may also occur (Figure 6.4). This complication was found in 1.3% of 538 children with primary TB [53]. Obstructive hyper-aeration, when it occurs, is generally present in children under 2 years of age, associated with wheezing and needs to be differentiated from foreign body aspiration. The obstruction usually resolves on its own [23], but corticosteroids have been used to speed resolution [54]. Segmental bronchial obstruction is the most common form of this complication. In this form, the X-ray reveals a fan-like density involving the segment containing the primary focus [55]. Called collapse-consolidation by some, the abnormality is actually a combination of the primary lung focus, the caseation from the eroded bronchus, the inflammation elicited by the caseous material and atelectasis [23]. Segmental lesions were reported to occur in 29% of Payne's 545 cases and in 43% of those 0–1 years of age [56]. Physical signs and symptoms of segmental obstruction are often minimal.

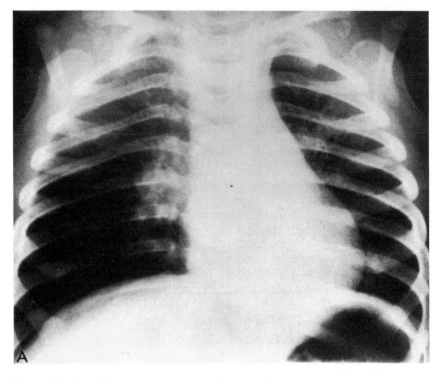

**Figure 6.4** Chest X-ray of an 8-month-old girl with obstructive emphysema of the right lower lobe due to TB. The heart and mediastinum are shifted to the left. Reproduced from [23] with permission of the publisher.

Permanent anatomic sequelae of these forms of obstruction are found in more than 50% of cases, even if no abnormality is seen on the chest X-ray [23]. Cylindrical bronchiectasis with or without stenosis is the most common. These lesions, usually in the middle or lower lobes, can predispose to recurrent bacterial infection as in the 'middle lobe syndrome' [57].

## 6.8 PLEURAL TUBERCULOSIS

Pleural involvement with effusion is a very common complication of primary infection in childhood. In fact, it is felt to be a component of the primary complex [23].

The effusion develops from the discharge of bacilli and/or antigenic material into the pleural cavity from a subpleural parenchymal focus or lymph node [58]. Pleural collections can be small or large, unilateral or bilateral. Bilateral effusions, which occur in less than 5% of cases, are related to primary parenchymal bilateral involvement [59]. Although TB equally affects both sexes, boys are more commonly affected by significant pleural involvement. Other clinical observations related to pleural TB [23] are relatively infrequent in children under 2 years of age and lack of association with segmental or miliary disease.

Many effusions have an insidious onset with minimal or no focal symptoms, but the disease may also be abrupt in onset with high fever and pleuritic chest pain. The fever may last for several weeks, resolving with the disappearance of the effusion. Thoracentesis, in clinically overt cases, reveals a bloody exudative fluid with a decreased glucose concentration. The cellular pleocytosis is usually lymphocytic, but neutrophils can predominate early. Since the number of AFB in the fluid is small, the yield on smear and culture is low. Pleural biopsy and culture produce a higher yield [60].

The prognosis of TB pleurisy in children has always been relatively good compared with other sites of the infection and with the same process in adults [60]. Restriction of chest wall movement resulting in pulmonary function compromise is quite uncommon, even if significant pleural thickening and adhesions are seen on X-ray. Very rarely, significant scoliosis may develop in a growing child related to respiratory splinting.

## 6.9 HEMATOGENOUS TUBERCULOSIS

Occult dissemination of TB via the blood occurs early in the course of the disease, usually before tuberculin reactivity develops. Using radiolabeled BCG organisms locally inoculated, systemic spread within hours was reported [61]. In addition, liver biopsies performed on asymptomatic skin test convertors [62] found hepatic involvement in four of 71 cases.

The spectrum of manifestations caused by this lymphohematogenous spread is related to the number of organisms released and to host susceptibility. Smith and Marquis [23] categorize cases into three distinct clinical forms. Occult dissemination remains asymptomatic until the development of a reactivation focus months or years later. This is the most common form of dissemination but is rarely recognized *per se*. Protracted multiform hematogenous disease is rarely seen in the therapeutic era. There is often hepatic and splenic enlargement with generalized lymph node involvement and panserositis [63]. In some, pulmonary apical nodular lesions (Simon foci), which may calcify, can develop [64]. In the pretherapeutic age, this form often ended with the development of TB meningitis.

The third, miliary disease, is analogous to bacteremia with pyogenic bacteria. It is the most commonly recognized form of disseminated infection, occurring when a large number of AFB invade the bloodstream from a caseating focus, often a lymph node, which ruptures into a blood vessel. It is often an early complication in infants and young children, occurring 3–6 months after the onset of primary TB. A review of miliary TB from South Africa found that children and adults with miliary disease accounted for 8.3% and 1.3% of TB cases, respectively [65]. More than half of the pediatric cases occurred in children under the age of 1 year.

Disease onset is insidious, but rapid progression may occur in an immunocompromised or malnourished child. The clinical manifestations are nonspecific, including low grade fever, anorexia, weight loss and night sweats. The patient may present with fever of unknown origin or failure to thrive. Hepatomegaly, splenomegaly and lymphadenopathy are common [66]. Cutaneous and ocular signs are uncommonly found but can suggest the diagnosis. Most young children with dissemination have radiological evidence of pulmonary primary TB prior to the X-ray changes of miliary infection.

The diagnosis of miliary TB may be difficult but can be made by liver and/or bone marrow biopsy [62]. Many patients are anergic to tuberculin. Most children with acute miliary TB develop meningitis and die if not treated promptly. Children who recover from miliary TB require close medical follow-up after treatment, since occult foci of infection may persist.

Focal extrathoracic manifestations of TB are often different in children compared with adults. Table 6.3 summarizes the relevant points regarding certain sites of extrapulmonary disease in children. More emphasis is given to areas that may be seen commonly in children and/or sites of infection not covered in Chapter 4.

## 6.10 TUBERCULOSIS OF THE CENTRAL NERVOUS SYSTEM

Meningitis is the most common cause of death in childhood TB. It causes significant morbidity, even when appropriately treated. TB of the central nervous system can be classified by location (meningeal or parenchymal, intracranial or spinal) and by type (diffuse meningitis, tuberculoma, abscess or focal cerebritis).

Tuberculous meningitis is estimated to occur in one of every 300 primary infections. It often develops 3–6 months after primary infection, mostly in children 6–24 months of age. The typical presentation is progressive fever and vomiting over a period of 2–3 weeks. These manifestations are non-specific and often lead to a delay in diagnosis. A history of TB exposure can be elicited in 50% of cases [67]. CSF examination usually reveals a leukocyte count of less than 500/mm$^3$. There is a predominance of poly-morphonuclear neutrophils (PMNs) early in the illness, which later changes to lymphocytes. The glucose level is low and the protein is significantly elevated, but each may be normal early in disease. Several methods for the

**Table 6.3** Selected extrapulmonary tuberculosis in children

---

**Central nervous system** (1.8%)[a]
Common cause of death in tuberculosis
May be meningeal or parenchymal, spinal or intracranial

**Superficial lymph node** (13.5%)
More indolent than pyogenic lymphadenitis
Can be associated with cutaneous inoculation sites

**Cutaneous disease** (< 0.1%)
Primary inoculation usually on the face or lower extremity
Hypersensitivity related involvement may occur

**Genitourinary** (0.3%)
Urinary infection is often not diagnosed until late in involvement
Genital involvement is rare before puberty

**Ocular involvement** (< 0.1%)
May result from direct involvement or hypersensitivity
Choroidal tubercles can be useful in diagnosing miliary disease

**Pericardium** (0.8%)
Often specific signs of pericardial disease are lacking
Diagnosis often made only at autopsy

**Skeletal** (1.6%)
Vertebrae account for 50% of bony sites
Dactylitis is an uncommon, usually resolving complication

**Intra-abdominal** (0.2%)
*M. bovis* may be involved
The disease may be insidious, presenting as chronic abdominal pain and
  obstruction

**Otomastoiditis** (< 0.1%)
Painless draining chronic otitis occurs
Facial nerve paralysis and deafness can result

---

[a]  Percentage rates based on 1991 CDC data [66a] with extrapulmonary disease constituting
    22.9% of all childhood cases, age 0–19 years.

rapid detection of CSF AFB have been reported. These include adenosine deaminase level, bromide partition and mycobacterial antigen and antibody detection. One report of the latex agglutination technique for TB antigen detection reported that all 18 patients with TB meningitis had antigen detected in the CSF, and 133 of 134 asymptomatic contacts tested negative [68]. More sophisticated methodology such as polymerase chain reaction may prove useful.

Early diagnosis and treatment of TB meningitis are essential to optimize the outcome. Treatment should never be delayed while waiting for the microbiologic confirmation. Chest X-ray evidence of TB can exist in about half of cases [67]. Although the tuberculin test is usually positive, only 50% of children had 10 mm or more of induration and an additional 13% had 5–9 mm of induration in one review [67]. Since clinical and laboratory findings can be nonspecific and an exposure history may be lacking, TB should be considered in the differential diagnosis of all patients with aseptic meningitis. Computerized tomography (CT) should be obtained in all cases of suspected or confirmed TB meningitis. Hydrocephalus seems to be the most consistent finding in the early stages of meningitis [67]. After appropriate therapy, the intracranial lesions associated with TB meningitis regress after many weeks in most patients, though hydrocephalus may persist and require shunting. Electrolyte abnormalities can contribute to the encephalopathy associated with TB meningitis. Inappropriate ADH secretion causes profound hyponatremia and vomiting with diminished fluid intake and can lead to severe dehydration with hypochloremia and hypokalemia. The fluid and electrolyte status of the patient should be carefully evaluated and managed.

Late sequelae include mental deficiency, seizures, cranial nerve palsies, hydrocephalus and blindness. The primary event responsible for these sequelae is the replacement of inflammatory exudate by fibrous tissue. Direct invasion by the granulomatous reaction and strictures around blood vessels may obstruct the blood supply to any area of the brain. Occlusion of these vessels can result in ischemia and infarction [69]. Obstruction of the CSF pathway leads to increased intracranial pressure and hydrocephalus. Sequelae are most likely in children younger than 3 years and those who develop significant neurologic abnormalities in the acute phase [70]. Choroidal tubercles and papilledema are poor prognostic signs [71]. The use of corticosteroids has been shown to be helpful in children in reducing morbidity and mortality in TB meningitis [69]. The steroids should be given for at least 4 weeks and withdrawn slowly over several weeks.

Intracranial tuberculomas [72] are usually solitary, but approximately 15–25% of cases have multiple lesions. These lesions are most often seen in children under 10 years of age, and are often located infratentorially. They may rupture into the meninges causing meningitis, manifest as space occupying lesions or be asymptomatic. Tuberculomas may appear during therapy of pulmonary or extrapulmonary TB and are usually treated medically, only occasionally needing surgical intervention.

In older patients TB brain abscesses occur more often than tuberculomas. The presentation is similar, however, with constitutional and focal neurologic symptoms [73]. Magnetic resonance imaging (MRI) has been shown to be more sensitive than CT in detection of such focal lesions [74]. Pathologically, an abscess is distinguishable from a tuberculoma by the absence of granulomas. Vascular granulation tissue in the lesion wall and the paucity of giant cells are also indicative of a TB brain abscess.

Serous TB meningitis has been reported in 13% of cases [75] from a TB focus close to the subarachnoid space inducing a lymphocytic pleocytosis in the CSF. The clinical features are similar to those of early TB meningitis, but the condition may resolve spontaneously.

Spinal intramedullary tuberculomas and leptomeningitis are rare. The presence of abdominal symptoms can cause diagnostic confusion.

## 6.11 TUBERCULOSIS OF THE HEART AND PERICARDIUM

Pericarditis is more common (0.4–4.0%) [76,77] than myocarditis, the latter is usually diagnosed only at autopsy. Pericarditis is more commonly found in males and results from direct extension from mediastinal lymph nodes or from hematogenous or lymphatic spread. Symptoms are nonspecific and include poor appetite, low grade fever and weight loss. Chest pain is typically absent. Physical examination reveals a pericardial friction rub in only a minority of cases. If a large effusion is present, signs of cardiac tamponade may be noted. Clinical signs and X-ray and electrocardiogram findings are indistinguishable from those found in pericardial effusions of other etiologies. In a recent study from South Africa [78], 44 of 105 children with pericardial disease were felt to be tuberculous in origin. Of the 44, 37 had effusions, four had constrictive pericarditis and three had effusive constrictive disease. Biopsy and culture yields for *M. tuberculosis* were low (18%). This entity usually responds to anti-TB chemotherapy. Corticosteroids may also be used. Surgery is indicated for pericardial tamponade. Constrictive pericarditis may develop as a late complication, but is unusual in children.

## 6.12 TUBERCULOUS SUPERFICIAL LYMPHADENITIS (SCROFULA)

In children, mycobacterial lymphadenitis is more often caused by non-TB AFB than by tubercle bacilli [79]. TB lymphadenitis often appears within 6 months of primary infection and develops in 5–15% of children with TB [80]. Lymphadenopathy is common in primary TB, with cervical adenopathy accompanying the primary lesions in the upper lung fields. Axillary and inguinal lymphadenopathy can result from primary TB skin lesions in the upper and lower extremities, respectively [23]. The skin lesions may seem trivial and the only clue to their significance is the concurrent lymph node enlargement. Preauricular adenitis accompanies a focus on the scalp or face. Parinaud's oculoglandular syndrome (conjunctivitis and preauricular lymphadenopathy) can be caused by TB. Generalized superficial lymphadenopathy can occur in the course of lymphohematogenous spread and localized or generalized adenitis may occur in asymptomatic infected adolescents during reactivation disease. Involvement of multiple groups of nodes are not uncommon in children, as one study found only 24% with one group affected [81].

Tuberculous lymphadenopathy is usually painless and accompanied by low grade fever. Early, the nodes are discrete and rubbery, becoming matted and adherent to the skin, which becomes erythematous or violaceous in color as the infection progresses. Occasionally, the patient presents with a fluctuant mass or draining sinus. Intercurrent viral or bacterial infections may exacerbate the symptoms of TB lymphadenitis, associated with high fever and increased pain.

The differential diagnosis of scrofula is substantial including viral, bacterial and fungal diseases as well as toxoplasmosis, neoplasia and sarcoidosis. Management of patients with adenitis, particularly of the cervical nodes, should always include assessment for TB with skin testing and chest X-ray. In TB lymphadenitis, the skin test is frequently greater than 15 mm in diameter [81,82]. One particular problem is the child with a borderline 5 TU PPD result who may have either a non-TB mycobacterial or TB adenitis. A history of TB exposure, evidence of extralymphatic disease and an elevated sedimentation rate are suggestive of TB [82]. An abnormal chest X-ray can be helpful but it is often normal even with TB cervical adenitis [81].

## 6.13 SKELETAL TUBERCULOSIS

Tubercle bacilli can reach skeletal sites via hematogenous or lymphatic spread or by direct extension from adjacent structures. Skeletal TB is seen in approximately 5% of overtly infected children. While many cases appear within 6 months after a recognized primary infection, skeletal involvement may be the first manifestation of TB. In a large group of children with primary TB followed at Bellevue Hospital in New York, skeletal involvement developed in 1% after 1 year or more of follow-up [83].

Disease onset is insidious following an incubation period which is 'characteristic' for the bone or joint involved. For example, the onset is 1 month for dactylitis developing primarily in infants and young children and more than 2 years for the hip joint. Younger children seem to be at increased risk for progressive skeletal infection because of higher blood flow in the growing bones. Areas with the largest blood supply, such as vertebrae and metaphyses of long bones, are most often affected. Weight bearing bones and joints are also prone to skeletal TB. TB of the facial bones and multifocal disease are uncommon [84]. While skeletal TB may be associated with trauma, it is unclear whether the local injury reactivates a latent lesion or simply draws attention to an active process. Symptoms vary according to the area affected and may include pain, swelling, decreased range of motion, fever and weight loss. Neurological deficits related to vertebral disease with cord compression and structural deformities can occur.

Approximately 50% of patients with skeletal TB have vertebral disease, most affected children are under 5 years of age [85]. The lower thoracic and upper lumbar vertebrae are the most common site of tuberculous spondylitis (Pott's disease) [83,85,86] which usually involves two adjacent vertebrae and the intervertebral disk. Children with spinal TB may have an unusual posture or gait due to muscle spasm and anticipation of pain caused by sudden movement which could be referred to other areas, such as the abdomen. Examination reveals tenderness on percussion of the spine, paraspinal guarding and/or neurologic deficits. Kyphosis and scoliosis are well known complications of spinal TB [85,87] and abscess formation (retropharyngeal, paravertebral, psoas) may develop.

The CT scan is a useful tool in the evaluation of vertebral involvement as it defines areas of destruction, compression, abscess formation and the extent of disease [86]. If needed, CT guided needle biopsy and abscess aspiration can be easily done. Although MRI does not show calcification as well as CT does, it is more sensitive in demonstrating inflammatory changes within the bone and soft tissue.

Tuberculous dactylitis occurs in 0.6–6% of pediatric TB cases [88]. Mainly in children less than 2 years of age, it can be the presenting feature. Dactylitis occurs eight times more frequently in the hands than in the feet. In the hands (Figure 6.5), the most commonly affected bones are the proximal phalanges and metacarpals [88]. The affected digit appears as a fusiform, indurated, painless swelling with overlying skin that is shiny, thin and discolored. X-rays show abnormalities ranging from minimal medullary changes with periosteal elevation to ballooning of the cortex and bony destruction. Even with dramatic clinical and X-ray disease, the dactylitis usually heals without therapy with only residual mild deformity or bone shortening. Radiographically, even extensive destructive lesions heal within 3 years [88]. Other conditions to be differentiated from tuberculous dactylitis include syphilis, sickle cell disease and juvenile rheumatoid arthritis.

## 6.14 CUTANEOUS TUBERCULOSIS

Involvement of the skin in TB was not common (3–5% of all patients) even before specific therapy became available [89]. Cutaneous TB is divided into four groups [90,91], related to direct exogenous inoculation, local extension, hematogenous spread and hypersensitivity.

Primary inoculation through traumatized skin is most common on the lower extremities and face of children. Miller [92] reported 20 cases in which sites were located on the lower extremity in ten and on the face in seven. The process is often overlooked because of its initially minor, nondescript brownish papular nature. Regional lymphadenopathy develops, but may be attributed to pyogenic infection or cat scratch disease [93].

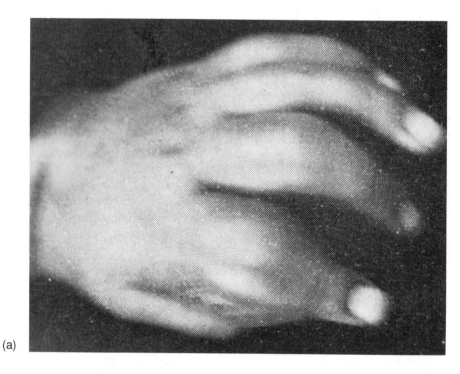

(a)

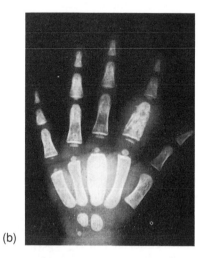

(b)

**Figure 6.5** Tuberculous dactylitis. (a) Shows the left hand of an 11-year-old girl with fusiform swelling of the index and middle fingers. (b) The corresponding X-ray with involvement of the proximal phalanx of the index finger and third metacarpal. Reproduced from [83].

A tender cord-like lymphangitis can develop [89]. The primary lesion develops into an indolent, non-tender ulcer or chancre, sometimes surrounded by satellite lesions. A wound which fails to heal in the presence of painless regional lymphadenopathy should raise the suspicion of TB. Some lesions can be impetiginous or ecthymatous in appearance [89]. Tuberculin tests are usually reactive, but aspiration or biopsy may be needed in some cases to confirm the diagnosis or to exclude other infections. The skin lesion heals within several weeks after initiation of therapy and, if treated promptly, results in minimal scarring. Traumatic inoculations of TB into the skin of a previously sensitized individual cause a more verrucous lesion called a prosector's wart [90,94]. This process, originally described by Laennec [94], is generally not associated with the substantial lymphadenopathy occuring in those not previously sensitized to tuberculin.

Lupus vulgaris is a chronic process most frequently found on a child's cheek. Moschella and Cropley [89] state that it is the most common, most serious and most variable type of cutaneous TB. It is felt to represent spread of TB to the skin from a remote internal source in the setting of a high degree of tuberculin sensitivity. These characteristic red or red–brown nodules have the appearance of apple jelly when compressed under a glass slide. The process is slowly progressive, may recede spontaneously [95] and is more frequent in females [89]. It is difficult to find AFB histopathologically in this entity which responds very slowly to therapy.

Scrofuloderma describes skin involvement caused by extension from an underlying focus, most frequently a cervical lymph node [90] (Figure 6.6). The first sign of cutaneous involvement is adherence of the node to the overlying skin, usually on the face or neck. The skin becomes erythematous or violaceous, and if untreated the underlying focus drains through the skin with an ulcer or fistula. Fistulous tracts draining at a mucosal orifice (orificial cutaneous TB) have been described. These lesions are usually ulcerative and painful and may occur at traumatized areas [90]. Infection responds promptly to medical treatment, preventing skin break down and subsequent scarring. Metastatic tuberculous abscess refers to scrofuloderma in which a subcutaneous nodule unrelated to any other focus initiates skin infection.

The typical lesions of hematogenous dissemination to the skin are discrete blue to red–brown papules. They can be located asymmetrically anywhere on the body, but are primarily found on extensor surfaces of the extremities and the lower part of the back [96]. Usually there are no more than 20–30 of the lesions [97]. The eruptions, often called tuberculosis cutis miliaris acuta generalista, may be difficult to differentiate from chickenpox, and vary in size from minute papules to 1 cm in diameter. Vesicular, pustular, umbilicated and encrusted lesions can appear simultaneously. Histologically, they are miliary tubercles and AFB are easily demonstrated in the necrotic tissue and blood vessels. Biopsy is the fastest test to differentiate this lesion from those caused by varicella, papular urticaria, histiocytosis X and molluscum contagiosum.

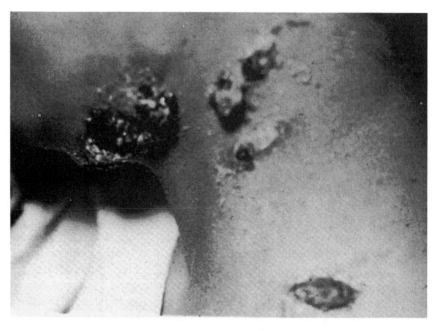

**Figure 6.6** Scrofuloderma in a child with cervical lymph node TB. Reproduced with permission from Moschella and Cropley (1992) in *Dermatology*, 3rd edn (eds Moschella and Hurley), W.B. Saunders, Philadelphia [89].

Several conditions are referred to as tuberculids or hypersensitivity reactions where no AFB bacilli are found, including papulonecrotic tuberculids, lichen scrofulosum and Bazin's erythema induratum [91]. Papulonecrotic tuberculids, classically occurring in children and adolescents, are thought to be due to an Arthus reaction followed by a delayed hypersensitivity reaction to TB antigens. The lesions resolve promptly with TB therapy [98]. Although some authors feel that it is not clear whether these entities have a true relationship to TB [90], using the polymerase chain reaction and primers specific for *M. tuberculosis*, TB DNA has been detected in tuberculid lesions including erythema induratum [99].

Erythema nodosum related to TB occurs mostly in teenage girls as an early manifestation of primary TB [100]. Other causes of erythema nodosum include group A streptococcal and fungal infections, sarcoidosis and drug reactions. The lesions are large, painful nodules occurring on the shins and occasionally on the arms. They appear soon after primary infection, may be the sole focal manifestation and are thought to be due to tuberculin hypersensitivity. The lesions disappear spontaneously even untreated within a few weeks. Biopsy is useless to confirm a diagnosis of TB, since histologic changes are nonspecific. In one report, however, culture of the biopsy yielded *M. tuberculosis* [90].

## 6.15 GASTROINTESTINAL TUBERCULOSIS

TB may involve any of the organs within the abdominal cavity. Abdominal TB lymphadenitis (tabes mesenterica) accompanies a primary intestinal focus. This form of TB was common before pasteurization of milk. It also occurs after swallowing respiratory secretions or via hematogenous spread. The tuberculous nodes may become adherent to the peritoneum and cause intestinal obstruction. Ascites and edema can develop when fibrosis involves the portal vein or inferior vena cava. Chylous ascites from compression on the thoracic duct has also been reported [101].

Tuberculous peritonitis can be localized or diffuse, developing by extension of infection from an abdominal lymph node or salpingitis. Pain is the most common complaint and is associated with fever, weight loss and/ or ascites [102]. The peritonitis is often insidious in onset with low grade fever the only symptom. In other patients, intestinal obstruction is the first indication, related to adherent omentum. The omentum may develop into a mass which on sonography may appear to be cystic with a small collection of fluid. If the diagnosis is made before 'plastic peritonitis' (also known as the frozen belly) develops, chemotherapy, sometimes combined with surgical lysis of adhesions, can prevent further complications.

Tuberculous ascites may develop by extension of primary infection in the intestinal wall or by hematogenous spread. Some patients may have pleural effusion and ascites at the same time. The ascitic fluid is usually yellow with a high content of protein and a variable number of cells, predominantly lymphocytes. Caseous peritonitis is rarely seen today but used to accompany protracted hematogenous TB. Chemotherapy is effective in all forms of peritonitis, and some authors have suggested the use of steroids for severe disease [101,103].

Gastrointestinal disease is further detailed in Chapter 4.

## 6.16 GENITOURINARY TUBERCULOSIS

Renal TB rarely occurs less than 5 years after primary infection and, therefore, is likely to be seen in adolescence [104,105]. It is a serious complication and may progress to destructive cavitary renal TB. Diagnosis may be difficult because symptoms are often minimal and the number of leukocytes in the urine may be small. Some patients will complain of dysuria, hematuria and pyuria, but most are asymptomatic. The disease may be active in one or both kidneys. Chemotherapy is effective and nephrectomy is usually not necessary. A urogram should be done to define the site and extent of renal, ureteral and bladder involvement. The diagnosis should be considered in any child with chronic and recurrent urinary tract infections which do not respond to antibacterial medication.

Genital tract TB is unusual before puberty. It is a hazard for adolescent girls with primary TB infection; the fallopian tubes are most commonly involved. TB of the external genitalia can be evidence of child abuse and primary TB of the penis has been reported after circumcision. Genitourinary TB is discussed in more detail in Chapter 4.

## 6.17 TUBERCULOUS OTOMASTOIDITIS

Prior to the therapeutic era, TB involvement of the middle ear and/or mastoid was frequently recognized. Turner and Fraser in 1915 [106] reported that most cases of middle ear drainage in children less than one year of age were tuberculous, but only a small number of cases in older children were. Tuberculous meningitis was a common outcome [23]. In 1942, TB was implicated in about 3% of cases of chronic otitis media [107]. In 1977, three new cases and 10 other cases reported since 1960 were reviewed [108]. Of these 13 children, eight were 3 years of age or less and five had bilateral disease.

Classically, the infection is associated with painless, watery otorrhea and enlarged periauricular lymph nodes. Early, severe hearing loss in the speech frequencies may occur and was noted in four of 13 cases in the therapeutic era [108]. Facial nerve involvement also occurs and may be permanent. Although TB rates have diminished in the chemotherapeutic era, TB otitis or otomastoiditis remains more common in infants and young children than in older children or adults [108].

## 6.18 OCULAR TUBERCULOSIS

Ocular TB is uncommon, but may occur as a primary process, postprimary infection or from a hypersensitivity reaction. Any part of the eye may be involved, with the more common sites of involvement being the conjunctiva and uveal tract. In a review of ocular disease in over 10 000 children and adults from a TB sanatorium collected over a 26 year period, 154 cases (1.5%) were identified [109].

The conjunctiva can be the site of an initial inoculation, especially following trauma. Primary conjunctival TB presents with unilateral redness and tearing, with small yellow gray nodules associated with a mucoid discharge and preauricular lymphadenopathy. Phlyctenular keratoconjunctivitis, however, represents an allergic reaction to TB or other stimuli. Phlyctenules (*phlyktaina* is Greek for blister) are small, grayish, jelly-like nodules on the bulbar conjunctiva or cornea near the limbus (Figure 6.7). Phlyctenules were seen in 10% of all children with untreated primary TB in one report [111]. It is stated [109] that local instillation of tuberculoprotein in sensitized individuals can produce phlyctenules. The lesions are well vascularized and are associated with significant photophobia and

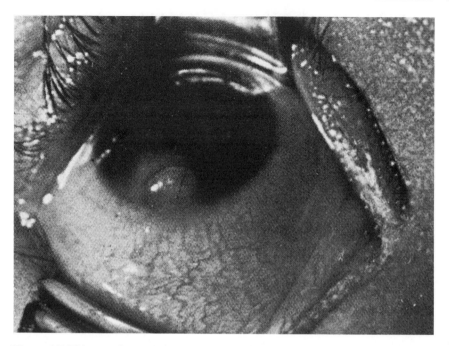

**Figure 6.7** Phlyctenular conjunctivitis. Reproduced from [110] with permission.

lacrimation. They usually heal, but may become necrotic, ulcerate and produce scarring.

Scleral involvement can occur as an episcleritis related to an immunologic reaction or as a deep scleritis directly related to TB. A reported case of scleral TB in an adult [112] is noteworthy in that topical anti-TB chemotherapy using subconjunctival streptomycin was necessary for resolution.

Uveitis is the most common ocular manifestation of TB. A recent report of a 3-year-old Spanish child [113] with tuberculous iridocyclitis resulting in loss of the eye illustrates its potential severity. In this case, the ocular infection was the first clinical manifestation of TB. Posterior TB uveitis is rarer. The diagnosis is based on examination, a reactive tuberculin test and a dramatic improvement from a therapeutic antituberculous trial [114]. Sterile uveitis can occur as well, as a reaction to a tuberculin test. Such a reaction is suggested by bilateral ocular involvement in the absence of miliary disease [115].

Choroidal tubercles occur, singly or multiply, usually around the macular area. These lesions are raised, whitish–gray masses which become hyalinized and leave atrophic scars. The lesions are valuable, easily obtainable, objective evidence of miliary TB. Healing of the lesions with therapy is also diagnostic [116]. A 1993 report in children re-emphasized the importance of these lesions in the diagnosis of TB [117].

## 6.19 PEDIATRIC ASPECTS OF ANTITUBERCULOUS CHEMOTHERAPY

The anti-TB agents are discussed in detail in Chapter 11, but certain aspects in children are stressed here. Pediatric doses of anti-TB drugs are shown in Table 12.4.

### 6.19.1 Dosage formulations of first line agents

INH is available in the USA as scored 100 mg and 300 mg tablets so a dose of 10 mg/kg can be obtained. An intramuscular dosage form of 10 mg/ml is also available. A liquid preparation of INH exists as a sorbitol based 10 mg/ml syrup. Starke [118] states, however, that this formulation is unstable at 37°C and can cause excess gastrointestinal symptoms, particularly diarrhea. Crushed INH tablets can be given in food, but there may be problems with absorption; crushed INH tablets in apple sauce produced substantially lower and delayed peak serum levels compared with the syrup [119]. This may be a significant problem in rapid INH acetylators.

Rifampin is available as 150 mg and 300 mg capsules as well as a fixed combination with 150 mg INH and 300 mg rifampin to obtain a dose of 20 mg/kg/day. These formulations are inconvenient to obtain a range of pediatric dosages. Therefore, an extemporaneously prepared suspension can be made using the capsule contents and a compounding syrup. It is usually produced as a 1% weight/volume 10 mg/ml suspension and is stable at room or refrigerator temperatures for 1 month [120]. The absorption can be erratic if taken with food [118]. An intravenous form of rifampin as a 600 mg ampule is also available.

Pyrazinamide is supplied as scored 500 mg tablets. Few studies in children are available to derive optimal dosage but a dose of 30 mg/kg daily produces adequate CSF levels and is well tolerated [118]. No liquid form of the drug exists, but the tablets can be crushed and given in food or as a suspension. There is no information regarding bioavailability of this form.

Ethambutol is produced as scored 100 mg and 400 mg tablets. No suspension is available. Although the pediatric risk of optic toxicity is unknown, the drug can be used in circumstances where therapeutic options are limited. Since it is not recommended in children at the ages when visual fields and acuity cannot be measured, a liquid form is not likely to be needed.

### 6.19.2 Pediatric toxicity of first line agents

INH hepatotoxicity is less common in children than in adults. Clinically relevant hepatitis from INH is more likely to occur in adolescents than in younger children and in children with more severe forms of TB [121,122]. Starke [118] states that, for most children, the toxicity of INH can be monitored using clinical signs and symptoms and that routine aminotransferase monitoring is not necessary. Kendig's group, however, follows liver function tests at the initiation of therapy, after 8–12 weeks and at its conclusion [123]. Asymptomatic mild elevations of serum aminotransferases occur less commonly in children as well, taking place in 4–10% of children receiving INH prophylaxis [121,124]. Pyridoxine supplementation to avoid INH neurotoxicity should be used in any child with an inadequate diet, those with limited or no intake of milk and meat, and breast fed babies [118].

Rifampin's effect on the metabolism of other drugs (Chapter 11) is less of a problem in children since they are often taking no other medication. Adolescent girls taking oral contraceptives, however, should be counseled regarding alternative forms of birth control while on a regimen containing rifampin. Likewise, those who use soft contact lenses should be warned about permanent staining of the lenses.

The side effects of pyrazinamide in children have not been well documented, especially those related to clinical effects of hyperuricemia. Ethambutol is generally not used in children in whom visual toxicity can not be adequately followed.

### 6.19.3 Recent clinical pediatric regimens for tuberculosis

The evaluation of therapy in pediatric TB is difficult because the establishment of a diagnosis and clinical success and failure are often imprecise [118]. This is because of the frequent lack of positive cultures and the natural history of primary TB which is often improvement without treatment. Moreover, trials done in developing countries are difficult to compare with those in developed areas and well controlled trials are rare, with most studies compared with historical controls.

Although short course TB treatment regimens have been mostly studied in adults, one of the earliest suggestions that a more abbreviated treatment schedule may be effective in children was made by Lorber [125], an English pediatrician. A 1984 report [126] found a 9 month course to be effective with daily INH and rifampin for 1 month and twice weekly for 8 months. In areas with substantial drug resistance, such a two drug treatment course is likely to fail. Several more recent pediatric studies have used 6 month courses with INH, rifampin and pyrazinamide for 2 months and INH and rifampin daily or intermittently for four additional months [127,128]. When an empiric four drug regimen is needed for children, if ethambutol cannot be used, streptomycin is likely the best alternative. Extrapulmonary non-life-threatening TB can be managed in the same way as pulmonary disease is treated. Compliance with therapy (Chapter 9) must always be considered in designing any treatment regimen.

## 6.20 TUBERCULOSIS AND PEDIATRIC HIV INFECTION

The rise in TB over the past decade has coincided with the HIV epidemic. A significant member of adults are co-infected by HIV and *M. tuberculosis* with the incidence varying widely depending on the location. Recommendations for the management of these patients have been published [129]. Because HIV-infected infants and children live in close proximity to their tuberculous parents, they are at particularly high risk of developing symptomatic TB once they are immunocompromised. Parents co-infected with TB and HIV pose multiple problems including an increased incidence of cavitary disease, higher mortality and multiply resistant strains (Chapters 3, 5, and 13).

In the absence of information on known or possible exposure to TB or demonstration of AFB in specimens, TB may elude the physician. Significant immunosuppression may cause poor reaction to tuberculin. In the immunocompromised, PPD reactions 5 mm or larger in size are considered positive [3]. Reactions smaller than 5 mm in the presence of exposure to and/or suspicion of TB based on clinical or X-ray findings should be interpreted carefully. The decision to provide prophylaxis for HIV-infected children in contact with persons at risk of acquiring TB is problematic. Through history in combination with known potential disease progression in the child, one should be able to determine a patient's need for prophylaxis. Infants and young children develop symptomatic and extrapulmonary infections rapidly. HIV-infected children are at even greater risk on both accounts [130,131].

The Brooklyn Pediatric AIDS Network has developed as yet unpublished guidelines for the management of TB in HIV-infected children. Anergic patients whose risk for TB infection is greater than 10% should be considered for prophylactic therapy for 12 months after excluding active infection. This includes those exposed to known active TB cases, foreign born children, those from endemic areas, and children living in high risk conditions such as shelters and with drug using family members.

The choice of anti-TB agents may be difficult since individuals with HIV infection are more likely to be infected with strains resistant to one or more first line agents [130,131]. Other risk factors are discussed in Chapters 3, 5 and 13. Rifampin can be used for prophylaxis in those known or expected to be infected with INH resistant strains [132]. There are no efficacy studies of preventive regimens against INH and rifampin resistant strains. The WHO recommends the use of BCG vaccine in asymptomatic HIV-infected infants who live in high incidence regions [133]. Symptomatic patients (i.e. those with AIDS) may develop disseminated BCG disease and should not receive the vaccine. In the USA, it is not given to infants with HIV infection but the emergence of resistant strains may change this practice. This issue is discussed in detail elsewhere [134]. Therapy for active disease is the same as discussed above but short course regimens may be inadequate in those with significant immunosuppression.

# REFERENCES

1. Lincoln, E.M. (1950) Course and prognosis of tuberculosis in childhood. *Am J Med*, **9**, 623–32.
2. Wallgren, A. (1948) The time-table of tuberculosis. *Tubercle*, **29**, 245–51.
3. Kochi, A. (1991) The global tuberculosis situation and the new control strategy of the World Health Organization. *Tubercle*, **72**, 1–6.
4. Starke, J., Jacobs, R. and Jereb, J. (1992) Resurgence of tuberculosis in children. *J Pediatrics*, **120**, 839–55.
5. Lee, S., Bloch, A. and Onorato, I. (1993) *Changes in reported tuberculosis cases in children <15 years old, U.S., 1988–1991.* Interscience Conference on Antimicrobial Agents and Chemotherapy, New Orleans, LA, American Society for Microbiology.
6. Bakshi, S.S., Alvarez, D., Hilfer, C.L. *et al.* (1993) Tuberculosis in human immunodeficiency virus-infected children. A family infection. *Am J Dis Child*, **147**, 320–4.
7. Dankner, W.M. Waeckner, N.J., Essig, M.A. *et al.* (1993) *Mycobacterium bovis*: a significant cause of childhood tuberculosis disease in San Diego. A clinicoepidemiologic study of 73 patients and a review of a forgotten pathogen. *Medicine*, **72**, 11–37.
8. Committee on Infectious Diseases (1994) Screening for tuberculosis in infants and children. *Pediatrics*, **93**, 131–4.
9. Schutze, G.E., Price, T.D. and Starke, J.R. (1993) Routine tuberculin screening of children during hospitalization. *Pediatr Infect Dis J*, **12**, 29–32.
10. Jacobs, R.F. and Starke, J.R. (1993) Tuberculosis in children. *Med Clin N Am*, **77**, 1335–51.
11. New York City Department of Health (1990) Tuberculosis in children. *City Health Information*, **9** (2), 1–3.
12. Starr, S. and Berkovich, S. (1964) Effects of measles, gamma globulin-modified measles and vaccine measles on the tuberculin test. *N Engl J Med*, **270**, 386–91.
13. Ormerod, L. and Garnett, J. (1988) Tuberculin response after neonatal BCG vaccination. *Arch Dis Child*, **63**, 1491–2.
14. Fox, A.S. and Lepow, M.L. (1983) Tuberculin skin testing in Vietnamese refugees with a history of BCG vaccination. *Am J Dis Child*, **137**, 1093–4.
15. Kröger, L., Katila, M.L., Korppi, M. and Pietikäinen, M. (1992) Rapid decrease in tuberculin skin test reactivity at preschool age after newborn vaccination. *Acta Paediatr Scand*, **81**, 678–81.
16. Tuberculosis prevention trial (1979) Trial of BCG vaccines in south India for tuberculosis prevention: First report. *Bull WHO*, **57**, 819–27.
17. Crawshaw, P. and Thomson, A. (1988) Heaf test results after neonatal BCG. *Arch Dis Child*, **63**, 1490–1.
18. Teale, C., Cundall, D.B. and Pearson, S.B. (1989) Heaf status after infant BCG immunization. *Thorax*, **44**, 843P.
19. Ormerod, L.P. and Garnett, J.M. (1992) Tuberculin skin reactivity four years after neonatal BCG vaccination. *Arch Dis Child*, **67**, 530–1.
20. Leung, A.N., Müller, N., Pineda, P. and FitzGerald, J.M. (1992) Primary tuberculosis in childhood: radiographic manifestations. *Radiology*, **182**, 87–91.
21. Medlar, E. (1955) Behavior of pulmonary tuberculous lesions: a pathological study. *Am Rev Tuberc*, **71**, 1–244.

22. Courtice, F.C. and Simmonds, W.J. (1954) Physiological significance of lymph drainage of the serous cavities and lungs. *Physical Rev*, **34**, 419–47.

23. Smith, M.H.D. and Marquis, J.R. (1987) Tuberculosis and other mycobacterial infections, in *Textbook of Pediatric Infectious Diseases* (eds R. Feigin and J. Cherry), W.B. Saunders, Philadelphia, pp. 1342–87.

24. Abadco, D.L. and Steiner, P. (1992) Gastric lavage is better than bronchoalveolar lavage for isolation of *Mycobacterium tuberculosis* in childhood pulmonary tuberculosis. *Pediatr Infect Dis J*, **11**, 735–8.

25. Lincoln, E.M. and Sewell, E.M. (1963) *Tuberculosis in Children*, McGraw-Hill, New York, pp. 49.

26. Jacobs, R.F. and Abernathy, R.S. (1988) Tuberculosis in children. *Sem Respir Med*, **9**, 474–80.

27. Giammona, S.T. and Zelkowitz, P.S. (1969) Superheated nebulized saline and gastric lavage to obtain bacterial cultures in primary pulmonary tuberculosis in children. *Am J Dis Child*, **117**, 198–200.

28. Hedvall, E. (1953) Pregnancy and tuberculosis. *Acta Med Scand*, **147** (Suppl 286), 1–101.

29. Flanagan, P. and Hensler, N.M. (1959) The course of active tuberculosis complicated by pregnancy. *JAMA*, **170**, 783–7.

30. Present, P.A. and Comstock, G. (1975) Tuberculin sensitivity in pregnancy. *Am Rev Respir Dis*, **112**, 413–6.

31. Snider, D.E., Layde, P.M., Johnson, M.W. and Lyle, M.A. (1980) Treatment of tuberculosis during pregnancy. *Am Rev Respir Dis*, **122**, 65–79.

32. Swartz, H.M. and Reichling, B.A. (1978) Hazards of radiation exposure for pregnant women. *JAMA*, **239**, 1907–8.

33. Bobrowitz, I.D. (1974) Ethambutol in pregnancy. *Chest*, **66**, 20–24.

34. Lewit, T., Nebel, L., Terracina, S. and Karman, S. (1974) Ethambutol in pregnancy: observations on embryogenesis. *Chest*, **66**, 25–6.

35. Wilson, E.A., Thelin, T.J. and Dilts, P.V. (1973) Tuberculosis complicated by pregnancy. *Am J Obstret Gynecol*, **115**, 526–9.

36. Anonymous (1980) Antituberculous drugs in pregnancy. *Lancet*, **2**, 1285–6.

37. Centers for Disease Control (1988) Use of BCG vaccine in the control of tuberculosis. A joint statement by the ACIP and the Advisory Committee for Elimination of Tuberculosis. *MMWR*, **37**, 663–4, 669–75.

38. Kendig, E.L. (1969) The place of BCG vaccine in the management of infants born of tuberculous mothers. *N Engl J Med*, **281**, 520–3.

39. Hageman, J., Shulman, S., Schreiber, M. *et al.* (1980) Congenital tuberculosis: critical reappraisal of clinical findings and diagnostic procedures. *Pediatrics*, **66**, 980–4.

40. McCray, M.K. and Esterly, N.B. (1981) Cutaneous eruptions in congenital tuberculosis. *Arch Dermatol*, **117**, 460–4.

41. Voyce, M. and Hunt, A. (1966) Congenital tuberculosis. *Arch Dis Child*, **41**, 299–300.

42. Cantwell, M.F., Shehab, Z., Costello, A.M. *et al.* (1994) Congenital tuberculosis. *N Engl J Med*, **330**, 1051–4.

43. Costello, A., Glasby, C., Cantwell, M. and Shehaab, Z. (1993) *Contact follow-up after exposure involving a newborn with congenital tuberculosis at 2 medical centers.* Interscience Conference on Antimicrobial Agents and Chemotherapy, New Orleans, LA, American Society for Microbiology.

44. Schaaf, H.S., Smith, J., Donald, P.R. and Stockland, B. (1989) Tuberculosis presenting in the neonatal period. *Clin Pediatrics*, **28**, 475.
45. Vallejo, J., Starke, J. and Ong, L. (1993) *Diagnosis and treatment of tuberculosis in infants*. Interscience Conference on Antimicrobial Agents and Chemotherapy, New Orleans, LA, American Society for Microbiology.
46. Schaaf, H.S., Gie, R.P., Beyers, N. *et al.* (1993) Tuberculosis in infants less than 3 months of age. *Arch Dis Child*, **69**, 371–4.
47. Lincoln, E.M. and Sewell, E.M. (1963) *Tuberculosis in Children*, McGraw-Hill, New York, p. 19.
48. Starke, J.R. and Taylor-Watts, K.T. (1989) Tuberculosis in the pediatric population of Houston, Texas. *Pediatrics*, **84**, 28–35.
49. Lincoln, E.M. (1940) The clinical picture of tuberculosis in children. *Am J Dis Child*, **60**, 371–83.
50. Lincoln, E.M. and Sewell, E.M. (1963) *Tuberculosis in Children*, McGraw-Hill, New York, pp. 14–15.
51. Daly, J.F., Brown, D.S., Lincoln, E.M. *et al.* (1952) Endobronchial tuberculosis in children. *Dis Chest*, **22**, 380–98.
52. Larmola, E. (1949) Two cases of sudden death in infants recovering from primary tuberculosis. *Acta Tuberc Scand*, **21** (Suppl), 67.
53. Walker, C.H.M. (1955) Pulmonary primary tuberculosis in childhood. *Lancet*, **1**, 218–24.
54. Nemir, R.L., Cardona, J., Lacoius, A. *et al.* (1963) Prednisone therapy as an adjunct in the treatment of lymph node-bronchial tuberculosis in childhood: A double-blind study. *Am Rev Respir Dis*, **88**, 189–98.
55. Morrison, J.B. (1973) Natural history of segmental lesions in primary pulmonary tuberculosis. *Arch Dis Child*, **48**, 90–8.
56. Payne, M. cited by Miller, F.J.W., Seale, R.M.E. and Taylor, M.D. (1963) *Tuberculosis in Children*, Little, Brown and Co., Boston.
57. Brock, R.C. (1950) Post-tuberculous bronchostenosis and bronchiectasis of the middle lobe. *Thorax*, **5**, 5–39.
58. Lincoln, E.M. and Sewell, E.M. (1963) *Tuberculosis in Children*, McGraw-Hill, New York, pp. 151–60.
59. Miller, F.J.W., Seale, R.M.E. and Taylor, M.D. (1963) *Tuberculosis in Children*, Little, Brown and Co., Boston, p. 214 .
60. Levine, H., Metzger, W., Lacera, S. *et al.* (1970) Diagnosis of tuberculous pleurisy by culture of pleural biopsy specimens. *Arch Intern Med*, **126**, 269–71.
61. Strom, L. (1949) On labeling tubercle bacilli with radioactive phosphorus. *Acta Tuberc Scand*, **23** (Supp 21), 98–101.
62. Choremis, C., Vlachos, J., Vlachos, C.A. *et al.* (1963) Needle biopsy of the liver in various forms of childhood tuberculosis. *J Pediatrics*, **62**, 203–7.
63. Grethman, W. (1936) Protracted multiform hematogenous tuberculosis. *Tr Nat Tuberc A*, **32**, 80–5.
64. Simon, G. (1930) Sekundaere streuherde der Lunge, in besondere die fruhen Spitzenherde, in *Handbuch Der Kindertuberkulose* (eds S. Engel and C. Pirquet), George Thieme, Leipzig, Germany.
65. Hussey, G., Chisholm, T. and Kibel, M. (1991) Miliary tuberculosis in children: a review of 94 cases. *Pediatr Infect Dis J*, **10**, 832–6.
66. Lincoln, E.M. and Sewell, E.M. (1963) *Tuberculosis in Children*, McGraw-Hill, New York, pp. 133–50.

66a. Division of Tuberculosis Control, Centers for Disease Control (1993) Tuberculosis Statistics in the United States, 1991, Atlanta, GA.

67. Waecker, N.J. and Connor, J.D. (1990) Central nervous system tuberculosis in children: a review of 30 cases. *Pediatr Infect Dis J*, **9**, 539–43.

68. Krambovitis, E., McIllmurray, M.B., Lock, P.E. *et al.* (1984) Rapid diagnosis of tuberculosis meningitis by latex particle agglutination. *Lancet*, **2**, 1229–31.

69. Girgis, N.I., Farid, Z., Kilpatrick, M.E. *et al.* (1991) Dexamethasone adjunctive treatment for tuberculous meningitis. *Pediatr Infect Dis J*, **10**, 179–83.

70. Delage, G. and Dusseault, M. (1979) Tuberculous meningitis in children: a retrospective study of 79 patients with an analysis of prognostic factors. *Canad Med Assoc J*, **120**, 305–9.

71. Lamba, P.A., Bhalla, J.S. and Mullick, D.N. (1986) Ocular manifestations of tubercular meningitis: a clinico-biochemical study. *J Pediatr Ophthalmol Strabismus*, **23**, 123–5.

72. Teoh, R., Humphries M.J. and O'Mahony, G. (1987) Symptomatic intracranial tuberculoma developing during treatment of tuberculosis: Report of 10 patients and review of the literature. *Quart J Med*, **63**, 449–60.

73. Henrickson, M. and Weisse, M.E. (1992) Tuberculous brain abscess in a three-year-old South Pacific Islander. *Pediatr Infect Dis J*, **11**, 488–91.

74. Tyler, B., Bennett, H. and Kim, J. (1983) Intracranial tuberculomas in a child: computed tomographic scan diagnosis and nonsurgical management. *Pediatrics*, **71**, 952–4.

75. Udani, P.M., Parekh, U.S.C. and Dastur, D.K. (1971) Neurological and related syndromes in CNS tuberculosis: clinical features and pathogenesis. *J Neurol Sci*, **14**, 341–57.

76. Lincoln, E.M. and Sewell, E.M. (1963) *Tuberculosis in Children*, McGraw-Hill, New York, pp. 249–54.

77. Boyd, G. (1953) Tuberculous pericarditis in children. *Am J Dis Child*, **86**, 293–300.

78. Hugo-Hamman, C.T., Scher, H. and DeMoor, M.M.A. (1994) Tuberculous pericarditis in children. *Pediatr Infect Dis J*, **13**, 13–18.

79. Lai, K.K., Stottmeier, K.D., Sherman, I.H. and McCabe, W.R. (1984) Mycobacterial cervical lymphadenopathy. Relationship of etiology to age. *JAMA*, **251**, 1286–8.

80. Lincoln, E.M. and Sewell, E.M. (1963) *Tuberculosis in Children*, McGraw-Hill, New York, pp. 207–15.

81. Jawahar, M.S., Sivasubramanian, S., Vijayan, V.K. *et al.* (1990) Short course chemotherapy for tuberculous lymphadenitis in children. *Brit Med J*, **301**, 359–62.

82. Schuit, K.E. and Powell, D.A. (1978) Mycobacterial lymphadenitis in children. *Am J Dis Child*, **132**, 675–7.

83. Lincoln, E.M. and Sewell, E.M. (1963) *Tuberculosis in Children*, McGraw-Hill, New York, pp. 184–206.

84. Halsey, J., Reeback, J. and Barnes, C. (1982) A decade of skeletal tuberculosis. *Ann Rheum Dis*, **41**, 7–10.

85. Bailey, H.L., Gabriel, M., Hodgson, A. and Shin, J.S. (1972) Tuberculosis of the spine in children. *J Bone Joint Surg*, **54-A**, 1633–57.

86. Omari, B., Robertson, J.M., Nelson, R.J. and Chiu, L.C. (1989) Pott's disease: a resurgent challenge to the thoracic surgeon. *Chest*, **95**, 145–50.

87.  Lachenauer, C.S., Cosentino, S., Wood, R.S. *et al.* (1991) Multifocal skeletal tuberculosis presenting as osteomyelitis of the jaw. *Pediatr Infect Dis J*, **10**, 940–4.

88.  Hardy, J.B. and Hartmann, J.R. (1947) Tuberculous dactylitis in childhood: a prognosis. *J Pediatrics*, **30**, 146–56.

89.  Moschella, S.L. and Cropley, T.G. (1992) Diseases of the mononuclear phago- cytic system (the so-called reticuloendothelial system), in *Dermatology*, 3rd edn, (eds S.L. Moschella and H.J. Hurley), W.B. Saunders, Philadelphia, pp. 1089–1100.

90.  Beyt, B.E., Ortbals, D.W., Santa Cruz, D.J. *et al.* (1980) Cutaneous mycobac- teriosis: analysis of 34 cases with a new classification of the disease. *Medicine*, **60**, 95–109.

91.  Fisher, J.R. (1977) Miliary tuberculosis with unusual cutaneous manifestations. *JAMA*, **238**, 241–2.

92.  Miller, F.J.W. (1953) Recognition of primary tuberculous infection of skin and mucosal. *Lancet*, **1**, 5–9.

93.  Fisher, I. and Orkin, M. (1966) Primary tuberculosis of the skin. *JAMA*, **195**, 174–6.

94.  Marmelzat, W.L. (1962) Laennec and the 'prosector's wart'. *Arch Dermatol*, **86**, 74–6.

95.  Case Report of the Massachusetts General Hospital. Case 43-1972. *N Engl J Med*, **287**, 872–8.

96.  Schermer, D.R., Simpson, C.G., Haserick, J.R. and van Ordstrand, H.S. (1969) Tuberculosis cutis miliaris acuta generalista. *Arch Dermatol*, **99**, 64–9.

97.  Kennedy, C. and Knowles, G.K. (1975) Miliary tuberculosis presenting with skin lesions. *Brit Med J*, **3**, 356.

98.  Held, J.L., Kohn, S.R., Silvers, D.N. and Grossman, M.E. (1988) Papulonecrotic tuberculid. *N Y State J Med*, **88**, 499–501.

99.  Penneys, N.S., Leonardi, C.L., Cook, S. *et al.* (1994) Indentification of *Mycobacterium tuberculosis* DNA in five different types of cutaneous lesions by the polymerase chain reaction. *Arch Dermatol*, **129**, 1594–8.

100.  Lincoln, E.M., Alterman, J. and Bakst, H. (1944) Erythema nodosum in chil- dren. *J Pediatrics*, **25**, 311–18.

101.  Lincoln, E.M. and Sewell, E.M. (1963) *Tuberculosis in Children*, McGraw-Hill, New York, pp. 224–32.

102.  Dineen, P., Homan, W.P. and Grafe, W.R. (1976) Tuberculous peritonitis: 43 years experience in diagnosis and treatment. *Ann Surg*, **148**, 717–22.

103.  Sioson, P.B., Stechenberg, B.W., Courtney, R. *et al.* (1992) Tuberculous peri- tonitis in a three-year old boy: case report and review of the literature. *Ped Infect Dis*, **11**, 409–12.

104.  Ehrlich, R.M. and Lattimer, J. (1971) Urogenital tuberculosis in children. *J Urol*, **105**, 461–5.

105.  Smith, A.M. and Lattimer, J.K. (1973) Genitourinary tract involvement in children with tuberculosis. *N Y State J Med,* **73**, 2325–8.

106.  Turner, A.L. and Fraser, J.S. (1915) Tuberculosis of the middle ear cleft in children: a clinical and pathological study. *J Laryngol Otol*, **30**, 209–47.

107.  Proctor, B. and Lindsay, J.R. (1942) Tuberculosis of the ear. *Arch Otolaryngol*, **35**, 221–49.

108.  MacAdam, A.M. and Rubio, T. (1977) Tuberculous otomastoiditis in children.

*Am J Dis Child*, **131**, 152–6.

109. Donahue, H.C. (1967) Ophthalmologic experience in a tuberculosis sanatorium. *Am J Ophthalmol*, **64**, 742–8.

110. Fedukowicz, H.B. and Stenson, S. (1985) *External Infections of the Eye*, 3rd edn, Appleton-Century-Crofts, Norwalk, CN, pp. 290–1.

111. Lincoln, E.M. and Sewell, E.M. (1963) *Tuberculosis in Children*, McGraw-Hill, New York, p. 245.

112. Bloomfield, S.E, Mondine, B. and Gray, G.F. (1976) Scleral tuberculosis. *Arch Ophthalmol*, **94**, 954–6.

113. Asensi, F., Otero, M.C., Pérez-Tamarit, D. *et al.* (1991) Tuberculous iridocyclitis in a three-year-old girl. *Clin Pediatrics*, **32**, 605–6.

114. Abrams, J. and Schlaegel, T.F. (1982) The role of the isoniazid therapeutic test in tuberculosis uveitis. *Am J Ophthalmol*, **94**, 511–5.

115. Lish, A. and Berman, D.H. (1993) Tuberculin-triggered panuveitis in a patient recently treated for active pulmonary tuberculosis. *Am J Ophthalmol*, **116**, 771–2.

116. Olazábal, F. (1967) Choroidal tubercles. A neglected sign. *JAMA*, **200**, 374–7.

117. Palacios, P.T. and Ramos, M.J.M. (1993) Ocular lesions of tuberculosis. *Ped Infect Dis J*, **12**, 884–5.

118. Starke, J.R. (1992) Current chemotherapy for tuberculosis in children. *Infect Dis Clin N Am*, **6**, 215–38.

119. Notterman, D.A., Nardi, M. and Saslow, J.C. (1986) Effect of dose formulation on isoniazid absorption in two young children. *Pediatrics*, **77**, 850–2.

120. Krukenberg, C.C., Mischler, P.G., Massad, E.N. *et al.* (1986) Stability of 1% rifampin suspensions prepared in five syrups. *Am J Hosp Pharm*, **43**, 2225–8.

121. Litt, I.F., Cohen, M.I. and McNamara, H. (1976) Isoniazid hepatitis in adolescents. *J Pediatrics*, **89**, 133–5.

122. Donald, P.R., Schoeman, J.F. and O'Kennedy, A. (1987) Hepatic toxicity during chemotherapy for several tuberculous meningitis. *Am J Dis Child*, **141**, 741–3.

123. Kendig, E.L. and Inselman, L.S. (1991) Tuberculosis in children. *Adv Pediatr*, **38**, 233–55.

124. Rapp, R.S., Campbell, R.W., Howell, J.C. and Kendig, E.L. (1978) Isoniazid hepatotoxicity in children. *Am Rev Respir Dis*, **118**, 794–6.

125. Lorber, J. (1954) Isoniazid and streptomycin in tuberculous meningitis. *Lancet*, **1**, 1149–51.

126. Abernathy, R.S., Dutt, A.K., Stead, W.W. and Moers, D.J. (1983) Short-course chemotherapy for tuberculosis in children. *Pediatrics*, **72**, 801–6.

127. Biddulph, J. (1990) Short-course chemotherapy for childhood tuberculosis. *Pediatr Infect Dis J*, **9**, 794–801.

128. Kumar, L., Dhand, R., Singhi, P.D. *et al.* (1990) A randomized trial of fully intermittent vs. daily followed by intermittent short-course chemotherapy for childhood tuberculosis. *Pediatr Infect Dis J*, **9**, 802–6.

129. Subcommittee of the Joint Tuberculosis Committee of the British Thoracic Society (1992) Guidelines on the management of tuberculosis and HIV infection in the United Kingdom. *Brit Med J*, **304**, 1231–3.

130. Jones, D.S., Malecki, J.M., Bigler, W.J. *et al.* (1992) Pediatric tuberculosis and human immunodeficiency virus infection in Palm Beach County, Florida. *Am J Dis Child*, **146**, 1166–70.

131. Khouri, Y.F., Mastrucci, M.T., Hutto, C. *et al.* (1992) *Mycobacterium tuberculosis* in children with human immunodeficiency virus type 1 infection. *Pediatr Infect Dis*, **11**, 950–5.

132. Steiner, P., Rao, M., Victoria, M.S. *et al.* (1983) A continuing study of primary drug-resistant tuberculosis among children observed at the Kings County Hospital Medical Center between the years 1961 and 1980. *Am Rev Respir Dis*, **128**, 425–8.

133. Special Program on AIDS and Expanded Program on Immunization (1987) Consultation on human immunodeficiency virus (HIV) and routine childhood immunization. *Wkly Epidem Rec*, **62**, 297–304.

134. Braun, M.M. and Cauthen, G. (1992) Relationship of the human immunodeficiency virus epidemic to pediatric tuberculosis and bacillus Calmette-Guérin immunization. *Pediatr Infect Dis*, **11**, 220–7.

# 7 | The microbiology of tuberculosis

Michael H. Levi

## 7.1 ORGANIZATION OF THE CLINICAL MYCOBACTERIOLOGY LABORATORY

The diagnostic mycobacteriology laboratory is an important participant in the control and eradication of TB [1–3]. Ironically, the long interval between specimen collection and results diminishes the impact of the laboratory and can create confusion among clinicians. With the recent increase in TB cases, some with multiple drug resistance, it has become even more important to understand the basic operation of the mycobacteriology laboratory.

This chapter will not describe the detailed microbiology performed in the mycobacteriology laboratory. Readers are referred elsewhere [4–6] for excellent resources in this regard. It will describe the organization and responsibilities of the laboratory in relation to diagnostic testing for TB and present material on the interpretation of these tests. Understanding this information should improve patient care and aid in the control of the disease.

### 7.1.1 Levels of laboratory operation

Any mycobacteriology laboratory can be classified at one of three levels of operation [7]:

1. Specimen collection and transport; acid-fast bacillus (AFB) smear preparation and examination; referral to reference laboratory for culture.
2. Level 1 procedures, and TB isolation and identification.
3. Level 1 and 2 procedures, and the identification of all AFB species. Susceptibility testing may be done at Level 2, but should be performed at Level 3.

The laboratory director must ensure that the physical structure of the laboratory meets the necessary safety requirements [8–10]. It is also useful to remember that the operation of a mycobacteriology laboratory is quite expensive, so that when the volume of test requests are low it may be more efficient and cost effective to send specimens, cultures and/or susceptibility testing to a reference laboratory.

### 7.1.2 Laboratory protocols

Since culture results may take up to 8 weeks (incubation time for a negative TB culture), the laboratory must establish protocols assuring that tests are promptly performed and reports are rapidly communicated to the clinical staff and appropriate health officials. Two publications [11,12] have made specific recommendations in this area, including the following.

- Specimens should be delivered to the laboratory rapidly.
- AFB smears should be examined within 24 hours of receipt using a fluorescent stain. Direct, unconcentrated AFB (other than those for solid tissue specimens) should only be performed on an emergency basis, and reported only if positive.
- Mycobacterial cultures, including a broth culture, should also be initiated within 24 hours of receipt and all cultures should be examined at least weekly.
- Upon observing adequate growth, the organisms should be confirmed as AFB and identified as *Mycobacterium tuberculosis* or not within four working days.
- Broth based susceptibility tests for *M. tuberculosis* should be set up rapidly. Direct tests should be initiated within 24 hours of a positive smear, indirect tests within 7 days of obtaining adequate growth.
- AFB positive smears, *M. tuberculosis* positive cultures and susceptibility results must be reported within 24 hours to a clinician involved in the patient's care, infection control personnel and the local health department.
- All laboratories must maintain records of standard operating procedures, quality control, proficiency testing and equipment maintenance.

## 7.2 BASIC MICROBIOLOGY

### 7.2.1 Mycobacteria

The genus *Mycobacterium* is composed of slow growing organisms which are acid fast and differ from other closely related genera (Table 7.1) [13]. Currently, at least 55 species of mycobacteria are recognized which are non-motile, slightly curved or straight rods, 0.2–0.6 × 1.0–10 μm, and occasionally demonstrate branching. Filamentous or mycelium-like growth

**Table 7.1** Differentiation of *Mycobacterium* from other genera

| Characteristics | Mycobacterium | Nocardia | Rhodococcus | Corynebacterium |
|---|---|---|---|---|
| Morphology | Rods, occasionally branched filaments; no aerial mycelium[a] | Mycelium, later fragmenting into rods and cocci; usually some aerial mycelium | Scanty mycelium, fragmenting into irregular rods and cocci; no aerial mycelium | Pleomorphic rods, often club-shaped; commonly in angular and palisade arrangement |
| Rate of growth: time for visible colonies | 2–40 days | 1–5 days | 1–3 days | 1–2 days |
| Degree of acid-fastness | Usually strongly acid-fast | Often partially acid-fast | Often partially acid-fast | Sometimes weakly acid-fast |
| Degree of staining in Gram stain | Weak | Usually strong | Usually strong | Strong |
| Reaction to penicillin | Resistant[b] | Resistant | Sensitive | Sensitive |
| Mycolic acids: number of carbons | 60–90 | 46–60 | 34–64 | 22–32 |

[a] Some species may occasionally produce aerial mycelia.
[b] Some species (e.g. *M. avium*) may be sensitive to penicillin.
Adapted from Sneath, 1986, *Bergey's Manual of Systematic Bacteriology*, Volume 2, Section 16, *Mycobacteria*, Williams & Wilkins, Baltimore [13].

sometimes occurs, but will easily break apart into rods and cocci. Organisms are aerobic and do not contain endospores, conidia or capsules. Although they do not Gram stain well, the organisms have Gram-positive cell walls.

Mycobacteria contain a lipid rich cell surface which includes true waxes and glycolipids accounting for about 60% of the cell as dry weight [14]. The long chain (60–90 carbons) mycolic acids in the cell wall, unique to the mycobacteria, are composed of saturated γ-alkyl, ß-hydroxyl fatty acids. This lipid rich cell surface is responsible for acid fastness, failure to react with Gram stain and probably for resistance to the bacteriocidal action of antibody and complement.

### 7.2.2 Acid-fast properties

Acid fastness, the most prominent feature of the genus, is related to the capacity of mycolic acids to form complexes with certain arylmethane dyes (i.e. carbol fuchsin), which cannot be removed with acidic ethanol or mineral acids (Figure 7.1). Several observations have led to a working model for the acid-fast stain [14]. First, mycobacteria with ruptured cell walls are weakly acid fast and treatment with alkaline ethanol renders them non-acid fast. Secondly, free mycolic acids bind fuchsin on a mole for mole basis. Additionally, after mycolic acids have formed complexes with the arylmethane dyes, the cell surfaces become extremely hydrophobic. It is thought, therefore, that the intense carbol fuchsin staining after decolorization with acid alcohol is produced by the portion of stain that has penetrated the interior of the mycobacterium which is protected by the hydrophobic complex of fuchsin and mycolic acids on the cell's exterior. *Corynebacteria*, *Nocardia* and *Rhodococcus* which may be acid fast after exposure to mineral acids, are unable to protect the interior of the cells from acid alcohol decolorization.

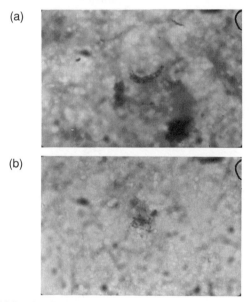

(a)

(b)

**Figure 7.1** Acid-fast bacilli in Kinyoun stained sputum smears later identified as *M. tuberculosis*. (a) Organisms demonstrating cording. (b) Organisms demonstrating beading. Magnification 1000×.

### 7.2.3 Growth characteristics

Slow growth is another central characteristic of the genus. Mycobacteria are divided into two groups, which either grow in less than 7 days (rapid growers) or require more than 7 days, usually 2–4 weeks or more, to grow (slow growers). This characteristic is not well understood, but is believed to be associated with a DNA dependent RNA polymerase initiating RNA synthesis and producing RNA in *M. tuberculosis* at a rate at least 10 times slower than in *Escherichia coli* [15]. The enzyme in *M. tuberculosis* is also

1000 times more sensitive to rifampin compared with the *E. coli* DNA dependent RNA polymerase [16].

The genus is defined by a combination of phenotypic and genetic characteristics. The basis for this classification was established in the 1950s by Runyon who utilized the ability of some mycobacteria to produce carotenoid pigments either in the absence or in the presence of light to separate the genus into groups [17]. A battery of biochemical tests and genetic probes have further expanded the identification of organisms within *M. tuberculosis* complex and mycobacteria within the Runyon classifications (Table 7.2) [4–6].

**Table 7.2** Classification of the genus *Mycobacterium*[a]

| Mycobacterial groups | Growth rate | Pigment formation in: Light | Dark | Typical species |
|---|---|---|---|---|
| TB complex | Slow | – | – | *M. tuberculosis* (see Table 7.3) |
| Photochromogens | Slow | + | – | *M. kansasii* *M. marinum* |
| Scotochromogens | Slow | + | + | *M. scrofulaceum* |
| Nonchromogens | Slow | – | – | *M. avium-intracellulare* complex |
| Rapid growers | Rapid | – | – | *M. fortuitum-chelonei* complex |

[a] Adapted from [17] and reproduced with permission.

### 7.2.4 *Mycobacterium tuberculosis* complex

The four species in the *M. tuberculosis* complex are virtually identical in terms of DNA homology, growth rate, lipid content, immunologic characteristics and antimicrobial susceptibility [16,18]. Nevertheless, the organisms of the *M. tuberculosis* complex can be separated by several phenotypic and epidemiologic characteristics (Table 7.3). *Mycobacterium bovis* rarely causes disease in areas of the world where animal husbandry includes TB screening and milk pasteurization [19]. *Mycobacterium microti* is believed to represent a transitional organism between *M. bovis* and *M. tuberculosis*, but is not known to cause disease in humans. The validity of *M. africanum* as a unique species has been questioned and in one study, most of the *M. africanum* strains were similar to either *M. bovis* or *M. tuberculosis* [20,21]. Bacillus Calmette-Guérin (BCG) was derived from a strain of *M. bovis*.

All these organisms react with commercially available DNA probes used

**Table 7.3** Features providing maximal resolution within the tuberculosis complex[a].
Positive strains (%)

| | Mycobacterium tuberculosis | M. microti | M. africanum | M. bovis | BCG |
|---|---|---|---|---|---|
| Nicotinamidase | 99 | 99 | 62 | 1 | 1 |
| Pyrazinamidase | 94 | 99 | 33 | 1 | 1 |
| Niacin | 99 | 99 | 50 | 1 | 29 |
| Nitrate reduction | 98 | 60 | 29 | 8 | 86 |
| Growth stimulated by glycerol | 98 | 33 | 1 | 1 | 99 |
| Resists 1 µg/ml thiophen-2-carboxylic hydrazide | 96 | 1 | 1 | 1 | 33 |
| Resists 44 µg/ml pyrazinamide | 1 | 1 | 7 | 99 | 99 |
| Lebek niveau (sub-surface growth in semisolid agar) | 10 | 1 | 93 | 92 | 1 |

[a] Adapted from [16] with permission.

to identify *M. tuberculosis*. This is the reason that laboratories which exclusively use these probes to identify *M. tuberculosis* must report *M. tuberculosis* complex as a final organism identification. Laboratories will use the nitrate and niacin tests, in addition to the DNA probe, to separate *M. tuberculosis* and *M. bovis*.

## 7.3 SPECIMEN SELECTION

A critical factor in the ability of the laboratory to isolate *M. tuberculosis* is obtaining appropriate specimens for AFB smear and culture [4]. Although 85% of TB cases are pulmonary, many patients cannot produce sputum spontaneously and alternative respiratory tract specimens (e.g. induced sputum, gastric lavage or fiberoptic bronchoscopy) may be needed [7]. The remaining 15% of cases involve other sites and specimens. It is important to provide adequate specimens from extrapulmonary sites as the proportion of patients with this form of TB is increasing [22]. Specimens sent to the laboratory for AFB stain and culture should conform to the rules listed in Table 7.4.

### 7.3.1 General recommendations for specimen collection and transport

- Collect specimen prior to use of antimicrobial agents. If this is not possible, indicate on the request that the patient is receiving TB therapy.

**Table 7.4** Specimen requirements for mycobacterial isolation and acid-fast stains[a]

| Specimen type | Specimen[b] requirements | Special instructions | Unacceptable specimens |
|---|---|---|---|
| Abscess contents, aspirated fluid | As much as possible in syringe with Luer tip cap | Cleanse skin with alcohol before aspirating sample. Laboratory may provide 7H9 broth for transport of small volumes of aspirates | Dry swab |
| Blood | 10 ml SPS (yellow top) blood collection tube or 10 ml Isolator tube or 5 ml inoculated directly into BACTEC 13A vial | Disinfect site as for routine blood culture. Mix tube contents immediately after collection. SPS is preferred anticoagulant. Heparinized blood is also acceptable | Blood collected in EDTA, which greatly inhibits mycobacterial growth even in trace amounts<br><br>Coagulated blood |
| Body fluids (pleural, pericardial, peritoneal) | As much as possible (10–15 ml minimum) in sterile container or syringe with Luer tip cap. Collect bloody specimens into SPS blood collection tubes | Disinfect site with alcohol if collecting by needle and syringe. Volumes of ≤ 10 ml may be directly inoculated into BACTEC 13A vial | |
| Bone | Bone in sterile container without fixative or preservative | | Specimen submitted in formalin |
| Bone marrow | As much as possible in SPS blood collection tube or 1.5 ml in pediatric Isolator tube or inoculate directly into BACTEC 13A vial | Collect aseptically. Mix SPS tube contents immediately following collection | |

| | | | |
|---|---|---|---|
| Bronchoalveolar lavage or bronchial washings | ≥ 5 ml in sterile container | Avoid contaminating bronchoscope with tap water. Saprophytic mycobacteria may produce false-positive culture or smear results | |
| Bronchial brushing | Sterile container or Middlebrook 7H9 broth | | |
| CSF | ≥ 2 ml in sterile container | Use maximum volume attainable | |
| Gastric lavage fluid | ≥ 5–10 ml in sterile container. Collect in the morning soon after patient awakens in order to obtain sputum swallowed during sleep | Collect fasting early morning specimen on three consecutive days. Use sterile saline. Adjust to neutral pH with 100 mg of sodium carbonate immediately following collection. Laboratory should provide collection tube containing sodium carbonate | Specimen that has not been neutralized |
| Lymph node | Node or portion in sterile container without fixative or preservative | Collect aseptically, and avoid indigenous microbiota. Select caseous portion if available. Do not immerse in saline or other fluid or wrap in gauze | Specimen submitted in formalin |
| Skin lesion material | Submit biopsy specimen in sterile container without fixative or preservative. Submit aspirate in syringe with Luer tip cap | Swabs in transport medium (Amies or Stuarts) are acceptable *only* if biopsy sample or aspirate is not obtainable. For cutaneous ulcer, collect biopsy | Dry swab |

*cont'd*

**Table 7.4**
*continued*

| | | | |
|---|---|---|---|
| | | sample from periphery of lesion, or aspirate material from under margin or lesion | |
| Smear on slides | Smear specimen over 1.5 by 1.5 cm area of clear slide | Heat fix smears. Transport in slide container taped closed and labeled BIOHAZARD[c] | |
| Sputum | 5–10 ml in sterile, wax-free, disposable container. Collect an early morning specimen from deep, productive cough on at least three consecutive days. Do not pool specimens. For follow-up of patients on therapy, collect at weekly intervals beginning three weeks after initiation of therapy | For expectorated sputum, instruct patient on how to produce sputum specimen as distinct from saliva or nasopharyngeal discharge. Have patient rinse mouth with water before collecting sputum to minimize contaminating specimen with food particles, mouthwash, or oral drugs, which may inhibit the growth of mycobacteria. For induced sputum, use sterile hypertonic saline. Indicate on request if specimen is induced sputum | 24 hour pooled specimens; saliva |
| Stool | ≥ 1 g in sterile, wax-free, disposable container | Collect specimen directly into container, or transfer from bedpan or plastic wrap stretched over toilet bowl. Wax from container may produce false-positive smear | Frozen specimen. Utility of culturing stool for acid-fast bacilli remains controversial |

| | | | |
|---|---|---|---|
| Tissue biopsy sample | 1 g of tissue, if possible, in sterile container without fixative or preservative | Collect aseptically, and avoid indigenous microbiota. Select caseous portion if available. Do not immerse in saline or other fluid or wrap in gauze. Freezing decreases yield | Specimen submitted in formalin |
| Transtracheal aspirate | As much as possible, in syringe with Luer tip cap or other sterile container | | |
| Urine | As much as possible (minimum 40 ml) of first morning specimen obtained by catheterization or of midstream clean catch in sterile container. For suprapubic tap, as much as possible in syringe with Luer tip cap or other sterile container | Collect first morning specimen on three consecutive days. Accept only one specimen/day. Organisms accumulate in bladder overnight, so first morning void provides best yield. Specimens collected at other times are dilute and are not optimal | 24 hour pooled specimens; urine from catheter bag; specimens of <40 ml unless larger volume is not obtainable |
| Wound material | See biopsy or aspirate | Swabs are acceptable *only* if biopsy or aspirate is not obtainable. If used, they must be placed in transport medium (Amies or Stuarts). Negative results are not reliable | |

[a] Adapted from [6] with permission.
[b] SPS, sodium polyanethol sulfonate.
[c] Sixty per cent of acid-fast bacilli present on smear will survive heating for 2 h at 65°C.

- Collect specimen in a sturdy sterile container. Never use wax containers since false-positive smears can occur.
- Specimens should not be batched for sending to the laboratory to avoid delay in detection.
- Swabs are usually unacceptable AFB specimens.
- Ensure prompt delivery of specimens to the laboratory. If specimens have to be mailed, follow Centers for Disease Control (CDC) recommendations for proper shipment [4].
- When possible, avoid contamination of specimen with normal microbial flora.
- Specimens, other than blood and other sterile body fluids, which cannot be processed immediately, should be stored at 4°C.

## 7.4 AFB SMEARS

An AFB smear is a clinically useful and cost effective test [4,5]. It can be done rapidly, provide an indication on how infectious a patient may be, offer an early indication of a response to therapy and can be used in the laboratory to confirm that growth on mycobacterial media is, in fact, an AFB. Sputum specimens must contain a large number of organisms, 5000–10 000 AFB/ml, to be detected by smear while culture can detect as few as 10–100 AFB [23]. It is important, therefore, that laboratories follow recommended protocols for the decontamination and concentration of specimens and always perform or refer a specimen for culture.

### 7.4.1 Decontamination

Proper decontamination of specimens containing normal microbial flora and concentration are crucial to AFB detection. Since most specimens for AFB smear and culture are from the respiratory tract, successful decontamination and concentration also requires the use of an agent to liquify mucus. Mucus will trap AFB and protect other organisms from decontamination. Most often this is done with a combination of 2% NaOH (decontaminant) with 0.5% N-acetyl-L-cysteine (mucolytic agent).

Contamination rates should be no more than 3–5%. Significantly lower rates indicate that the procedure may be too harsh and vice versa [4]. Specimens obtained from sterile sites, such as CSF, peritoneal or pleural fluid do not need decontamination. The methods and details of these procedures are fully described in several current manuals [4–6].

### 7.4.2 Maximizing the AFB smear

The crucial factors in maximizing smear sensitivity and specificity are listed below.

- Centrifugation of digested or fluid specimens at a minimum of $3000 \times g$ [4,24].
- The smear should be prepared on a new, clean and undamaged slide over an area of $1 \times 2$ cm.
- A fluorescent AFB technique should be used to screen slides, (i.e. auramine-rhodamine) which allows the scan of a larger area of the slide, demonstrating brightly stained organisms against a dark background. About 18% of positive specimens will be missed if these stains are not used [25,26].
- Scanning of slides should be done so that at least 300 fields are examined.
- Smear results should be reported quantitatively according to the number of AFB per field at 1000 times magnification and the method of staining. The CDC recommended method of reading and reporting AFB smears stained with carbol fuchsin is shown in Table 7.5. If fluorescent stains are used exclusively, the results of these smears can be converted [4]. In my laboratory, a Kinyon stain is performed directly on the positive fluorescent smear providing better AFB morphology and CDC quantitation.

**Table 7.5** Reporting acid-fast stains

| Number of acid-fast bacilli (AFB) observed with a carbol fuchsin stain | Patient report |
|---|---|
| None | No AFB observed |
| 1–2/300 fields | ± Doubtful; please repeat |
| 1–9/100 fields | 1+ |
| 1–9/10 fields | 2+ |
| 1–9 field | 3+ |
| >9/field | 4+ |

Smears with fewer than three AFB per slide account for about 85% of false-positive smear reports and are therefore considered 'doubtful' and a repeat specimen requested [27]. A sizable proportion of ± and 1+ AFB smears will be observed from patients with TB [27,28]. *Mycobacterium tuberculosis* infection must, therefore, be considered for any patient with an AFB positive smear regardless of quantity.

### 7.4.3 Smears from pulmonary specimens

Lipsky reviewed over 3000 specimens submitted for AFB smear and culture and found the smear sensitivity to be 33% [27]. If only patients with positive TB cultures (removing all patients with cultures for mycobacteria other than *M. tuberculosis*) are considered, however, 65% were AFB smear positive and multiple numbers of specimens increased the smear positivity rate to 96%. Several other papers support the value of an AFB smear in both known TB patients [28–31] and general hospital populations [32,33]. Overall, the sensitivity of an AFB sputum smear in patients with confirmed cases of pulmonary TB has been 50–80% [7].

Cavitary TB is associated with a markedly increased number of AFB within the lesion, probably because of the aerobic requirements of *M. tuberculosis*. It has been estimated that the number of organisms is 5–6 logs greater in cavitary lesions than noncavitary ones [34]. Patients with active TB cavities have an AFB smear positivity rate of 98% [31].

False-positive smears are usually caused by specimens from patients being treated for TB (specimens contain non-viable organisms), smear reader inexperience or overall poor quality control of staining techniques. When patients being treated are removed from the analysis, the positive and negative predictive values for AFB smears are greater than 95% [33,35].

In patients who do not produce spontaneous early morning sputum, specimens can be acquired by either sputum induction, fiberoptic broncho-scopy or gastric washings. Induced sputum is the preferred method for acquisition as it is the least invasive and does not significantly alter the specimen [4]. Gastric washings, which sample the stomach for swallowed respiratory tract secretions, are acceptable for AFB [36–38]. However, *M. tuberculosis* is isolated more frequently from induced sputa than from gastric washings and does not require neutralization of the specimen [39,40]. Fiberoptic bronchoscopy is an effective method to increase the yield of AFB positive specimens from 20% to 50% [41–47]. To ensure the safety of the health care provider from aerosolized *M. tuberculosis*, sputum induction and bronchoscopy require adequate ventilation and appropriate protective equipment [9].

Young children (particularly those under 3 years of age), the elderly and HIV-infected persons may not produce cavitary lesions, granulomas or sputum. This can significantly lower AFB smear positivity. In a recent study on the use of the AFB smear in the elderly, only one of 19 patients had cavitary disease and two of 19 (10%) were smear positive [48]. Although only 6% of HIV-infected patients with TB demonstrate cavitation, 85% will have a chest X-ray suggestive of infection with *M. tuberculosis* and a smear positivity rate of 31–82% [49]. In one case control study, HIV-infected patients with TB had a significantly lower rate of AFB positive smears (45%) compared with controls (81%) [50]. In general, the HIV disease host response to *M. tuberculosis* is directly related to the level of immunosuppression [49]. When immunosuppression is mild, TB disease is similar to that seen in the normal host, while increasing immunosuppression increases the risk of atypical presentation of TB and dissemination [22].

There has been some concern regarding the value of an AFB sputum smear in populations where the incidence of *M. avium-intracellulare* (MAI) infection is high. In HIV-infected patients, MAI mainly produces an infection of nonpulmonary tissue with the gut a more important portal of entry than the respiratory tract [51]. MAI pneumonia is only present in 4% of patients with disseminated MAI disease. In a recent study of sputum specimens from San Francisco, 248 of 450 (55%) smears were AFB positive in specimens which grew TB, while only 15 of 232 (6%) smears were positive in the MAI group [52]. This was significantly different (p< 0.001) with a positive predictive value of 92%. We have seen similar results at Montefiore Medical Center, Bronx, NY [53]. Therefore, despite the large number of MAI-infected patients, an AFB positive sputum smear is still predictive of *M. tuberculosis*.

### 7.4.4 Smears from nonrespiratory tract specimens

Since almost any organ can be TB infected, the value of direct smears from tissue and various fluids must be considered. For a discussion on the clinical aspects of extrapulmonary disease, the reader is referred to Chapter 4. It is best to obtain tissue from the organ involved, if available, since both AFB and granulomas may be observed. Sputum or other respiratory tract specimens may also be helpful, since co-existing pulmonary infection may exist.

The sensitivity of smears from extrapulmonary sites is lower than from sputa. A negative AFB smear should, therefore, not rule out the clinical diagnosis of extrapulmonary TB [19]. In miliary disease, a form of TB where significant numbers of tubercle bacilli shower both extrapulmonary and pulmonary sites, only 31% of sputum smears were AFB positive [54]. TB lymphadenitis is the most common extrapulmonary form of infection, but biopsy demonstrates AFB in only 50% of peripheral nodes while culture can be positive in almost all specimens [19]. Pleural infection is the second most common site. Smears of pleural fluid are usually negative with culture only positive in about a third of cases. Diagnosis is usually confirmed by stain and culture of pleural biopsy.

AFB positive smears from tissues or usually sterile body fluids are generally due to either *M. tuberculosis* or MAI. Although the differentiation of TB and disease produced by MAI is often made on clinical features, there are times when the two diseases cannot be separated [49]. Additionally, patients can be infected with both organisms [55]. The CDC has recommended that all patients with HIV infection and a positive smear receive treatment for TB, at least until the bacilli can be identified. This is a diagnostic area that will be greatly improved when sensitive and specific genetic probes which are used directly on specimens for the recognition of *M. tuberculosis* become more available (see below).

It is important in the evaluation of the AFB stain to distinguish between those tests performed on tissue sent to microbiology and those done on fixed pathology material. The yield of the former is higher since a concentrate of more material is able to be stained. It is not unusual for surgical biopsies, which histologically show granulomas, not to be sent for TB culture. This occurs primarily when TB is not considered as a diagnostic possibility. This will obviously profoundly affect the ability to isolate *M. tuberculosis* and evaluate drug sensitivities. The primary physician must be vigilant in assuring that proper handling of surgical specimens is accomplished.

## 7.5 CULTURE AND IDENTIFICATION

In 1882, Koch reported the *in vitro* isolation of *M. tuberculosis* on enriched bacteriologic media. The modern mycobacteriology laboratory has sophisticated bacteriological media available to it, but in many respects TB isolation is carried out in a similar way to that pioneered by Koch.

An ideal isolation medium would be able to produce rapid and abundant growth, enhance phenotypic characteristics, inhibit the growth of contaminants and could be used for antimicrobial drug testing. Unfortunately despite advances, the isolation of *M. tuberculosis* is still a slow process requiring from 10 days to 8 weeks. Considering the current TB resurgence, the most important aspects are the time to isolation and the sensitivity of the medium for *M. tuberculosis* [12,56]. These criteria make the solid media systems the least desirable and the radiometric system the most effective.

### 7.5.1 Identification methodology

Great progress has been made in the rapid identification of the tubercle bacillus. Each laboratory must choose not only an isolation media but also an identification technique which meets the needs of the population being served. This may be different for a reference and a primary care hospital laboratory. There are four methods available for TB identification: biochemical tests such as niacin, nitrate and urease; radiometric NAP (nitro-α-acetylamino-ß-hydroxypropiophenone) test; nucleic acid probes; and fatty acid analysis by liquid chromatography (HPLC). The details of these procedures are well described [4–6].

Biochemical testing is slow, requiring about 3 weeks to identify an isolate as *M. tuberculosis*. On the other hand, the Bactec NAP test can be done in about 4–5 days [57] and DNA probes and HPLC are done in hours [5,6]. The use of commercially available bioluminescent DNA probes which are directed at highly conserved ribosomal RNA of *M. tuberculosis* (Bioluminescent DNA probe system, Gen-Probe, San Diego, CA) has made identification of *M. tuberculosis* complex accurate, extremely rapid and relatively inexpensive [5,6]. The probes have been coupled with isolation systems to improve the speed of *M. tuberculosis* identification.

### 7.5.2 Isolation techniques

*(a) Solid media*

Solid media for *M. tuberculosis* isolation have improved steadily since the early part of the 1900s. Two basic media types are currently used, both of which perform best when incubated in 10% $CO_2$.

Egg-potato based (Lowenstein–Jensen type) medium produces a slightly higher rate of TB isolation, but is prone to slant contamination and is a poor drug testing medium [4,58]. It is relatively non-selective but can be made highly selective by the addition of antibiotics.

Agar based medium (Middlebrook formulations: non-selective and selective) is transparent, which allows for quicker examination of colony morphology. It is more resistant to contamination and produces growth of *M. tuberculosis* faster than the Lowenstein–Jensen based medium [4]. Middlebrook formulations are also easier to prepare in the routine laboratory and can be used in Petri dishes for isolation of mixed cultures and drug susceptibility testing.

When laboratories rely primarily on solid media, it will take a minimum of 3 weeks to produce colonies of *M. tuberculosis*. Additionally, neither of these solid media is ideal for all strains of AFB. For primary isolation, therefore, many laboratories use a non-selective Lowenstein–Jensen medium with selective Middlebrook medium.

*(b) Liquid media*

Liquid media have been developed for enrichment of growth of small numbers of mycobacteria [59]. These media, either Middlebrook 7H9 or Dubos Tween albumin broth, have been used to isolate mycobacteria from uncontaminated specimens where the number of AFB tend to be low, such as cerebrospinal, pleural and peritoneal fluids. The use of DNA probes to identify *M. tuberculosis* from broth cultures and the increased growth rate of *M. tuberculosis* in these broths, has led to a recommendation that all mycobacterial cultures should include broth [12].

*(c) Biphasic media*

Biphasic media are commercially available (Becton–Dickinson, Cockeysville, MD). This system employs a modified Middlebrook 7H9 broth bottle attached to a media paddle which has one side of non-selective Middlebrook 7H11 and on the other side has chocolate agar and a modified Lowenstein–Jensen medium. After inoculation, the broth is periodically inverted to seed the solid media. This system maintains the appropriate $CO_2$ environment, does not require a special incubator, and has increased the total yield of *M. tuberculosis* by about 10%, producing colonies about 5–6 days earlier than culture on solid media [60,61]. The biphasic system is, however, more costly than conventional cultures and cannot be used for antimicrobial drug testing.

### (d) Radiometric media

The radiometric broth method for AFB isolation was developed in the late 1970s and represents the most significant improvement for the rapid isolation of *M. tuberculosis* and other mycobacteria [1,62]. This system is commercially available from Becton–Dickinson, Towson, MD, USA, as the Bactec 460, and utilizes a 7H11 broth with $^{14}$C-palmitic acid as a substrate. As mycobacteria multiply, $^{14}CO_2$ is liberated into the bottle and can be detected. Detection time is directly proportional to the number of metabolically active mycobacteria present. The metabolic rate is influenced by the type of specimen, number of organisms, therapy status of the patient, decontamination procedure and incubation temperature. The growth of AFB, subsequently identified as *M. tuberculosis*, in smear positive specimens can be detected in about 9 days [63], and in smear negative specimens in about 14 days [64]. These data compare with 20 days or more for 7H11 agar. Once growth is detected within a Bactec bottle, organisms can be identified from a centrifuged pellet with either DNA probes or HPLC [6,65].

A survey of reference mycobacteriology laboratories reported on coupling of this radiometric method with rapid identification methodology. The time to reporting the isolation and identification of *M. tuberculosis* was 22 ± 9 days compared with 31 ± 8 days for solid media with rapid identification [56]. The time to detection was somewhat longer than expected, probably because results from laboratories which performed DNA probe identifications were not separated from NAP users. In another study in which the radiometric system was coupled with commercially available DNA probes for *M. tuberculosis* complex, positive cultures in AFB smear positive specimens were reported in an average of 8 days and AFB smear negative specimens in 23 days [66].

Although isolation of *M. tuberculosis* from blood is rare, a specialized radiometric bottle (Bactec 13A medium) can be used for the isolation of mycobacterium from blood. This medium has been shown to be superior to lysis–centrifugation for isolation of TB and MAI [67].

This information clearly indicates the advantages of using the radiometric system, especially in areas where TB is a significant problem. Despite this, there are some caveats on the routine use of the radiometric system: it is more labor intensive; it requires use and disposal of $^{14}$C; some tubercle bacilli isolates and specimens with mixed mycobacterial species will only be detected on agar slants, therefore some laboratories still use Lowenstein–Jensen slants as backup to the Bactec; and though rare, false-positive cultures have been found due to improper sterilization of needles [68].

## 7.6 *MYCOBACTERIUM TUBERCULOSIS* SUSCEPTIBILITY TESTING

Resistance to TB agents was recognized soon after their introduction, and by the early 1960s standardized methods for antimicrobial susceptibility testing were developed [34,69]. It is now established that any population of *M. tuberculosis* has a defined number of spontaneous drug-resistant mutants and that these chromosomal mutations cannot be transferred from strain to strain [70]. The chromosomal changes responsible for isoniazid (INH) and rifampin resistance have recently been described [71–73]. In clinical practice, the use of a single agent increases the chance of selection for a resistant mutant and, accordingly, multiple drug therapy is recommended [74].

The probability of selection for an INH and rifampin resistant mutant is in the order of $10^{14}$ which exceeds the number of organisms found in a TB cavity ($\pm 10^{10}$) [75]. This means that, within a cavitary lesion, the chance of one *M. tuberculosis* carrying resistance mutations to both these agents is extremely low unless there has been selection pressure of ineffective treatment. This selection is demonstrated by the cases of multi-drug-resistance in New York City where previous treatment was significantly associated with drug resistance [76]. For a more detailed discussion of these issues, see chapters 3, 12 and 13.

### 7.6.1 Indications for susceptibility testing

Routine laboratory susceptibility testing of primary TB isolates had not generally been suggested unless drug resistance in a particular community exceeded 5% [4,74]. The American Thoracic Society recommended susceptibility testing on TB isolates from persons thought to be at high risk of infection with drug resistant organisms; patients with a history of previous TB chemotherapy; foreign-born patients; contacts of known or suspected resistant cases and from persons with life threatening forms of TB [7].

These suggestions, however, were made prior to the current increases in resistant TB as prominently demonstrated in New York City. There, between 1989 and 1993, TB drug resistance rose from 6% to 26% for INH, from less than 1% to 22% for rifampin and from 5% to 19% for combined INH and rifampin resistance [75–78]. Accordingly, CDC has recently recommended that susceptibility tests should be performed on all primary isolates [77]. Clinicians should also ensure *M. tuberculosis* susceptibility tests are carried out for patients:

- who fail to respond after 3 months of treatment;
- who do not convert to having negative smears after 3 months of treatment with regimes that include INH and rifampin or 5 months for treatment without INH and rifampin;

- whose smears demonstrate increasing numbers of AFB after an initial decrease;
- whose cultures do not become negative after 4–6 months;
- who relapse.

### 7.6.2 Defining drug resistance

TB susceptibility testing has three main goals. It provides data on which drugs should be used in treatment; screens for drug resistance; and measures the incidence and prevalence of resistance within a community. To utilize the laboratory results of susceptibility tests better, it is necessary to understand the terms used in defining resistance.

Resistance of TB to a particular drug is defined as 'a decrease in sensitivity of sufficient degree to be reasonably certain that the strain concerned is different from a sample of wild strains of human type that have never come into contact with the drug' [75]. Resistance of an isolate from a patient who has not received treatment is called primary drug resistance (PDR). Resistance of isolates from a patient who received or is receiving therapy is termed acquired resistance. The latter is usually caused by ineffective or noncompliant use of chemotherapy. Wild TB strains have never been in contact with treatment agents and these exhibit very little variation in minimum inhibitory concentrations to a particular agent.

Critical proportion is the proportion of organisms within a population which exhibit resistance to a particular agent. This proportion has been set at 1% or more, which is determined by quantitative culture of a strain in media with and without antimycobacterial agents. Critical concentrations for each agent are defined as the amount of drug which inhibits the wild strains. Although these concentrations are above the usual minimum inhibitory concentrations, they are not related to serum or tissue levels. Therefore a resistant strain of *M. tuberculosis* is defined as one which demonstrates 1% or more growth in the presence of an antimycobacterial agent which is at or above the critical concentration.

### 7.6.3 Susceptibility methodology

Susceptibility tests can be performed either directly, from a smear positive specimen, or indirectly, from the growth of colonies from the specimen. The former has the advantage of measuring the sensitivity prior to cultivation on laboratory media. The direct method also produces results more rapidly but because of uncertainty on the species of mycobacterium, less control of the viable inoculum size and results that require confirmation with an indirect test, the direct test is not generally utilized.

Three methods make use of critical concentrations to define resistance and can be performed directly or indirectly [4,5,76].

The absolute concentration method determines if 1% or more of an inoculum will grow after being cultured on media containing critical concentrations of a drug on the plate. It requires growth of the patient strain on drug free medium to demonstrate the viability but does not compare the colony numbers on drug free and drug containing media so that the inoculum must be carefully standardized.

The resistance ratio is similar to the absolute concentration method except that the patient strain is compared with the growth of a standard laboratory strain. Results are reported as the ratio of the MIC of the patient strain to that of the laboratory strain. A patient strain with a ratio of 8:1 is considered resistant, while 4:1 is suggestive of resistance. This method is more tolerant to variations in concentrations of drugs within different batches of media.

The proportion method compares the growth of a patient strain in the presence and absence of a drug. If 1% or more of the inoculum produces colonies on media that contains an agent at the critical concentration compared with controls, the isolate is considered to be resistant. This method is the most popular in the USA and is relatively simple to perform and interpret.

A Bactec based adaptation for the proportion method has been shown to correlate well with the agar based test for susceptibility to INH, streptomycin, ethambutol, rifampin and pyrazinamide [5,74]. This method compares the growth of a patient isolate in the presence of the agent to a 1:100 dilution of the same strain in which no drug is present. If the difference in growth index values between two consecutive days in the drug containing vial is less than that in the control, the strain is susceptible (< 1% of control); if it is greater than the control it is resistant (< 1% of control) and if it is equal to the control it is borderline (=1% of control). Pyrazinamide susceptibility testing is also available in this system compared with an undiluted control. Methods to test other drugs have been supplied by the manufacturer [74]. The susceptibility results using this method are available in about 10 days.

A multicenter Bactec trial has been reported showing that the susceptibility results were completed in 11–23 days compared with 33–42 days for conventional susceptibility tests [62]. A study of state health department facilities demonstrated a completion time of $31 \pm 11$ days when isolation and susceptibility testing was done exclusively on the Bactec. This compares favorably with the completion time of $36 \pm 9$ days for Bactec isolation of *M. tuberculosis* with agar based susceptibility tests and $48 \pm 13$ days for exclusively agar based testing [56]. Although these results are slower than previous reports of completion time for isolation and susceptibility testing of 21 days, the Bactec is faster overall than conventional testing.

Susceptibility testing based on the critical concentration and critical proportion is more qualitative and may not be sensitive enough to detect emerging resistance or to guide a clinician who is treating a patient with multi-drug-resistant TB [75]. In these settings, an MIC determination should be requested. This can be done in the USA through the Myco-bacteriology Laboratory at the National Jewish Center for Immunology and Respiratory Medicine, 1400 Jackson Street, Denver, CO 80206. In other countries, consultation should be made through local health officials.

### 7.6.4 Drug levels

There may also be a need to monitor the drug levels of anti-TB agents in the serum or urine. This is necessary when there is doubt about the absorption or elimination of the drugs (e.g. kidney or gastrointestinal disease), if the therapeutic range of a drug is very close to the toxic range (e.g. cycloserine), or if there is doubt about a patient's compliance with drug therapy. This can also be requested at the National Jewish Center through the Infectious Disease Pharmacokinetics Laboratory (telephone 800 423-8891 extension 1427). In other countries, consultation should be made through local health officials.

## 7.7 RAPID METHODS FOR THE LABORATORY DIAGNOSIS OF TUBERCULOSIS

### 7.7.1 Antigen/antibody tests

Many studies on the rapid diagnosis of TB have focused on the detection of mycobacterial antigens or antibodies [79,80]. Generally, these sero-logical tests have shown mixed results and the assays have found little application in the routine mycobacteriology laboratory. Nonetheless, in the developing world, where the prevalence of TB infection may be very high, these methods may be of value. In these settings, tests can be designed to be performed simply and with high positive predictive value [81–83]. Especially for TB meningitis, where smears are usually negative and culture has been shown to be only 50% successful, a sensitive and specific serological assay would be significant [79]. More recently, a number of new antigens for use in the serodiagnosis of TB have been described. These include antigens referred to as P32, 85B and antigen 5. P32 antibody has been reported to be potentially useful in discriminating active from treated pulmonary TB [84] as was reported for 85B [85]. Using a combination of antigen 5 and 3 glycolipid antigen antibody assays, any one positive was found in 58% of smear positive cases, 32% of smear negative culture positive cases, 9% of inactive cases and 0.7% of normals [86].

A test for tuberculostearic acid, a constituent of the mycobacteria cell wall, has been used to detect *M. tuberculosis* in CSF specimens and shown to have sensitivity and specificity of 95% and 91%, respectively [87]. Unfortunately this test requires sophisticated and expensive equipment. Requests for tuberculostearic acid testing can be made in the USA to the CDC (telephone 404 639-3421). Pang *et al.* [88] reported the use of a tuber-culostearic acid assay of bronchial aspirate or bronchoalveolar lavage fluid as a tool for rapid diagnosis of smear negative pulmonary TB. The test was positive in 26 of 29 eventually culture positive patients but could not distinguish between species of mycobacteria.

A surrogate marker, adenosine deaminase, an enzyme produced by lymphocytes, has been shown to predict TB meningitis and pleural infections [89,90]. The test is easy to perform, inexpensive, but is by definition nonspecific. Despite sensitivity and specificity above 90%, the test is not widely available.

### 7.7.2 Nucleic acid tests

Nucleic acid probes and amplification of specific DNA or RNA sequences are providing a new opportunity to identify *M. tuberculosis* rapidly [91,92]. Amplification of specific nucleic acid sequences can be accomplished by various combinations of polymerase enzymes. Within hours, thousands of copies of genus or species specific nucleic acid sequences can be produced which are easily detected as TB markers. At least six systems are currently under commercial development. The Roche PCR system for identification of *M. tuberculosis* is commercially available through the Roche Center for Molecular Biology (telephone 800 872-5727). A preliminary report demonstrated an overall sensitivity and specificity of 85% and more than 95%, but detected only 63% in smear negative culture positive sputa [93].

Gen-Probe has developed a transcriptional amplification technique which uses highly conserved *M. tuberculosis* ribosomal RNA as probe targets that are amplified by interaction of their probe with reverse transcriptase and RNA polymerase [94]. This system should be able to produce $10^5$ copies of the rRNA within 15 minutes compared with 1.5 hours for PCR to produce an equivalent amount of product. Preliminary studies on this system (currently submitted to the FDA) demonstrated sensitivity and specificity in the 90% and over 95% ranges, respectively [95,96]. A Swiss report confirms the high sensitivity and specificity of this assay used directly on respiratory specimens [96a]. Discrepant positivity seems to occur with the newly described species *M. celatum* in which eight of 20 strains resulted in a cross reactive gene probe assay [97]. PCR development has led to other amplification techniques and the literature contains many papers specifically on the identification of *M. tuberculosis*. Performance characteristics have varied widely [98–101].

This information emphasizes that for any of the nucleic acid amplification techniques to be readily adopted by the mycobacteriology laboratory, there is a need to: optimize all steps of the assay including sample preparation, reaction conditions and quality control; establish standard operating procedures; and perform large clinical studies so that sensitivity and specificity of the test can be established. It is not surprising, therefore, that a blind comparison of seven laboratories using PCR resulted in substantial ranges of sensitivity and specificity [102].

### 7.7.3 Sensitivity testing

Novel approaches to perform rapid *M. tuberculosis* susceptibility testing have also been reported. Jacobs *et al.* have developed a method which enables the laboratory to test a patient isolate of *M. tuberculosis* against any drug and obtain results in hours [103]. In their approach, *M. tuberculosis* is infected with mycobacteriophage that have been constructed to contain the firefly luciferase gene. Within minutes of infecting the *M. tuberculosis* strain with these phage, luciferase activity can be detected. A growing *M. tuberculosis* produces light, while an inhibited organism does not. Preliminary data has shown this system can detect resistance or susceptibility of TB strains to rifampin, INH or streptomycin.

Other groups have localized specific *M. tuberculosis* mutations, responsible for resistance to INH and rifampin. These sites may be used as amplification targets and provide a rapid method for testing the susceptibility of an isolates to these drugs [71–73].

### 7.8 CONCLUSION

The worldwide problem of TB along with advances in nucleic acid technology have made it possible to envision dramatic changes in the laboratory diagnosis of this disease [22,89,104]. Within sight are diagnostic tests to identify *M. tuberculosis* which can be done rapidly with results in hours or days, have excellent sensitivity and specificity and can be performed in a cost effective manner. In all likelihood, within the total clinical microbiology area, the mycobacteriology laboratory will be at the forefront in the applications of molecular diagnostics.

### REFERENCES

1. Good, R.C. and Mastro, T.D. (1989) The modern mycobacteriology laboratory. How it can help the clinician. *Clin Chest Med*, **10**, 315–22.
2. Centers for Disease Control (1989) A strategic plan for the elimination of tuberculosis in the United States. *MMWR*, **38 (S-3)**, 9–15.
3. Centers for Disease Control (1992) National action plan to combat multidrug-resistant tuberculosis. *MMWR*, **41 (RR-11)**, 1–71.
4. Kent, P.T. and Kubica, G.P. (1985) *Public Health Mycobacteriology – A Guide for the Level III Laboratory*, U.S. Department of Health and Human Services/Public Health Service/Centers for Disease Control, Atlanta, GA.
5. Roberts, G.D., Koneman, E.W. and Kim, Y.K. (1991) *Mycobacterium*, in *Manual of Clinical Microbiology*, 5th edn (eds A. Balows, W. Hausler *et al.*), *American Society for Microbiology*, Washington, DC, pp. 304–33.
6. Isenberg, H.D. (1992) *Mycobacteriology. Clinical Microbiology Procedures Handbook*, American Society for Microbiology, Washington, DC, pp. 3.0.1–3.16.4.

7. Bass, J.B., Farer, L.S., Hopewell, P.C. *et al.* (1990) Diagnostic standards and classification of tuberculosis. *Am Rev Respir Dis*, **142**, 725–35.

8. Richardson, J.H. and Barkley, W.E. (eds) (1988) *Biosafety in Microbiological and Biomedical Laboratories*, U.S. Department of Health and Human Services, Washington, DC.

9. Dooley, S.W., Castro, K.G., Hutton, M.D. *et al.* (1990) Guidelines for the prevention of transmission of tuberculosis in health care settings with special focus on HIV related issues. *MMWR*, **39 (RR-17)**, 1–29.

10. Bauer, S., Alpert, L.I., DiSalvo, A.F. *et al.* (1991) *Protection of Laboratory Workers from Infectious Disease Transmitted by Blood, Body Fluids, and Tissue*, National Committee for Clinical Laboratory Standards Laboratory Safety, **11**(14), pp. 1–214.

11. New York City Department of Health Codes, Article 13, Clinical Laboratories, Section 13.25–13.28, 1992.

12. Tenover, F.C., Crawford, J.T., Huebner, R.E. *et al.* (1993) The resurgence of tuberculosis: is your laboratory ready? *J Clin Microbiol*, **31**, 767–70.

13. Sneath, P.H. (1986) *Bergey's Manual of Systematic Bacteriology Volume 2, Section 16 Mycobacteria*, Williams & Wilkins, Baltimore, MD.

14. Barksdale, L. and Kim, K.S. (1977) Mycobacterium. *Bacteriol Rev*, **41**, 217–372.

15. Harshey, R.M. and Ramakrishnan, T. (1977) Rate of ribonucleic acid chain growth in *Mycobacterium tuberculosis* H$_{37}$R$_v$. *J Bacteriol*, **129**, 616–22.

16. Wayne, L.G. (1982) Microbiology of tubercle bacillus. *Am Rev Respir Dis,* **125**, 31–41.

17. Levinson, W.E. and Jawetz, E. (eds) (1992) *Medical Microbiology and Immunology, Mycobacteria*, 2nd edn, Appleton & Lange, East Norwalk, CT, p. 113.

18. Gross, W. and Wayne, L.G. (1970) Nucleic acid homology in the genus *Mycobacterium. J Bacteriol*, **104**, 630–4.

19. Des Prez, R.M. and Heim, C.R. (1991) Mycobacterium tuberculosis, in *Principles and Practice of Infectious Diseases*, 3rd edn (eds G.L. Mandell, R.G. Douglas and J.E. Bennett), Churchill Livingstone, New York, pp. 1877–1906.

20. David, H.L., Jahan, M.T., Jumin, A. *et al.* (1978) Numerical taxonomy analysis of *Mycobacterium africanum. Int J Syst Bacteriol*, **28**, 464–73.

21. Braunstein, H., Hicks, L. and Konyn, C. (1990) *Mycobacterium africanum* and other members of the *Mycobacterium tuberculosis* complex. American Society of Clinical Pathology – Microbiology No. MB 90-4, **33**, 1–5.

22. De Cock, K.M., Soro, B., Coulibaly, I.M. *et al.* (1992) Tuberculosis and HIV infection in sub-Saharan Africa. *JAMA*, **268**, 1581–7.

23. Hobby, G.L., Holman, A.P., Iseman, M.D. *et al.* (1973) Enumeration of tubercle bacilli in sputum of patients with pulmonary tuberculosis. *Antimicrob Agents Chemother*, **4**, 94–104.

24. Rickman, T. and Moyer, N. (1980) Increased sensitivity of acid-fast smears. *J Clin Microbiol*, **11**, 618–20.

25. Bogen, E. (1941) Detection of tubercle bacilli by fluorescence microscopy. *Am Rev Tuberc*, **44**, 267–71.

26. Richards, O.W., Kline, E.K. and Leach, R.E. (1941) Demonstration of tubercle by fluorescence microscopy. *Am Rev Tuberc*, **44**, 255–66.

27. Lipsky, B.A., Gates, J., Tenover, F.C. *et al.* (1984) Factors affecting the clinical value of microscopy for acid fast bacilli. *Rev Infect Dis*, **6**, 214–22.

28. Levy, H., Feldman, C., Sacho, H. *et al.* (1989) A reevaluation of sputum microscopy and culture in the diagnosis of pulmonary tuberculosis. *Chest*, **95**, 1193–7.

29. Blair, E., Brown, G., Tull, A. *et al.* (1976) Computer files and analyses of laboratory data from tuberculosis patients. II. Analyses of six years' data on sputum specimens. *Am Rev Respir Dis*, **113**, 427–32.

30. Kim, T., Blackman, R., Heatwole, K. *et al.* (1984) Acid fast bacilli in sputum smears of patients with pulmonary tuberculosis. *Am Rev Respir Dis*, **129**, 264–8.

31. Barnes, P.F, Verdegem, T.D., Vachon, L.A. *et al.* (1988) Chest roentgenogram in pulmonary tuberculosis: new data on an old test. *Chest*, **94**, 316–20.

32. Strumpf, I., Tsang, A., and Sayre, J. (1979) Re-evaluation of sputum staining for the diagnosis of pulmonary tuberculosis. *Am Rev Respir Dis*, **119**, 599–602.

33. Murray, P.R., Elmore, C. and Krogstad, D.J. (1980) The acid fast stain: a specific and predictive test for mycobacterial disease. *Ann Intern Med*, **92**, 512–13.

34. Canetti, G. (1965) Present aspects of bacterial resistance in tuberculosis. *Am Rev Respir Dis*, **92**, 687–703.

35. Boyd, J. and Marr, J. (1975) Decreasing reliability of acid fast smear techniques detection of tuberculosis. *Ann Intern Med*, **82**, 489–92.

36. Saslaw, S. and Perkins, R.L. (1962) Gastric smear for AFB with presumptive diagnosis of tuberculosis. *Am J Med Sci*, **243**, 470–7.

37. Strumpf, I.J., Tsang, A.Y., Schork, M.A. *et al.* (1976) Reliability of gastric smears by auramine-rhodamine stain for diagnosis of tuberculosis. *Am Rev Respir Dis*, **114**, 971–6.

38. Berean, K. and Roberts, F.J. (1988) The reliability of acid fast stained smears of gastric aspirate specimens. *Tubercle*, **69**, 205–8.

39. Elliot, R.C. and Reichel, J. (1963) The efficacy of sputum specimens obtained by nebulization versus gastric aspirates in the bacteriologic diagnosis of pulmonary tuberculosis. *Am Rev Respir Dis*, **88**, 223–7.

40. Jones, F.L. (1966) The relative efficacy of spontaneous sputa, aerosol-induced sputa and gastric aspirates in the bacteriologic diagnosis of pulmonary tuberculosis. *Dis Chest*, **50**, 403–8.

41. Danek, S.J. and Bower, J.S. (1979) Diagnosis of pulmonary tuberculosis by flexible fiberoptic bronchoscopy. *Am Rev Respir Dis*, **119**, 677–9.

42. Wallace, J.M, Deutsch, A.L., Harrel, J.H. *et al.* (1981) Bronchoscopy and transbronchial biopsy of patients with suspected active tuberculosis. *Am J Med*, **70**, 1189–94.

43. de Fracia, J., Curuil, V., Vidal R. *et al.* (1988) Diagnostic value of bronchoalveolar lavage in suspected pulmonary tuberculosis. *Chest*, **93**, 329–32.

44. Chan, H., Sun, A. and Hoheisel, G. (1990) Bronchoscopic aspiration and bronchoalveolar lavage in the diagnosis of sputum smear-negative pulmonary tuberculosis. *Lung*, **168**, 215–20.

45. Al-Kassimi, F.A., Azhar, M., Al-Majed, S. *et al.* (1991) Diagnostic role of fiberoptic bronchoscopy in tuberculosis in the presence of typical X-ray pictures and adequate sputum. *Tubercle*, **72**, 145–8.

46. Kennedy, D., Lewis, W. and Barnes, P. (1992) Yield of bronchoscopy for the diagnosis of tuberculosis in patients with human immunodeficiency virus infection. *Chest*, **102**, 1040–4.

47. Salzman, S., Schindel, M., Aranda, C. *et al.* (1992) The role of bronchoscopy in the diagnosis of pulmonary tuberculosis in patients at risk for HIV infection. *Chest*, **102**, 143–6.

48. Morris, C.D.W. (1991) Sputum examination in the screening and diagnosis of pulmonary tuberculosis in the elderly. *Quart J Med*, **296**, 999–1004.

49. Barnes, P., Bloch, A., Davidson, P. *et al.* (1991) Tuberculosis in patients with human immunodeficiency virus infection. *N Engl J Med*, **324**, 1644–50.

50. Klein, N., Duncanson, F., Lenox, T. *et al.* (1989) Use of mycobacterial smears in the diagnosis of pulmonary tuberculosis in AIDS/ARC patients. *Chest*, **95**, 1190–2.

51. Horsburgh, R.C. (1991) *Mycobacterium avium* complex infection in the acquired immunodeficiency syndrome. *N Engl J Med*, **324**, 1332–38.

52. Yajko, D.M., Sanders, C.K., Nassos, P.S. *et al.* (1993) *Predictive Value of the Acid-fast Smear for Tuberculosis in a Setting where Mycobacterium avium Complex is a Common Isolate,* American Society for Microbiology, Atlanta, GA.

53. Klein, R. and Motyl, M. (1991) *Frequency of pulmonary tuberculosis in patients undergoing sputum induction for diagnosis of suspected Pneumocystis carinii pneumonia.* 7th International Conference on AIDS, Florence, Italy, World Health Organization.

54. Munt, P.W. (1972) Miliary tuberculosis in chemotherapy era with clinical review in 69 American adults. *Medicine*, **51**, 139–55.

55. Kiehn, T.E. and Cammarata, R. (1986) Laboratory diagnosis of mycobacterial infections in patients with acquired immunodeficiency syndrome. *J Clin Microbiol*, **24**, 708–11.

56. Huebner, R.E., Good, R.C. and Tokars, J.I. (1993) Current practices in mycobacteriology: results of a survey of state public health laboratories. *J Clin Microbiol*, **31**, 771–5.

57. Laszlo, A. and Siddiqi, S.H. (1984) Evaluation of a rapid radiometric differentiation test for the *Mycobacterium tuberculosis* complex by selective inhibition with p-nitro-a-acetylamino-B-hydroxy-propiophenone. *J Clin Microbiol*, **19**, 694–8.

58. Iseman, M.D. (1992) *Mycobacteriology. Syllabus of the Clinical Management and Control of Tuberculosis, 28–30 October 1992.* New York City Department of Health, New York.

59. Martin, T., Cheke, D. and Natyshak, I. (1989). Broth culture: the modern 'guinea pig' for the isolation of mycobacteria. *Tubercle*, **70**, 53–4.

60. D'Amato, R.F., Isenberg, H.D., Hochstein, L. *et al.* (1991) Evaluation of the Roche Septi-chek AFB system for recovery of mycobacteria. *J Clin Microbiol*, **29**, 2906–8.

61. Isenberg, H.D., D'Amato, R.F., Heifets, L. *et al.* (1991) Collaborative feasibility study of a biphasic system (Roche Septi-chek AFB) for rapid detection and isolation of mycobacteria. *J Clin Microbiol*, **29**, 1719–22.

62. Middlebrook, G., Reggiardo, Z. and Tigerit, W.D. (1977) Automatable radiometric detection of growth of *Mycobacterium tuberculosis* in selective media. *Am Rev Respir Dis*, **115**, 1066–9.

63. Roberts, G.D., Goodman, N.L., Heifets, L. *et al.* (1983) Evaluation of the BACTEC radiometric method for recovery of *Mycobacterium tuberculosis* from acid fast smear-positive specimens. *J Clin Microbiol*, **18**, 689–96.

64. Morgan, M.A., Horstmeier, C.D., DeYoung, D.R. *et al.* (1983) Comparison of a radiometric method (BACTEC) and conventional culture media for recovery of mycobacteria from smear-negative specimens. *J Clin Microbiol*, **18**, 385–8.

65. Ellner, P.D., Kiehn, T.E., Cammarata, R. *et al.* (1988) Rapid detection and identification of pathogenic mycobacteria by combining radiometric and nucleic acid probe methods. *J Clin Microbiol*, **26**, 1349–52.

66. Callihan, D.R., Christie, J.D., Ware, T.R. *et al.* (1993) *Growth in BACTEC 12B Medium with Direct GenProbe Identification Permit Timely Identification of Mycobacterium tuberculosis and M. avium Complex*, American Society for Microbiology, Atlanta, GA.

67. Witebsky, F.G., Keiser, J.F., Conville, P.S. *et al.* (1988) Comparison of BACTEC 13A medium and Du Pont isolator for detection of mycobacteremia. *J Clin Microbiol*, **26**, 1501–5.

68. Small, P.M., McClenny, N.B., Singh, S.P. *et al.* (1992) Molecular strain typing of *Mycobacterium tuberculosis* to identify cross-contamination in the mycobacteriology laboratory and identification of procedures to minimize occurrence of false-positive cultures. *J Clin Microbiol*, **31**, 1677–82.

69. Canetti, G., Froman, S., Grosset, J. *et al.* (1963) Mycobacterial laboratory methods for testing drug sensitivity and resistance. *Bull WHO*, **29**, 565–78.

70. David, H.L. (1980) Drug resistance in *M. tuberculosis* and other mycobacteria. *Clin Chest Med*, **1**, 227–30.

71. Zhang, Y., Heym, B., Allen, B. *et al.* (1992) The catalase-peroxidase gene and isoniazid resistance of *Mycobacterium tuberculosis*. *Nature*, **358**, 591–3.

72. Banerjee, A., Dubnau, E., Quemard, A. *et al.* (1994) *inhA*, a gene encoding a target for isoniazid and ethionamide in *Mycobacterium tuberculosis*. *Science*, **263**, 227–30.

73. Telenti, A., Lowrie, D., Matter, L. *et al.* (1993) Detection of rifampicin resistance mutations in *Mycobacterium tuberculosis*. *Lancet*, **341**, 647–50.

74. Mitchison, D.A. (1979) Basic mechanisms of chemotherapy. *Chest*, **76**, 771–84.

75. Heifets, L.B. (1991) *Drug Susceptibility Tests in the Management of Chemotherapy of Tuberculosis*, CRC Press, London, pp. 89–121.

76. Frieden, T.R., Sterling, T., Pablos-Mendez, A. *et al.* (1993) The emergence of drug-resistant tuberculosis in New York City. *N Engl J Med*, **328**, 521–6.

77. New York City Department of Health (1990) *Bureau of Laboratories Survey of Mycobacteriology Laboratories in New York City*.

78. Centers for Disease Control (1993) Initial therapy for tuberculosis in the era of multidrug resistance: Recommendations of the Advisory Council for the Elimination of Tuberculosis. *MMWR*, **42** (**RR-7**), 1–8.

79. Daniel, T.M. (1987) New approaches to the rapid diagnosis of tuberculous meningitis. *J Infect Dis*, **155**, 599–602.

80. Daniel, T.M. (1989) Rapid diagnosis of tuberculosis: Laboratory techniques applicable in developing countries. *Rev Infect Dis*, **11**, 471–8.

81. Daniel, T.M., De Murillo, G.L., Sawyer, J.A. *et al.* (1986) Field evaluation of enzyme-linked immunosorbent assay for serodiagnosis of tuberculosis. *Am Rev Respir Dis*, **134**, 662–5.

82. Mehta, A., Rodrigues, C., Bhatt, T.R. *et al.* (1993) *LAM Antigen and Antigen 60 in Serological Diagnosis of Mycobacterial Infection*, American Society for Microbiology, Atlanta, GA.

83. Banica, D., Algeorge, G. and Balasoiu, M. (1993) *Evaluation of an Immunoblot Test for the Serological Diagnosis of Tuberculosis*, American Society for Microbiology, Atlanta, GA.

84. Drowart, A., Huygen, K., De Bruyn, J. *et al.* (1991) Antibody levels to whole culture filtrate antigens and to purified P32 during treatment of smear-positive tuberculosis. *Chest*, **100**, 685–7.
85. Van Vooren, J.-P., Drowart, A., De Bruyn, J. *et al.* (1992) Humoral responses against the 85A and 85B antigens of *Mycobacterium bovis* BCG in patients with leprosy and tuberculosis. *J Clin Microbiol*, **30**, 1608–10.
86. Chan, S.L., Reggiardo, Z., Daniel, T.M. *et al.* (1990) Serodiagnosis of tuberculosis using an ELISA with antigen 5 and a hemagglutination assay with glyco-lipid antigens. *Am Rev Respir Dis*, **142**, 385–90.
87. Brooks, J.B., Daneshvar, M.I., Haberberger, R.L. *et al.* (1990) Rapid diagnosis of tuberculous meningitis by frequency-pulsed electron-capture gas-liquid chromatography detection of carboxylic acids in cerebrospinal fluid. *J Clin Microbiol*, **28**, 989–97.
88. Pang, J.A., Chan, H.S., Chan, C.Y. *et al.* (1989) A tuberculostearic acid assay in the diagnosis of sputum smear-negative pulmonary tuberculosis. *Ann Intern Med*, **111**, 650–4.
89. Banales, J.L., Pineda, P.R., Fitzgerald, J.M. *et al.* (1991) Adenosine deaminase in the diagnosis of tuberculosis pleural effusions. *Chest*, **99**, 355–7.
90. Ribera, E., Martinez-Vazquez, J.M., Ocana, I. *et al.* (1987) Activity of adenosine deaminase in cerebrospinal fluid for the diagnosis and follow-up of tuberculous meningitis in adults. *J Infect Dis*, **155**, 603–7.
91. Desmond, E.P. (1992) Molecular approaches to the identification of myco-bacteria. *Clin Microbiol Newsletter*, **14**, 145–2.
92. Wolcott, M.J. (1992) Advances in nucleic acid-based detection methods. *Clin Microbiol Rev*, **5**, 370–86.
93. Tevere, V., Hocknell, J., Taurence, K. *et al.* (1993) *Direct Detection of Mycobacteria in Sputum using the PCR and Species Identification by a Colorimetric Microwell Plate Assay*, American Society for Microbiology, Atlanta, GA.
94. Jonas, V., Alden, M., Endozo, T. *et al.* (1993) *Rapid Direct Detection of Mycobacterium tuberculosis in Respiratory Specimens*, American Society for Microbiology, Atlanta, GA.
95. Curry, J.I., Wolfe, J.M. and Moore, D.F. (1993) *Detection and Identification of Mycobacterium tuberculosis Directly from Induced Sputum Specimens using Amplification of Ribosomal RNA*, American Society for Microbiology, Atlanta, GA.
96. Della-Latta, P., Waithe, E., Sorondo, G. *et al.* (1993) *RapidDetection of Mycobacterium tuberculosis Directly from Sputum by the Gen-Probe Amplified Mycobacterium tuberculosis Test*, American Society for Microbiology, Atlanta, GA.
96a. Phyffer, G.E., Kissling, P., Wirth, R. and Weber, R. (1994) Direct detection of *Mycobacterium tuberculosis* complex in respiratory specimens by a target-amplified test system. *J Clin Microbiol*, **32**, 918–23.
97. Butler, W.R., O'Connor, S.P., Yakrus, M.A. and Gross, W.M. (1994) Cross-reactivity of genetic probe for detection of *Mycobacterium tuberculosis* with newly described species *Mycobacterium celatum*. *J Clin Microbiol*, **32**, 536–8.
98. Eisenach, K.D., Sifford, M.D., Cave, M.D. *et al.* (1991) Detection of *Mycobacterium tuberculosis* in sputum samples using a polymerase chain reaction. *Am Rev Respir Dis*, **144**, 1160–3.
99. Savic, B., Sjobring, U., Alugupalli, S. *et al.* (1992) Evaluation of polymerase

chain reaction, tuberculostearic acid analysis, and direct microscopy for the detection of *Mycobacterium tuberculosis* in sputum. *J Infect Dis*, **166**, 1177–80.

100. Soini, H., Skurnik, M., Liippo, K. *et al.* (1992) Detection and identification of mycobacteria by amplification of a segment of the gene coding for the 32-kilodalton protein. *J Clin Microbiol*, **30**, 2025–8.

101. Forbes, B.A. and Hicks, K.E. (1993) Direct detection of *Mycobacterium tuberculosis* in respiratory specimens in a clinical laboratory by polymerase chain reaction. *J Clin Microbiol*, **31**, 1688–94.

102. Noordhoek, G.T., Kolk, A.H.J., Bjune, G. *et al.* (1994) Sensitivity amd specificity of PCR for detection of *Mycobacterium tuberculosis*: a blind comparison study using seven laboratories. *J Clin Microbiol*, **32**, 277–84.

103. Jacobs, W.R, Barletta, R.G., Udani, R. *et al.* (1993) Rapid assessment of drug susceptibilities of *Mycobacterium tuberculosis* by means of luciferase reporter phages. *Science*, **260**, 19–22.

104. Eisenach, K.D., Cave, M.D. and Crawford, J.T. (1993) PCR detection of *Mycobacterium tuberculosis*, in *Diagnositic Molecular Microbiology, Principles and Applications* (eds D.H. Persing *et al.*), American Society for Microbiology, Washington, DC, pp. 191–6.

# Tuberculin skin testing  8

Larry I. Lutwick

## 8.1 HISTORY

In 1891, Robert Koch, following his identification of the human tubercle bacillus, observed a skin reaction in animals that he felt could culminate in the development of an agent to treat TB [1]. Koch observed that animals already infected with *Mycobacterium tuberculosis* developed a self limited nodule at a skin inoculation site which differed from the progressive lesions produced in those animals not previously infected. He noted the same reaction with both live and killed bacilli and also with a concentrated, heat killed filtrate of organisms. This filtrate became referred to as old tuberculin (OT). Despite Koch's initial optimism, little success resulted using OT as a therapy in TB infections.

Snider [2] credits several early 20th century veterinarians as among the first to characterize the potential diagnostic use of OT. Eber, a German worker, found that more than 80% of cattle reacting to OT had lesions of TB at autopsy and more than 80% of those with no reaction had no lesions. Similar information was produced by Pearson in the USA. OT testing and prompt removal and slaughter of all reactors aided in the diminution of the disease in cattle.

An Austrian physician, Clemens von Pirquet, also represents an important figure in the use of tuberculin and delayed type hypersensitivity testing [3]. He coined the term allergy to describe the reaction to OT. He derived it from the Greek words for altered energy (*allos ergos*) and used the term anergy to refer to the lack of an immune reaction ('without energy'). Von Pirquet also suggested that anergy to OT could be caused by measles or develop during rapidly progressive TB.

A problem that eventually became obvious was lack of adequate standardization of the diagnostic tuberculin reagent. In 1934, Florence

Seibert developed a more purified, nonsensitizing product obtained by ammonium sulfate precipitation of OT. This material became referred to as purified protein derivative (PPD). Several years later, Seibert and Glenn [4] reported the preparation of a large lot of PPD (lot 49608) from the single strain of *M. tuberculosis*. This material became the international standard for PPD, referred to as PPD-S (for standard).

In addition to the standardization, both antigen dose and route needed uniformity. Furcolow and coworkers [5] found that a dose of 0.1 µg of PPD best distinguished the true positive (based on more than 5 mm of induration). This dosage is now referred to as 5 TU (tuberculin units). After the evaluation of a variety of tuberculin administration routes including cutaneous, percutaneous, conjunctival and subcutaneous, the Mantoux test (an intracutaneous test developed by the French physician Charles Mantoux) gradually became the preferred method. Here, the dose of PPD could be easily controlled and the degree of reaction readily quantitated.

## 8.2 CURRENTLY AVAILABLE SKIN TESTS FOR TUBERCULOSIS

There are two available techniques in general use for the application of a tuberculin test, the percutaneous multiple puncture and the intracutaneous Mantoux methods.

### 8.2.1 Percutaneous multiple puncture test

*(a) Administration forms*

This method delivers tuberculin into the skin by puncture with a device having points either coated with dried tuberculin or by application through a film of liquid tuberculin. A common form of this test is described by Rosenthal [6]. The test applicator (Figure 8.1) is a plastic handle attached to a stainless steel metal disc. Projecting from the disc are four 2 mm long prongs, or tines. Each prong has been dipped into OT-containing gum arabic and lactose as stabilizers and glycerin to prevent the OT film from flaking off. This method is usually referred to as the tine test. It is now available with either OT or PPD as the tuberculin antigen.

Other multiple puncture tests that have been used include the Sterneedle modification of the Heaf test and the MONO-VACC test [7]. The former uses a spring loaded gun with a sterile cartridge that delivers liquid tuberculin solution into the skin with six points. The latter uses a nine plastic point ring and liquid tuberculin. Liquid tuberculin is more concentrated and care must be taken not to inadvertently use it for Mantoux testing.

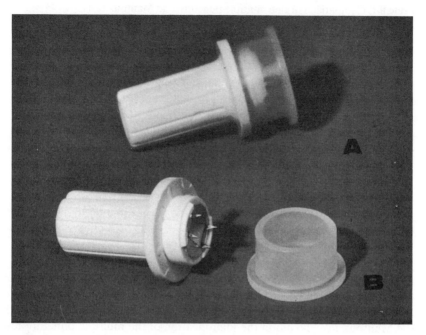

**Figure 8.1** The tuberculin tine test applicator: (A) unopened, (B) opened. Reproduced with permission of Professional Services, Lederle Laboratories, Pearl River, New York. © 1980, Lederle Laboratories. All rights reserved.

*(b) Advantages and disadvantages*

The advantages of these tests include ease of administration, stability and a very short administration time. The test can be easily used, therefore, in large scale screening programs, and may be used by less trained personnel. The comparisons of the tine test with the Mantoux test are shown in Table 8.1.

Because the amount of antigen which is inoculated cannot be precisely controlled, it is not considered to be as useful as other methods as a diagnostic test [8]. The variable delivery of tuberculin by a tine test may in part be explained by examining the tines using a scanning electron micrograph [9]. Substantial variation in the thickness of the tuberculin coating occurs and thickly coated tines do not deliver adequate antigen as reflected by smaller areas of induration. The time over which the applicator is in contact with the skin could also be a variable. Skin contact must be maintained for at least 1 second; 5 second applications do not seem to cause a real change in reactivity [10].

*(c) Measurement and reliability*

The multiple puncture test reaction is measured 48–72 hours after inoculation. If individual papules occur, the diameter of the largest single papule is

**Table 8.1** Comparison of tine multiple puncture and Mantoux tests

|  | Tine test | Mantoux test |
|---|---|---|
| Ease of administration | +++ | + |
| Time to prepare and give | < 10 seconds | 1–2 minutes |
| Cost | 99c | 35c |
| Technical skill needed | Minimal | Moderate |
| Hypodermic needle needed | – | + |
| Use | Large scale screening | Diagnosis of *Mycobacterial tuberculosis* exposure |
| Controlled antigen administration | ± | + |
| Need for light/heat protection | – | + |

recorded. If there is coalescence of individual papules, the longest diameter of coalescence is recorded. If a vesicular reaction occurs, it is recorded as such. Any reaction to a multiple puncture test should by confirmed with the Mantoux test. To aid in the identification of the multiple puncture test reaction, a card illustrating the kind of reactions that may occur can be distributed. Using this card and targeted instruction, a reporting compliance can be maximized with few false-negative tests [11].

Despite less control of the antigen inoculated, studies have compared this test with the intradermal Mantoux test relatively favorably. Badger, Breitwieser and Muench, using PPD positivity of more than 5 mm and tine positivity of 3 mm or more, found 90% agreement [12]. Sinclair and Johnston compared parallel tests in 190 subjects at 48, 72 and 96 hours. Of 1010 readings, 55% were Mantoux positive and 52% tine test positive [13]. The Tuberculin Subcommittee of the Research Committee of the British Thoracic Association [14], however, using identical definitions of reactivity in 307 subjects, found that only 32% of those who reacted to the Mantoux test had a positive tine test. The authors raised concern regarding the high proportion of presumed false-negative results in their study. This discordance compared with others was not clearly explained since Sinclair and Johnston present and cite data on almost 3000 subjects with 87–97% agreement of positives.

In 1977, a US Food and Drug Administration panel on skin test antigen recommended that multiple puncture tests provide no false-negative results in individuals shown to have a reactive Mantoux test. Sbarbaro subsequently stated that it would be unwise to use these devices unless there was adequate documentation that the sales lot of multiple puncture devices has been proved to have identified 100% of persons with a history of confirmed, culture positive TB who were simultaneously reactive to 5 TU PPD [15].

The American Academy of Pediatrics no longer recommends multiple puncture testing in children [15a].

### 8.2.2 Intracutaneous Mantoux test

*(a) Dosage forms*

Five TU has been defined as the delayed hypersensitivity activity contained in 0.1 μg of PPD-S delivered in 0.10 ml. Commercial PPD-S is standardized as the dosage of the product that is biologically equivalent to that in 5 TU PPD-S. That is, the induration is of equivalent size (+ 20%).

There are two other dosage forms of PPD available along with the 5 TU or Intermediate Strength form. These forms, First Strength (1 TU) and Second Strength (250 TU), respectively, do not contain 1/5 and 50 times the bioactivity of 5 TU. Rather they contain 1/5 and 50 times the antigen strength which is bioequivalent to 5 TU of PPD-S. Neither the 1 TU nor 250 TU dose forms require commercial evaluation of their activity. Likewise, neither of these products is particularly useful in the diagnosis of TB.

The 1 TU dose has been touted to be useful as an initial test in those who may be extraordinarily sensitive to tuberculin. These rare occurrences are not clearly diminished by the use of 1 TU. Reaction to 1 TU cannot be adequately interpreted because of the lack of standardization [8]. In addition, using a 1 TU PPD in an attempt to diminish cross reactions, it was reported that only half of 139 children with active TB had a 5 mm or greater induration and 25 of 35 children under the age of 2 years had no reaction [16].

The 250 TU dose reaction, likewise, cannot be adequately interpreted. Some individuals with active TB who are acutely ill and/or debilitated have a nonreactive 5 TU test yet still react to the 250 TU dose. Although Riebel [17] feels that this circumstance warrants its continued use in selected patients, some patients with TB can have a selective anergy to tuberculin. In other words, they will be nonreactive to any dose of tuberculin and still react to other antigens. In one study of 200 patients with active TB, 19 had a negative 250 TU but only three were completely anergic [18]. Therefore, a negative 250 TU cannot exclude TB. Care must be taken to ensure that neither the 1 TU nor 250 TU dosage form is inadvertently substituted for 5 TU.

*(b) Nontuberculous PPDs*

Other forms of PPD exist which are prepared from non-TB mycobacteria. These products include PPD-B (for Battey bacillus or *M. avium-intracellulare*), PPD-T (*M. bovis*), PPD-G (*M. scrofulaceum*) and PPD-Y (*M. kansasii*). They have not been found to be very useful as diagnostic tools.

Even using antigens felt to be bioequivalent to PPD-S, these preparations had too low a sensitivity and specificity to be useful [19].

### (c) Physical modifications of tuberculin

Tuberculin can adsorb on to glass and plastic, which may decrease the administered dose. To minimize this, PPD should not be transferred between containers and administration should be done as soon as possible once aspirated into a syringe. To further assist in minimizing adsorption, the non-ionic detergent Tween-80 (polysorbate 80) is added at 5 parts per million. The use of the detergent can not only minimize the adsorption of $^{14}$C-labeled PPD to syringes [20] but also decrease the 'false-negative' reaction rate of patients with active TB [21] using a 5 mm cutoff. In another study, a 5 TU dose without Tween-80 was reduced to 3 TU after standing in a syringe for 1 hour, 1.25 TU after 8 hours and less than 0.5 TU at 24 hours [22].

Tuberculin vials should be refrigerated, not frozen, and kept away from light. The antigen is thought to be more sensitive to the effect of light than heat. The effect can be seen with daylight and both fluorescent and UV light [23]. Comstock feels that storage of tuberculin in the refrigerator is based more on the fact that the light goes out when the door is closed, than on degradation at ambient temperatures [24].

### (d) Mantoux test administration

The Mantoux test should be done by a trained individual to ensure adequate inoculation. The test should be performed by the intradermal injection of 0.1 ml (5 TU) of PPD into the volar or dorsal surfaces of the forearm. Other areas can be used but the forearm is preferred using a site free from skin lesions and away from surface veins. The inoculation is made using a short, bluntly beveled 27 gauge needle (¼ to ½ inch long) and a tuberculin syringe. The fluid is delivered (Figure 8.2) with the bevel upward just below the surface of the skin. Care must be taken to maintain as flat an angle as possible to ensure intradermal administration. When performed correctly, a 6–10 mm wheal will appear at the time of injection. If an inadequate sized wheal develops or ecchymosis occurs, it is recommended that the test should be repeated at a separate site.

Although it is taught that errors in technique can be common causes for false-negative tests, this is not necessarily the case. Rhoades and Bryant [25] found that, in adults, not only were cutaneous reactions to 0.05 ml and 0.1 ml similar, but also differences in the sizes of reactions elicited by intradermal and subcutaneous tests were small. Subcutaneous tests, in fact, were often found to produce larger reactions (Figure 8.3). The borders of the reaction, however, may be less distinct and difficult to quantitate. Similar data on the subcutaneous route are available in children [26].

(a)

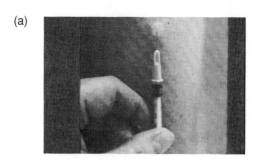

(b)

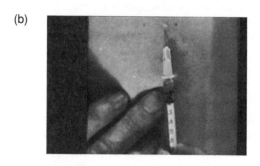

(c)

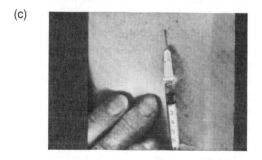

**Figure 8.2** Performance of the Mantoux test. (a) Inserting the filled tuberculin syringe into the volar surface of the forearm. (b) Using the tip of the needle to elevate the skin to maintain as flat an angle as possible while advancing the needle, beveled side up. (c) A wheal (6–10 mm) should develop at the time of injection. Reproduced with permission from *Journal of Respiratory Disease*, **11**(3), Cliggett Publications, Greenwich, CT, copyright 1990 [29].

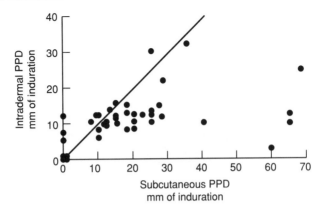

**Figure 8.3** Comparison of sizes of reactions in simultaneous testing with intradermal and subcutaneous injections of intermediate-strength tuberculin. Reproduced from *Chest* with permission of the American College of Chest Physicians, Northbrook, Illinois, copyright 1980 [25].

*(e) Techniques in reading the Mantoux test*

The test should be evaluated 48–72 hours after injection, though induration beyond this point is significant. The reading should be done using adequate lighting with the forearm partially flexed at the elbow. Measurements are based on induration, not erythema. The diameter of the induration is assessed transversely to the long axis of the arm. The results should be recorded as the dates of the inoculation and reading, name and strength of antigen and size of induration. The lot number of the antigen may also be recorded. A recorded result of negative or positive without the size of induration is never appropriate.

The degree of induration may be determined by inspection using side lighted palpation or the ballpoint pen technique. The latter has been advocated by Sokal [27] and proposed by a number of authors [28,29] as being superior to palpation and more reproducible than other methods. It is performed (Figure 8.4) by placing a pen away from the margin of the reaction and drawing toward the center of the reaction with enough pressure to indent the skin slightly. The pen should stop at the edge of the induration. The same procedure is repeated from the other side of the reaction. The amount of induration is then measured between the inside ends of the two lines. In a study of 806 healthy individuals [30], however, the pen technique may result in smaller degrees of induration than the palpation method. Strong conclusions regarding the reliability of either method are difficult to make since a true gold standard does not exist.

Tuberculin reactions can be measurable earlier than 48 hours. Although decisions are best made on results measured at 48–72 hours, strict adherence to this time restraint may result in prolonging hospitalization or allowing patients to interpret their own test results. It has been reported that the

(a)

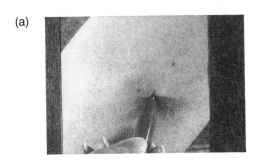

(b)

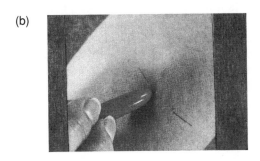

(c)

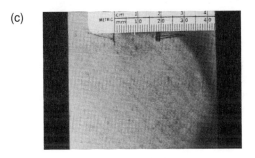

**Figure 8.4** Measuring the Mantoux reaction using the pen method. (a) Using the pen with enough pressure to slightly indent the skin drawing towards the induration. The pen will stop at the edge of the induration. (b) Marking the other side. (c) Measuring the reaction in millimeters. Reproduced with permission from *Journal of Respiratory Disease* 11(3), Cliggett Publications, Greenwich, CT, copyright 1990 [29].

degree of induration at 24 hours was a valuable measurement and correlated well with readings taken later in time [30]. In Indonesia, hospital workers with frequent occupational exposure to TB, in fact, developed a much more rapid reaction to tuberculin with reactions at 6 hours after inoculation that histopathologically appeared to be a typical tuberculin response [31].

The tuberculin test should be read by a trained health care professional. The ability of subjects to decipher their response is limited. In one study involving actively employed health care workers [30], only 79 of 212 (37.2%) with an observer positive Mantoux test thought that any induration was present. Even measurements done by appropriate personnel may be problematic. An audit at a community teaching hospital [32] demonstrated poor compliance related to reading and recording of the results. As few as 19% of the test results were, in fact, recorded.

Variability in Mantoux test reading has been demonstrated. Using four readers of two simultaneously applied tests involving over 1000 persons, agreement between observers was about 70% [33]. In fact, the differences recorded by experienced readers was found to be as variable as those of inexperienced readers [34]. This variability further underscores that the test is a diagnostic aid and not a definitive conclusion. Sbarbaro [35] clearly emphasizes this, stressing the importance of clinical judgement.

### (f) Interpretation of the Mantoux test

Although the substance used in this diagnostic test for TB has basically not been changed over the greater part of the 20th century, the interpretation of the test has and will likely continue to evolve. Indeed, significant reactivity has become substantially more flexible since that proposed by Mantoux himself as the 'erythema and induration the size of a two franc coin'. The criteria for positivity are linked to the relative risk of developing active TB, the immunocompetence of the host and the prevalence of non-TB mycobacteria (NTM).

It is known that subclinical infections with NTM (including BCG vaccination) will cause some reactivity but usually of a smaller diameter than one related to TB [36]. A significant amount of overlap in the size of the reaction to tuberculin between *M. tuberculosis* and NTMs does exist. Because of this overlap, any single cutoff for positivity will produce errors in classification. A small cutoff (for example, 5 mm) will include most of the reactions due to *M. tuberculosis* but also a large number of cross sensitization reactions will be classified as positive. This gives the test a high degree of sensitivity (few false-negatives) but a low degree of specificity (many false-positives). As the cutoff for a positive test is increased, many of the NTM induced reactions (including those related to BCG vaccination) will be no longer considered to be positive but a larger number of reactions induced by *M. tuberculosis* will be excluded. This larger cutoff, therefore, trades increasing specificity for lower sensitivity.

The definition of significant reactivity of the tuberculin test should vary depending on how important it is to detect the maximum number of true positive results. In individuals in whom a high risk of the development of active TB exists (for example, immunoincompetent hosts and close household contacts of active cases), the cutoff should be low. In individuals without a high risk of TB and the potential of harm from isoniazid (INH) therapy, the cutoff should be correspondingly higher.

In June 1989, the most recent classification of reactions to the 5 TU Mantoux test was adopted by the American Thoracic Society (ATS). They have been published as a joint statement of this organization and the Center for Disease Control (CDC) [37]. These guidelines were an attempt to optimize the appropriate use of this diagnostic test (Table 8.2).

**Table 8.2** American Thoracic Society classification of tuberculin reactions

---

**Tuberculin reactor**
An individual whose degree of induration from a 5 TU Mantoux test satisfies the cutoff requirements for the individual's risk factors

**Tuberculin convertor**
An individual whose degree of induration from a 5 TU Mantoux test qualifies as a reactor, was previously known or likely to be a non-reactor and has increased by 6 mm of induration or more

**Risk groups classified with ≥ 5 mm induration as a positive reaction**
- those with close recent contact with infectious tuberculosis cases
- those with chest X-rays consistent with old healed tuberculosis
- those with HIV infections or with risk factors for HIV acquisition with an unknown HIV status

**Risk groups classified with ≥ 10 mm induration as a positive reaction**
Risk factors other than those above which increase tuberculous risk. These include:
- foreign-born persons from high risk areas in Asia, Africa and Latin America
- intravenous drug users
- medically underserved populations including high risk racial or ethnic minorities such as Blacks, Hispanics and Native Americans
- residents of long-term care facilities such as prisons, nursing homes and psychiatric institutions
- medical risk factors including chronic renal failure, diabetes mellitus, gastrectomy, leukemia, lymphoma or other malignancies, jejuno-ileal bypass, silicosis and being ≥ 10% below ideal body weight

**Risk groups classified with ≥ 15 mm induration as a positive reaction**
- those not classified in other groups

---

[a] Reproduced with permission from the American Lung Association [37].

A reaction of 5 mm or more of induration is classified as positive in three groups, each with a substantial risk of the development of active TB. Two of the groups have long been known to be of high risk, those who have had recent close contact with an infectious TB case and those who have chest X-rays consistent with old, healed TB. The third in this category is of more recent vintage, those known to be infected with HIV or in a risk group for HIV with an unknown status. Although not formally mentioned in this category, individuals who live in areas where there is little if any environmental NTM may benefit from being placed in this grouping. Alaskan Eskimos are such a group [38]. It is likely that any amount of induration to a 5 TU tuberculin test in an HIV-infected individual should be interpreted as reactive.

A reaction of 10 mm or more of induration is classified as positive in those who do not meet the criteria for the 5 mm cutoff but who have other risk factors for the acquisition of TB. This would include the groups listed in Table 8.2. In addition to these groups, other high risk populations can also be included, based on the evaluation of public health officials. Workers in facilities where a person with active pulmonary TB could present a hazard to substantially large numbers of people (schools, child care facilities and facilities providing health care) may be considered positive at this level. Intravenous drug abusers in areas of significant HIV prevalence would be best placed in the smallest cutoff group. Depending on the level of cellular immune system depression, some immuno-suppressed subjects usually represented in this grouping might likewise be better in the 5 mm cutoff.

A reaction of 15 mm or more of induration is classified as positive in all other people who cannot be placed in a high risk group. Any individual whose tuberculin test is positive based on his or her population group and who has a history of BCG inoculation should be considered to be infected with *M. tuberculosis*. BCG induced induration in the order of 10–12 mm may occur especially if the vaccination had been recent but most reactions are less than 10 mm and often show no induration. Additionally, an accelerated reaction to BCG vaccination has been suggested to be a useful diagnostic test for TB [39] but it is not clear if a similar reaction would occur in those infected with NTM.

Several groups have reported discrepancies in tuberculin test results comparing different commercial products. This has been found in both intravenous drug users, particularly those infected with HIV [40], and hospital workers [41]. The significance of these discrepancies is not entirely clear but emphasizes the importance of interpreting the skin test results in a clinical context.

## 8.3 FALSE-NEGATIVE TUBERCULIN TESTS

A substantial number of factors have been associated with a variable degree of decreased reactivity to tuberculin (Table 8.3). It is important to note that the mere presence of such circumstances should not be an indicator that tuberculin testing should not be done or is contraindicated. Even in the presence of one or more of these factors, significant tuberculin reactions may occur. These factors must be considered in individuals who

**Table 8.3** Some factors causing decreased ability to respond to tuberculin[a]

**Factors related to the test subject**
- Infections
  Viruses (measles, varicella, mumps, rubella, influenza, HIV)
  Bacteria (typhoid, brucellosis, typhus, pertussis)
  Mycobacteria (tuberculosis, especially recent or overwhelming infection, leprosy)
  Fungi (South American blastomycosis)
- Live virus vaccination (measles, mumps, polio)
- Metabolic derangements (chronic renal failure, hypothyroidism, cirrhosis)
- Nutritional factors (severe protein depletion)
- Diseases affecting lymphoid organs (lymphoma, lymphocytic leukemia, sarcoidosis)
- Drugs (corticosteroids and other immunosuppression agents, warfarin)
- Age (newborn, elderly subjects with 'waned' sensitivity)
- Stress (surgery, burns, graft *versus* host reaction)
- Psychological factors (suggestion, mental illness)

**Factors related to the test reagent**
- Improper storage (exposure to light and heat)
- Improper dilutions
- Chemical degradation
- Contamination
- Adsorption (partially controlled by adding Tween-80)

**Factors related to the administration**
- Injection of too little antigen
- Delayed inoculations after drawing into a syringe
- Improper injection

**Factors related to reading and recording the test results**
- Inexperienced reader
- Conscious or unconscious bias
- Error in or no recording

[a] Adapted from [37] with permission of the American Lung Association.

had a negative tuberculin test associated with one or more of these factors and a subsequent positive one when the factor has been removed.

It has long been appreciated that some patients, even those with active TB, will have non-reactive tuberculin tests. Certainly progressive TB itself may produce non-reactivity. In one study from Detroit's Maybury Sanatorium [42], the characteristics of the tuberculin negative patients included progressive, extensive lung disease with cavitation, large numbers of organisms in the sputum and critically ill, emaciated patients. The tuberculin anergy could be reversed with adequate chemotherapy.

In HIV-infected individuals with low CD4 cell counts, anergy is common as the disease progresses [43]. Such anergic individuals should be considered for preventive therapy as if they were PPD reactive if they reside in areas of significant TB prevalence [44].

Since individuals may have a condition limiting the ability to react to skin test antigens, it may be useful to co-administer one or more antigens to which the individual may have been sensitized. Table 8.4 lists a number of antigens that can be used. Commercial multitest 'anergy' batteries exist where liquid antigens are applied by prongs. Standardization of such panels is difficult.

**Table 8.4** Delayed type hypersensitivity skin test antigens

| Agent | Dilution | Comments |
|---|---|---|
| Candida (Dermatophytin O) | 1:100 | Produced from a filtrate from a 21 day *Candida albicans* culture |
| Coccidiodin (Mycelial phase) antigen [a] | 1:100 | May be used at 1:10 Tissue phase (spherulin) antigen also available Contains thiomerosal |
| Histoplasmin[a] | 1:100 | Contains phenol and Tween-80 May elevate histoplasma serology |
| Mumps | 2 CFU/0.1 ml | Contains thiomerosal Do not use in those with avian protein hypersensitivity Read as area of erythema |
| Tetanus toxoid | 1:5 | Assess immunity, repeat after immunization |
| Trichophyton (Dermatophytin) | 1:30 | Mixture of filtrates from three *Trichophyton* species |
| Multi-test battery | | Contains tetanus toxoid, diphtheria toxoid, OT and filtrates of *Streptococcus* (Group C), *Candida, Trichophyton* and *Proteus mirabilis* |

[a] Useful in an 'anergy panel' only in patients who are from endemic areas.

### 8.3.1 Viral infections and immunizations

Some viral infections can transiently suppress the tuberculin reaction. The relation of measles infection and inhibition of this reaction was the first to be recognized. Most of the early studies involving measles and the tuberculin reaction used methodology for tuberculin testing not in use today. With the Mantoux test, however, dramatic decreases in induration occur shortly before the rash begins and persist for an average of 18 days but for as long as 42 days [45]. Similar, milder effects were noted in $\gamma$-globulin modified measles and after the live, attenuated measles vaccine. The same authors [46] described a milder depression of tuberculin reactivity during chickenpox. Whether this depression occurs during reactivation varicella-zoster is not known. Mumps may also transiently decrease the response to tuberculin. During a rubella outbreak, suppression of the tuberculin reaction also occurred [47] starting just before the rash and extending up to 4 weeks after the disease onset. Subclinical rubella suppressed the tuberculin reaction as well. Serologically proven influenza also produced hyporeactivity to skin test antigens but noninfluenza respiratory illnesses did not [48].

Vaccinations against mumps and polio may also be tuberculin suppressive. The suppression following polio vaccination has occurred with both live, attenuated [49] and killed [50] vaccine and the live, attenuated yellow fever vaccine as well [50]. The killed influenza vaccine did not suppress reactivity [48]. Vaccinia vaccination can also suppress tuberculin reactivity [51]. Despite these reports, in a study of 110 Canadian children known to be tuberculin positive, only 3% of children reverted to negative related to viral vaccination [52]. Importantly, there was no difference in this transient reversion rate in control, nonvaccinated children. The most recent ATS/CDC statement [37] does not recommend the avoidance of tuberculin testing at the time of vaccination but in the past the suggestion of administration and reading of the tuberculin test before or 30 days after live virus vaccination has been made [53]. Recent vaccination should be kept in mind, however, in interpreting skin test responses.

### 8.3.2 Corticosteroids

As a class of medications known to have immnosuppressive effects, exogenous corticosteroids should modify the response to tuberculin. The effect appears to be related to systemic steroids, not from topical use. A controlled trial in Alaska [54] found no decrease in induration associated with the use of hydrocortisone ointment compared with control. Another study [55] found no effect on the tuberculin reaction using a more potent halogenated steroid even when applied for 3 days prior to the skin test at the test site. The injection of steroids, however, into the tuberculin reaction consistently reduces induration compared with controls [56,57].

Although there is conflicting evidence, the data generally reveal a depressive effect of systemic corticosteroids. Comparison of various studies is difficult because of variation in the dose and type of steroid used. In patients with active TB [58], adrenocorticotrophic hormone (ACTH) was found to produce a significant decrease in induration which returned to control levels after the ACTH was discontinued (Figure 8.5). The increased induration during treatment for TB as noted has been reported previously [59] studying serial tuberculin reactions in pulmonary TB. It could represent a booster effect (see below) or increased immunologic competence produced by appropriate TB treatment. The degree of tuberculin reactivity in one study [60] was found to be indirectly related to urinary 17-ketosteroid excretion, suggesting that endogenous steroid production may modify the tuberculin reaction. In this regard, corticosteroid use restored tuberculin reactivity in 20 of 24 patients with adrenal insufficiency [61].

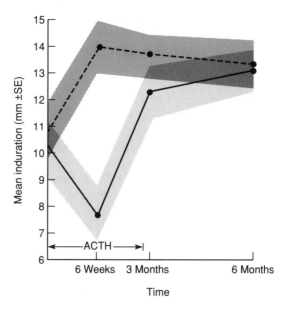

**Figure 8.5** The changes in the mean diameter of the tuberculin reaction during a course of adrenocorticotrophic hormone (ACTH) (solid line); control (dashed line). One standard deviation is shown as shaded areas. Reproduced from *American Review of Respiratory Disease* with permission of the American Lung Association, New York, NY, copyright 1961 [58].

### 8.3.3 The booster phenomenon

Over time, some tuberculin reactors will lose this reactivity. Known as skin test reversion, one study estimated that it occurs in as many as 6.8% of adults per year [62]. A 19-year follow-up of 22 tuberculin reactors [63] found three lost reactivity (13.7% or 0.7% per year). Surveys of tuberculin reactivity usually show lower prevalence of positivity in older adults. The change is greater than any expected mortality rate in the reactors and likely reflects skin test reversion. Administration of serial tuberculin tests in an individual who has reverted may produce what appears to be a new conversion, the so-called booster phenomenon. This effect, which is also noted with the histoplasmosis skin test [64], may be the equivalent of the anamnestic response in humoral immunity, that is, immunologic recall.

A landmark study describing this phenomenon was reported by Ferebee and Mount [65] based on studies in chronic care psychiatric hospitals. The work has been highlighted by Comstock [24]. An apparent dramatic tuberculin conversion rate over a year in three facilities (range 16–25%) was noted. In one institution, an apparent 47% conversion rate over 1 month was found. It was found that the positive test could manifest as early as 1 week following a negative one. If the reaction to the first test is classified as not significant, an additional test should be administered 1 week subsequently. If the second test is still below the cutoff point for positivity for the individual's risk group, the subject should be classified as having a nonsignificant reaction. If, however, the reaction is significant to the second test, this most likely represents the booster phenomenon. Not only can the immunologic recall increase the size of the tuberculin reaction but it may also produce induration more rapidly [66]. The reaction is more common in individuals over 55 years of age. In a group of Canadian health care students, booster phenomena were found in about 5% [67]. It may be difficult to distinguish new skin test conversions from booster effects. The use of other serial skin tests at the same time as the tuberculin tests may help. No correlation, however, between a booster response to tuberculin and one to *Candida* was found [68].

In a nursing home, tuberculin reversions occurred in about one quarter of a cohort of 258 subjects over a 3 year interval (8.3% per year) [69]. Interestingly, 16 of 21 individuals who had a significant tuberculin reaction only after boosting at the beginning of the study did not boost 3 years later. Further investigations by the same group [70] have questioned the significance of these reactions. It has yet to be shown that individuals who react only to the booster test are at risk of an increased development of active TB as patients with an initially reactive tuberculin test are. Stead and To [71] agree, stating that elderly individuals are able to mount a reaction to tuberculin if they remain infected with viable tubercle bacilli, albeit as yet asymptomatically. Those with waned responses may harbor only dead organisms.

The ATS/CDC recommendations from 1990 [37] recommend the sequential two step procedure in selected individuals. It has been reported in a cohort of subjects 85 years of age and older, however, that booster effects may continue after four tests at weekly intervals (72). Especially in the elderly, a better test is needed to identify those at risk for the development of active TB. It is not necessarily the case that those who manifest the booster phenomenon fall into this group.

### 8.3.4 Miscellaneous causes of low tuberculin reactivity

In examining delayed hypersensitivity in hospitalized patients [73], it was found that hyporeactivity was associated with leukocytosis, anemia and fever. Although strongly interrelated, these factors related independently to anergy. The effect between leukocytosis and anergy seemed to be a transient effect on lymphocyte function rather than a direct depression of the inflammatory response [74].

Reactivity to tuberculin can, in part, be modified by suggestion. It has been shown [75] that both the induration and erythema of the reaction could be decreased to non-reactive by direct suggestion under hypnosis. The effect seemed related to vascular reactivity since the degree of cellular accumulation in the skin biopsy was unchanged. Another study using direct suggestion and guided imagery during hypnosis found the subjects could produce an average of 35% more induration [76].

Prolongation of the prothrombin time by warfarin has been found to be related to a reduction in reactivity. Using a variety of skin test antigens [77], the number of reactions 10 mm or more decreased by 55% and reactions 5 mm or more decreased by 39%. The number of individuals who reacted to none of the four skin tests rose from two to 14.

Although pregnancy has generally been considered to depress cellular immunity, a study of 452 women found no clear effect of pregnancy in tuberculin reactivity [78]. No significant effect occurred even when examined by trimester in which the skin test was applied. These authors reviewed previous studies in pregnancy which had produced variable results regarding skin test suppression.

## 8.4 ADVERSE REACTIONS TO TUBERCULIN

Although the intradermal immunization route can be used successfully for certain vaccines [79], it is important to emphasize that although the PPD reaction may be enhanced in individuals whose sensitivity has waned over time, the repetition of tests in a truly tuberculin negative individual does not induce sensitization. This is true even when the same area of skin is used for repeated tuberculin tests [80] or if large amounts of tuberculin are used [81].

Immediate type reactions during tuberculin testing are very rare but well described. Such reactions were reported to occur within 20 minutes after injection of 10 TU PPD in 76 (2.3%) of 3248 individuals in an allergy clinic [82]. They occurred in all age groups and were more frequent in individuals with atopy. Interestingly, only three of 76 developed a delayed hypersensitivity reaction. The antigenic cause of the immediate reaction is unclear and the ATS felt that these reactions had no epidemiologic importance and did not indicate infection with TB.

An individual with a history of atopy and previously nonreactive PPD tests has been reported who developed both a local wheal, bronchospasm and syncope within 5 minutes of the application of a PPD tine test [83]. Evaluation revealed no IgE directed against tuberculin. The antigen responsible for the reaction was thought to be acacia (gum arabic) but was unproven. A severe reaction has been reported beginning 3 hours after administration of a 1 TU Mantoux test in a patient with TB lymphadenitis [84]. The reaction consisted of rigors with myalgias, fever and hypotension with no immediate reaction at the test site. Subsequently, the patient developed a markedly reactive delayed type hypersensitivity reaction. The antigen responsible for the reaction was undetermined. These reactions have been called paraphylactic shock or systemic tuberculin shock [85] and are manifest within 24 hours of inoculation. Symptoms include fever and chills, nausea and vomiting, icterus, bronchospasm, adrenal insufficiency and renal failure. Although the reaction may have been related to contaminating substances such as endotoxin, these reactions apparently continued despite using more purified tuberculin. A military recruit has been reported to have died minutes after a tine test but whether the tuberculin test was the cause was unclear [86].

Rarely, apparently extraordinarily sensitive individuals can develop necrotizing local reactions, regional lymphadenitis, lymphangitis and fever from tuberculin testing. Morrison in 1984 reported 12 cases of significant reactions with lymphangitis over 5 years after not seeing any in 39 years. Five occurred following Mantoux tests and seven after multipuncture tests [87]. The cause of the severe reactions was unclear. Increased potency of the Mantoux test was suggested but tests on guinea pigs could not substantiate this. An incidence of such reactions of 1 in 500 000 using 5 TU was reported from Athens, Greece [88].

The occurrence of such a reaction, albeit rare, should be minimized but the ATS [37], because of the inadequate standardization of the 1 TU Mantoux test, does not suggest preliminary testing of individuals with suspected TB using 1 TU. The reaction is apparently not dose related in the usual dosage range. Therapy of such a reaction is symptomatic including antipyretics and covering the lesion to prevent secondary infections. In certain high risk individuals, especially in the presence of erythema nodosum or phlyctenular conjunctivitis, some suggest that a lower strength PPD be used for initial evaluation [89]. Although some individuals have advocated topical steroids with an occlusive dressing as a therapeutic modality [90], trials have not shown this to be useful [91]. Systemic or intralesional steroids may be of value in severe tuberculin reactions.

In investigating these reactions, care must be taken to make sure that the inoculation was correct in quantity and quality. Severe reactions have been reported with an inadvertent PPD dose of 200 µg instead of 0.02 µg of PPD [81] and when diphtheria–tetanus–pertussis vaccine was accidentally substituted for PPD [92]. It should be noted that even the 10 000 times normal dose accidentally administered did not sensitize the previous tuberculin nonreactors to subsequent tuberculin doses.

## 8.5 CONCLUSION

In patients who are infected without clinical disease or who have not yet been found to be positive by an acid-fast bacillus (AFB) stain or culture, the tuberculin skin test is a very important modality to assess who may or has already developed actively infectious disease. This chapter summarizes the utility of the test, but results must be interpreted appropriately. As amply stated by Edwards [93]: 'Like any diagnostic test, the test result must be considered in context. Test material, method of administration and the condition of the person tested are all of consequence to the reaction. Of what value would an electrocardiogram be if the clinical history were unknown, the leads improperly placed, the stylus faulty, or the reader inexperienced or improperly trained?'

## REFERENCES

1. Koch, R. (1891) Weitere mitteilungen uber ein Heilmittel gegen Tuberculose. *Dtsch Med Wschr*, **17**, 101–2.
2. Snider, D.E. (1982) The tuberculin skin test. *Am Rev Respir Dis*, **125** (Supplement), 108–18.
3. Bothamley, G.H. and Grange, J.M. (1991) The Koch phenomenon and delayed hypersensitivity: 1891–1991. *Tubercle, 72*, 7–11.
4. Seibert, F.B. and Glenn, J.T. (1941) Tuberculin purified protein derivative: preparation and analyses of a large quantity for standard. *Am Rev Tuberc*, **44**, 9–25.
5. Furcolow, M.L., Hewell, B., Nelson, W.E. and Palmer, C.E. (1941) Quantitative studies of the tuberculin reaction. I. Titration of tuberculin sensitivity and its relation to tuberculous infection. *Pub Health Rep*, **56**, 1082–100.
6. Rosenthal, S.R. (1958) The disc-method tuberculin test. *Am Rev Tuberc*, **77**, 778–88.
7. MacLean, R.A. (1975) Tuberculin testing antigens and techniques. *Chest*, **68** (supplement), 455–9.
8. American Thoracic Society (1981) The tuberculin skin test. *Am Rev Respir Dis*, **124**, 356–63.
9. Herzog, C. (1981) Multiple-puncture tuberculin testing: reason for variable response to tine test. *Tubercle*, **62**, 249–56.
10. Schwartz, E. and Leibowitz, S. (1963) Tuberculin tine test. *Am Rev Respir Dis*, **88**, 97.
11. Asnes, R.S. and Magbook, S. (1975) Parent reading and reporting of children's tuberculin skin test results. *Chest*, **68** (Supplement), 459–62.
12. Badger, T.L., Breitwieser, E.R. and Muench, H. (1963) Tuberculin tine test. Multiple-puncture intradermal technique compared with PPD-S, intermediate strength. *Am Rev Respir Dis*, **87**, 338–53.
13. Sinclair, D.J.M. and Johnston, R.N. (1979) Assessment of tine tuberculin test. *Brit Med J*, **1**, 1325–6.
14. Lunn, J.A. and Johnson, A.J. (1978) Comparison of the tine and Mantoux tuberculin tests. *Brit Med J*, **1**, 1451–3.
15. Sbarbaro, J.A. (1979) The FDA's final decision concerning the tuberculin multiple puncture test. *Am Rev Respir Dis*, **120**, 1390–1.
15a.Committee on Infectious Diseases (1994) Screening for tuberculosis in infants and children. *Pediatrics*, **93**, 131–4.
16. Murtagh, K. (1980) Unreliability of the Mantoux test using 1 TU PPD in excluding childhood tuberculosis in Papua New Guinea. *Arch Dis Child*, **55**, 795–9.
17. Riebel W. (1983) The 250 TU and second-strength skin tests. *N Engl J Med*, **309**, 246.
18. Nash, D.R. and Douglass, J.E. (1980) Anergy in active pulmonary tuberculosis:

a comparison between positive and negative reactors and an evaluation of 5 TU and 250 TU skin test doses. *Chest*, **77**, 32–7.

19. Huebner, R.E., Schein, M.F., Cauthen, G.M. *et al.* (1992) Evaluation of the clinical usefulness of mycobacterial skin test antigens in adults with pulmonary mycobacteriosis. *Am Rev Respir Dis,* **146**, 1160–6.

20. Landi, S., Held, H.R., Hauschild, A.H.W. *et al.* (1966) Adsorption of tuberculin PPD to glass and plastic surfaces. *Bull WHO*, **35**, 593–602.

21. Holden, M., Dubin, M.R. and Diamond, P.H. (1971) Frequency of negative intermediate-strength tuberculin sensitivity in patients with active tuberculosis. *N Engl J Med*, **285**, 1506–9.

22. Landi, S., Held, H.R. and Tseng, M.C. (1971) Disparity of potency between stabilized and non-stabilized dilute tuberculin solutions. *Am Rev Respir Dis*, **104**, 385–93.

23. Landi, S. and Held, H.R. (1975) Effect of light on tuberculin purified protein derivative solutions. *Am Rev Respir Dis*, **111**, 52–61.

24. Comstock, G.W. (1975) False tuberculin test results. *Chest*, **68** (supplement), 465–9.

25. Rhoades, E.R. and Bryant, R.E. (1980) The influence of local factors on the reaction to tuberculin. 1. The effect of injection. *Chest*, **77**, 190–3.

26. Victoria, M.S., Steiner, P. and Rao, M. (1977) The effect of intradermal and subcutaneous route of administration variation in PPD sensitivity. *Clin Ped*, **16**, 514–5.

27. Sokal, J.E. (1975) Measurement of delayed skin test response. *N Engl J Med*, **293**, 501–2.

28. Jordan, T.J., Sunderman, G., Thomas, L. *et al.* (1987) Tuberculin reaction size measurement by the pen method compared to traditional palpation. *Chest*, **92**, 234–6.

29. Seibert, A.F. and Bass, J.B. (1990) Tuberculin skin testing: guidelines for the 1990s. *J Respir Dis*, **11**(3), 225–34.

30. Howard, T.R. and Solomon, D.A. (1988) Reading the tuberculin skin test. Who, when and how? *Arch Intern Med*, **148**, 2457–9.

31. Gibbs, J.H., Grange, J.M., Beck, J.S. *et al.* (1991) Early delayed hypersensitivity responses in tuberculin skin tests after heavy occupational exposure to tuberculosis. *J Clin Path*, **44**, 919–24.

32. Bryan, C.S. (1980) Unread tuberculin tests. *JAMA*, **244**, 1126.

33. Chaparas, S.D., Vandiviere, H.M., Melvin, I. *et al.* (1985) Tuberculin test. Variability with the Mantoux procedure. *Am Rev Respir Dis*, **132**, 175–7.

34. Loudon, R.G., Lawson, R.A. and Brown, J. (1963) Variation in tuberculin test reading. *Am Rev Respir Dis*, **87**, 852–61.

35. Sbarbaro, J.A. (1985) Tuberculin test. A re-emphasis on clinical judgement. *Am Rev Respir Dis*, **132**, 177–8.

36. Gottlieb, J.E. and Pauker, S.G. (1989) When is a positive purified protein derivative test falsely positive? A new look at old tuberculin. *Sem Respir Med*, **10**, 218–26.

37. American Thoracic Society (1990) Diagnostic standards and classification of tuberculosis. *Am Rev Respir Dis*, **142**, 725–35.

38. Reichman, L.B. (1979) Tuberculin skin testing. The state of the art. *Chest*, **76** (Supplement), 764–70.

39. Long, L., DeJesus, L., Rondilla, W. *et al.* (1993) Correlation of accelerated BCG response with positive AFB smear in adult PTB. *Chest*, **104**, 138S.

40. Lifson, A.R., Watters, J.K., Thompson, S. *et al.* (1993) Discrepancies in tuberculin skin test results with two commercial products in a population of intravenous drug users. *J Infect Dis*, **168**, 1048–51.

41. Rupp, M.E., Schultz, A.W. and Davis, J.C. (1994) Discordance between tuberculin skin test results with two commercial purified protein derivative preparations. *J Infect Dis*, **169**, 1174–5.

42. Howard, W.L., Klopfenstein, M.D., Steininger, W.J. and Woodruff, C.E. (1970) The loss of tuberculin sensitivity in certain patients with active pulmonary tuberculosis. *Chest*, **57**, 530–4.

43. Blatt, S.P., Hendrix, C.W., Butzin, C.A. *et al.* (1993) Delayed-type hypersensitivity skin testing predicts progression to AIDS in HIV-infected patients. *Ann Intern Med*, **119**, 177–84.

44. Moreno, S., Baraia-Etxaburu, J., Bouza, E. *et al.* (1993) Risk for developing tuberculosis among anergic patients infected with HIV. *Ann Intern Med*, **119**, 194–8.

45. Starr, S. and Berkovich, S. (1964) Effects of measles, gamma-globulin modified measles and vaccine measles on the tuberculin test. *N Engl J Med*, **270**, 386–91.

46. Starr, S. and Berkovich, S. (1964) The depression of tuberculin reactivity during chickenpox. *Pediatrics*, **33**, 769–72.

47. Ueda, K., Nishima, S., Sasak, F. *et al.* (1979) Suppression of tuberculin reactivity during natural rubella. *Clin Pediat*, **18**, 101–7.

48. Reed, W.P., Olds, J.W., and Kisch, A.L. (1972) Decreased skin-test reactivity associated with influenza. *J Infect Dis*, **125**, 398–402.

49. Berkovich, S. and Starr, S. (1966) Effect of live type 1 poliovirus vaccine and other viruses on the tuberculin test. *N Engl J Med*, **274**, 67–72.

50. Brody, J.A., Overfield, T. and Hammers, L.M. (1964) Depression of the tuberculin reaction by viral vaccines. *N Engl J Med*, **271**, 1294–6.

51. Smithwick, E.M., Steiner, M. and Quick, J.D. (1972) Vaccinia virus and tuberculin reactivity. *Pediatrics*, **50**, 660–1.

52. Brickman, H.G., Beaudry, P.H. and Marks, M.I. (1975) The timing of tuberculin tests in relation to immunization with live viral vaccines. *Pediatrics*, **55**, 392–6.

53. American Thoracic Society Committee on Diagnostic Skin Testing (1970) The place of tuberculin testing in relation to live virus vaccines. *Am Rev Respir Dis*, **102**, 469.

54. Hanson, M.L. and Comstock, G.W. (1968) Efficacy of hydrocortisone ointment in the treatment of local reaction to tuberculin skin tests. *Am Rev Respir Dis*, **97**, 472–3.

55. Thestrup-Pederson, K., Ahlburg, H., Hansen, P. *et al.* (1982) The influence of topical steroid application on tuberculin skin reactions in healthy persons. *Acta Dermatovener*, **62**, 43–6.

56. Vollmer, H. (1951) The local effect of cortisone on the tuberculin reaction. *J Pediat*, **39**, 22–32.

57. Goldman, L., Preston, R.H., Rockwell, E.M. *et al.* (1952) Inhibition of tuberculin reaction by local injection of compound F. *JAMA*, **150**, 30–1.

58. Solomon, H. and Angel, J.H. (1961) Corticotropin-induced changes in the tuberculin skin test. *Am Rev Respir Dis*, **83**, 235–42.

59. Ellis, M.G. (1956) The pattern of sensitivity in chronic pulmonary tuberculosis. *Tubercle*, **37**, 32–5.

60. Lane, J.J., Clarke, E.R. and Holmes, T.H. (1956) The relationship of tuberculin

sensitivity and adrenocortical function in humans. *Am Rev Tuberc*, **73**, 795–801.

61. Truelove, L.H. (1957) Enhancement of Mantoux reaction coincident with treatment with cortisone and prednisolone. *Brit Med J*, **2**, 1131–5.

62. Gryzbowski, S. and Allen, E.A. (1964) The challenge of tuberculosis: a study based on the epidemiology of tuberculosis in Ontario, Canada. *Am Rev Respir Dis*, **90**, 707–20.

63. Havlin, D.V., van der Kuyp, F., Duffy, E. *et al.* (1991) A 19-year follow-up of tuberculin reactors. Assessment of skin test reactivity and in vitro lymphocyte responses. *Chest*, **99**, 1172–6.

64. Ganley, J.P., Smith, R.E., Thomas, D.B. *et al.* (1972) Booster effect of histoplasmin skin testing in an elderly population. *Am J Epidemiol*, **95**, 104–10.

65. Ferebee, S.H. and Mount, F.W. (1963) Evidence of booster effect in serial tuberculin testing. *Am Rev Respir Dis*, **88**, 118.

66. Duboczy, B.O. (1964) Repeated tuberculin tests at the same site in tuberculin-positive patients. *Am Rev Respir Dis*, **90**, 77–86.

67. Menzies, R., Vissandjee, B., Racher, I. and St. Germain, Y. (1994) The booster effect in two-step tuberculin testing among young adults in Montreal. *Ann Intern Med*, **120**, 190–8.

68. Burstin, S.J., Muspratt, J.A. and Rossing, T.H. (1986) The tuberculin test. Studies of the dynamics of reactivity to tuberculin and *Candida* antigens in institutionalized patients. *Am Rev Respir Dis*, **134**, 1072–4.

69. Perez-Stable, E.J., Flaherty, D., Schecter, G. *et al.* (1988) Conversion and reversion of tuberculin reaction in nursing home residents. *Am Rev Respir Dis*, **137**, 801–4.

70. Gordin, F.M., Perez-Stable, E.J., Reid, M. *et al.* (1991) Stability of positive tuberculin tests: are boosted reactions valid? *Am Rev Respir Dis*, **144**, 560–3.

71. Stead, W.W. and To, T. (1987) The significance of the tuberculin skin test in elderly persons. *Ann Intern Med*, **107**, 837–42.

72. Van den Brande, R. and Demedts, M. (1992) Four stage tuberculin testing in elderly subjects induces age-dependent progressive boosting. *Chest*, **101**, 447–50.

73. Palmer, D.L. and Reed, W.P. (1974) Delayed hypersensitivity skin testing. II. Clinical correlates and anergy. *J Infect Dis*, **130**, 138–43.

74. Heiss, L.I. and Palmer, D.L. (1974) Anergy in patients with leukocytosis. *Am J Med*, **56**, 323–32.

75. Black, S., Humphrey, J.H. and Niven, J.S.F. (1963) Inhibition of Mantoux reaction by direct suggestion under hypnosis. *Brit Med J*, **1**, 1649–52.

76. Zacharie, R., Bjerring, P. and Arendt-Nielson, L. (1989) Modulation of type I immediate and type IV delayed immunoreactivity using direct suggestion and guided imagery during hypnosis. *Allergy*, **44**, 537–42.

77. Edwards, R.L. and Rickles, F.R. (1978) Delayed hypersensitivity in man: Effects of systemic anticoagulation. *Science*, **200**, 541–3.

78. Present, P.A. and Comstock, G.W. (1975) Tuberculin sensitivity in pregnancy. *Am Rev Respir Dis*, **112**, 413–16.

79. Burridge, M.J., Baer, G.M., Sumner, J.W. and Sussman, O. (1982) Intradermal immunization with human diploid rabies vaccine. *JAMA, 248*, 1611–4.

80. Stead, W.W. (1977) No local skin sensitization by repeated tuberculin tests. *N Engl J Med*, **297**, 225–6.

81. Egsmore, T. (1970) The effect of an exorbitant intracutaneous dose of 200 micro-

grams PPD tuberculin compared with 0.02 micrograms PPD tuberculin. *Am Rev Respir Dis*, **102**, 35–42.

82. Tarlo, S.M., Day, J.H., Mann, P. and Day M.P. (1977) Immediate hypersensitivity to tuberculin. In vivo and in vitro studies. *Chest*, **71**, 33–7.

83. Wright, D.N., Ledford, D.K. and Lockey, R.F. (1989) Systemic and local allergic reactions to the tine test purified protein derivative. *JAMA*, **262**, 2999–3000.

84. Spiteri, M.A., Bowman, A., Assefi, A.R. and Clarke, S.W. (1986) Life threatening reaction to tuberculin testing. *Brit Med J*, **293**, 243–4.

85. Besredka, A. (1940) La tuberculine, l'anaphylaxie et le phénomène de Koch. *La Presse Medicale*, **48**, 973–6.

86. DiMaio, V.J.M. and Froeode, R.C. (1975) Allergic reactions to the tine test. *JAMA*, **233**, 769.

87. Morrison, J.B. (1984) Lymphangitis after tuberculin tests. *Brit Med J*, **289**, 413.

88. Bouros, D., Niotis, M. and Blatsios, V. (1991) Lymphangitis after tuberculin test. *Eur Respir J*, **4**, 235.

89. Sewell, E.M., O'Hare, D. and Kendig, E.L. The tuberculin test. *Pediatrics*, **54**, 650–2.

90. Plaut, T.F. (1976) Prevention of skin necrosis caused by PPD. *N Engl J Med*, **295**, 1263.

91. Hanson, M.L. and Comstock, G.W. (1968) Efficacy of hydrocortisone ointment in the treatment of local reactions to tuberculin skin tests. *Am Rev Respir Dis*, **97**, 472–3.

92. Graham, D.R., Dan, B.B., Bertagnoll, P. and Dixon, R.E. (1981) Cutaneous inflammation caused by inadvertent intradermal administration of DTP instead of PPD. *Am J Public Health*, **71**, 1040–3.

93. Edwards, P. (1972) Tuberculin negative? *N Engl J Med*, **286**, 373–4.

# Infection control issues in tuberculosis | 9

Suzanne M. Lutwick

## 9.1 INTRODUCTION

The recent resurgence of tuberculosis (TB) has provoked a crisis in which the modern health care system is being forced to reassess the efficacy of many of its traditional TB control measures. Economic factors such as the decline of US federal funds for TB control projects from $20 million in 1969 to $1 million in 1982 [1] no doubt aggravated the problem. It is time to return to vigilance in the use of prudent infection control methodology. To quote Dr Michael Iseman from a recent perspective regarding the transmission of TB:

> Existentialist Soren Kierkegaard, confronted with the unprovable in his quest for philosophical understanding concluded that to survive in a threatening world one might have to suspend one's critical nature and simply affirm. On a grand scale, we in medicine are sometimes confronted with imminent problems for which minimal or imperfect data exists to guide us in seeking solutions. Classically, in the scientific model wherein we deal with material matters, we have been taught to defer action until we can conduct studies that document the preferable pathway. Unfortunately, we are currently encountering an urgent problem for which an ideal data set and a rapid scientific resolution are not available: the intra-institutional transmission of tuberculosis to patients, health care workers and staff [2].

This eloquent commentary describes the dilemma which has become a disturbing consequence of the recent resurgence of TB in the USA. The rising incidence of multi-drug-resistant TB has created new concerns about how to prevent transmission of this disease to health care workers. Recently called 'down, but not out' by Murray [3], the disease is clearly returning with a vengeance. The methodology described here addresses the control measures against this disease. The cycle of infection is kept going by smear positive cases resulting from exogenous infection or endogenous reactivation and requires a multifaceted approach for containment.

## 9.2 SOURCE CONTROL

### 9.2.1 Case finding

Case finding and effective treatment are the ultimate forms of source control. Early detection of patients with infectious pulmonary TB and the subsequent institution of appropriate isolation and chemotherapy are vital in achieving the broad objectives of control of the epidemic, to diminish both the prevalence of infection and the incidence of disease [4]. The keys to making the diagnosis of TB in a timely manner are to suspect the infection in any person with signs and symptoms compatible with the disease and to obtain appropriate specimens for examination [5]. More specifically, any patient presenting for care with pulmonary symptoms such as cough or chest pain for more than 3 weeks or those with weight loss or hemoptysis should be evaluated for TB. Relying on passive case finding, such as this, is commonly the only method of identification used [6], but it will not necessarily identify infectious cases quickly nor find those with poor access to the health care system. It is important to have a heightened awareness that, in the presence of underlying risk factors, there will be those cases presenting with an atypical examination or history.

In the hospital setting, the failure to identify TB patients will increase the risk of transmission to hospital personnel. A 1.65% skin test conversion rate in those exposed to initially unsuspected TB patients was found [7], more than six times higher than those without such contacts. Kantor, Poblete and Pusateri [8], reported a 17.8-fold increase in TB infection rate in those exposed to an unrecognized case.

One of the most important activities in any TB control program is to identify people with TB by evaluating the contacts of cases with pulmonary infection. The contacts most at risk are those who live in the same household as the index cases or spend a significant time in the same indoor space. In 1990, the overall rate of active TB in evaluated contacts in the USA was 700 per 100 000 (0.7%) [5]. Case contact evaluations are also valuable in hospitals, correctional facilities, nursing homes and schools.

Contact investigations should be designed with as few steps as possible and should identify those with both tuberculin positivity and active disease. Evaluations should be done at the convenience of the contact, to improve compliance. Examples include skin testing and sputum collection done in the field and mobile X-ray units. Evaluation of household contacts or others with prolonged indoor contact with smear positive pulmonary TB will find as many as 9–12% who develop active disease with substantially lower risks in smear negative index cases [9]. Important guidelines for an effective contact investigation are given in Table 9.1.

**Table 9.1** Guidelines for tuberculosis contact investigation

- Initiate the investigation with close contacts.
- If no transmission is found in close contacts, extending to other contacts is usually not needed.
- Those with a high risk of significant disease (HIV-infected, newborns) need a high priority for investigation.
- If evidence of recent infection is found in close contacts, progressively lower risk contacts should be evaluated until the level of infection approximates the community risk (concentric circle investigation).
- A contact investigation may be carried out to find the source of the infection as well as individuals infected by the index case.

In addition to contact investigations, routine screening for TB in high prevalence situations, such as in the homeless and certain immigrant and refugee populations, is useful. Table 9.2 lists groups of individuals in whom routine screening is reasonable. In a milieu such as a shelter for the homeless, case finding can be aided by the distribution of educational material to shelter clients, employees and volunteers. Shelter staff and others providing services can greatly assist in the identification of potential cases by ensuring that appropriately symptomatic individuals are medically evaluated [10]. Overall increased public awareness of the extent of the TB problem by local and national health care agencies via the print and broadcast media is important in case finding as well [11].

**Table 9.2** Tuberculosis screening

**Groups at high risk for tuberculosis**
- Close contacts of infectious tuberculosis
- Individuals with medical conditions including
  gastrectomy
  silicosis
  diabetes
  renal failure
  immunosuppression
- HIV-infected persons
- Foreign born people from high prevalence areas
- Health care workers
- Residents of long-term care facilities
- Correctional institution inmates
- Substance abusers
- Homeless persons
- Children from higher prevalence areas (> 1%)

**Areas where there is a high risk of spread**
- Nursing staff
- Day care center
- Hospital oncology unit

Although routine chest X-ray screening of all high risk individuals is not generally considered to be cost effective, it was reported to be useful in a hospital where the rate of TB in admitted patients was 6.25 per 1000 [12]. Purified protein derivative of tuberculin (PPD) test conversion rates in hospitals, particularly comparing rates in various areas in the facility, can be useful in identifying clusters. In areas of low TB prevalence, routine screening of patients at the time of admission and yearly screening of hospital employees is of lower yield [13].

A mechanism for reporting cases to appropriate public health officials should include private physicians, public and private hospitals, clinics, substance abuse programs, nursing homes, laboratories and correctional facilities. By rapidly reporting newly diagnosed smear positive TB cases or those highly suspicious following chest X-ray, local TB control personnel can quickly evaluate household contacts even before sputum cultures are positive. The speed of this evaluation is invaluable in HIV-infected household contacts since clinical disease has been reported to occur with intervals as short as 3 weeks [5]. Another group where rapid evaluation is vital is that with unstable housing (migratory workers, intravenous drug users, the homeless) where delays in contact evaluations will cause the contact to be lost to follow-up.

### 9.2.2 Effects of chemotherapy

Chemotherapy can cure almost any patient and can rapidly render a smear positive case noninfectious, thereby reducing disease transmission and accelerating the infection's decline. Not only does adequate treatment sterilize the sputum, it will also, within 2 weeks, significantly decrease the frequency of cough, thus decreasing the production of droplets [14].

Routine lifelong follow-up of individuals with inactive TB who have received adequate therapy and demonstrated satisfactory clinical, radiographic and bacteriologic responses is not recommended once treatment has been finished [15]. Those, however, currently inactive who have never been treated or were known not to have been compliant with therapy, benefit from routine follow-up. All individuals discharged from follow-up should be counseled regarding return if symptoms compatible with TB occur.

### 9.2.3 Segregation of patients at home or in institutions

The need for restriction of activities in non-hospitalized patients will depend on the degree of infectiousness, the response to treatment, the activity and the kind of individuals exposed to the index patient [5]. Once identified, the patient should be educated to minimize transmission by covering the nose and mouth when coughing or sneezing. Some patients are not infectious and therefore do not need restrictions. Most infectious patients can remain in their home environment with household members who have already been exposed prior to the diagnosis, since the increase in transmission after treatment has begun is minimal. In some settings, patients may be able to continue work activities providing the setting is not conducive to transmission, for example those who work predominantly out of doors [5]. No special precautions are needed for bed linen, dishes, glasses and eating utensils or other fomites [9]. Educational information, when combined with suitable attention to the individual patient's socio-economic situation, will maximize the effects of identification and control.

When patients are institutionalized, additional precautions are necessary to prevent nosocomial transmission. In the stationary setting, once isolation has been implemented, the door to the TB isolation room should remain closed and the patient should not be transported outside the room except for procedures that cannot be done in the room. Patients should wear a surgical mask when being transported. Efforts should be made to schedule such transportation for times when procedures can be carried out rapidly and waiting areas are less crowded. A consistent level of isolation must be maintained even when the patient is outside the isolation room. Because the mask on the patient serves more as a physical barrier than a filter, fit and filtration are less critical than for masks used for personal protection [5]. Although the amount of time it takes for a patient to be no longer infectious can be difficult to define, three properly collected negative smear sputum samples from separate days indicate an extremely low potential for transmission [5]. Smear positive patients should not be placed in indoor environments where infection can be easily spread (for example homeless shelters) nor in areas where highly susceptible people, such as those with HIV infection, are present.

## 9.3 PRINCIPLES OF ENVIRONMENTAL CONTROL

Wells, beginning by studying textile mill air in the 1930s, characterized the behavior of droplets in the air [16] and distinguished between dust, droplets and droplet nuclei. The myriad of tiny droplets produced during sneezing, coughing, speaking and singing, evaporate quickly to form smaller droplet nuclei which may contain viable pathogens. Most droplet nuclei originate in the secretions pooled in the anterior oropharynx, which may contain coughed up material [17]. These droplet nuclei are small enough to have minimal settling potential and are rapidly dispersed throughout a room, remaining a significant source of infection until removed, diluted or inactivated. Once outdoors, the droplet nuclei are eliminated by radiation from sunlight and by the infinite dilution in the outside air.

The likelihood of TB transmission relates to the infectious droplet nuclei level in the room air and the length of exposure to that air [5]. Substantial variability occurs in the concentration of TB containing droplet nuclei generated by different patients with as little as 1/11 000 ft$^3$ to 1/70 ft$^3$ of air from highly infectious individuals [5]. Living in premises previously occupied by active TB patients does not place individuals at risk for infection, showing the minimal role played by fomites in TB transmission [18]. It has been estimated that the probability of becoming infected with TB during a 1 hour exposure will range between 1 in 4 and 1 in 600 [5]. Generally, prolonged exposures over months are needed for infection to occur. Riley calculated that it would take about 12 months for a nurse breathing tuberculous air to become tuberculin positive [19]. This is similar to what was observed in the pretherapeutic era. Transmission has been documented, however, from exposures as brief as 2 hours [5]. To minimize transmission, control measures include source control, ventilation, air irradiation and filtration. The methods discussed in this chapter have been shown to interrupt the transmission of multi-drug-resistant TB [20].

### 9.3.1 Ventilation

Standards for indoor air quality in health care facilities have been established by the American Society of Heating, Refrigerating and Air Conditioning Engineers (ASHRAE) [21] and by the Federal Health Resources and Service Administration [22]. Compliance with these standards should decrease the risk of TB transmission but will not reduce the rate to zero. Application of these guidelines to TB has been made by both the US Public Health Service [23] and the California Department of Health [24].

Room ventilation works by two mechanisms; dilution and removal. Dilution diminishes the number of infectious droplet nuclei by adding noninfectious air. Removal is by an exhaust system, either directly to the outside or recirculating after appropriate air filtration or UV irradiation. Exhausted air contaminated by infectious droplets must not be discharged close to intake vents, people or animals.

The direction of the ventilated air flow is as important as dilution in the control of TB. With TB, the air should flow into the patient's room from adjacent inside areas by differences in air pressure producing a room under negative pressure. In localities with fire codes prohibiting negative pressure rooms, to prevent smoke entry in case of fire, an anteroom can be supplied with air pressure to make it slightly positive compared with both isolation room and corridor. Maintaining air pressure differentials is best done in completely closed rooms, minimizing short circulating of air and optimizing air mixing. Current US standards for hospital rooms housing patients with TB [23] advise negative pressure rooms with a minimum of six air exchanges per hour (ACH). Iseman [2] emphasizes that not only is implementation of appropriate isolation rooms costly, since many facilities do not have adequate negative pressure rooms, but ventilation patterns are difficult to maintain. A Center for Disease Control (CDC)/American Hospital Association survey found that over 200 (27%) of the hospitals surveyed had no rooms meeting acid-fast bacillus (AFB) isolation criteria [25]. Poorly ventilated patient rooms clearly contribute to nosocomial TB transmission even to hospital employees with little or no direct patient contact [26].

Certain hospital areas require more ventilation than the patient room. ASHRAE has recommended that the ventilation in hospital intensive care units provides a minimum of 6 ACH including, as with patient rooms, at least two outside air changes per hour [21]. Emergency department waiting rooms, because of a congregate setting of as yet undiagnosed patients, should have at least 10 ACH and autopsy suites 12 ACH [21]. In bronchoscopy rooms, where a very large number of infectious droplet nuclei may be produced, 20 ACH have been recommended [24]. Even high levels of ventilation may offer only limited protection with such a degree of infection potential [5]. Other procedures that can increase the risk of nosocomial transmission include endotracheal intubation and suctioning [27], open abscess irrigation [28], autopsy [29] and sputum induction and aerosol treatment [30]. Table 9.3 shows the effect of air exchange on the ability to remove airborne contaminants.

**Table 9.3** Air exchanges and the removal of airborne contaminants[a]

| Air changes per hour | Minutes required for a removal efficiency of | | |
|---|---|---|---|
| | 90% | 99% | 99.9% |
| 1 | 138 | 276 | 414 |
| 3 | 46 | 92 | 138 |
| 6 | 23 | 46 | 69 |
| 10 | 14 | 28 | 41 |
| 15 | 9 | 18 | 28 |
| 20 | 7 | 14 | 21 |
| 40 | 3 | 7 | 10 |

[a] Adapted from [31], reproduced with permission. Adler, J.J. (1993) Hospital-acquired tuberculosis: addressing the challenge. *Hospital Practice*, **28**(9), 112.

Isolation ventilatory conditions can be facilitated by the use of enclosed negative pressure structures, such as a tent or booth. These can be used to provide isolation in areas such as an emergency department or medical diagnostic procedure area. They also can be used to provide supplementary isolation in designated rooms.

### 9.3.2 Filtration

In general use areas, such as emergency rooms and waiting areas, and patient rooms that do not have adequate ventilation systems built in, the use of a high efficiency particulate air (HEPA) filtration device should be considered. These filters can be used as part of central air units, as whole wall filtration systems with laminar air flow or as portable units. A portable HEPA unit, which directly filters the room air rather than the incoming or outgoing air, can be used as an interim system while retrofitting inadequate areas [23]. It should not be considered as a permanent solution in deference to other standard methodology. The effectiveness of the portable unit will vary, based on the configuration of the room, furniture, individuals in the room and placement of the unit. Some units may not be able to circulate air adequately because of insufficient air flow capacity.

HEPA filters can be expensive and require proper testing and regular filter replacement. These devices can remove as many as 99.97% of particles greater than 0.3 μm in size and can remove *Aspergillus* spores which are in 2–6 μm in size [32]. Since TB containing droplet nuclei are similar in size, they should also be removed from the air. Inappropriate design, installation and maintenance can cause infectious droplet nuclei to circumvent the filtration system. Meticulous maintenance and testing of the devices must be continuous [33].

### 9.3.3 Ultraviolet air disinfection

Wells first reported the utility of 254 nm UV light to inactive organisms suspended in droplet nuclei [34]. Since such radiation is irritating to eyes and skin, it is generally used inside ventilatory duct work or in the room space between the ceiling and people's heads. Lamps should be no lower than 7 ft from the floor [5] with the bottom shielded so that the radiation is directed upwards. Air currents produced by ventilation, drafts and heating are generally adequate to produce enough air mixing so that the droplet nuclei will be exposed to the UV light [35].

The degree of inactivation varies based on factors including the intensity of radiation, specific microorganism and ambient relative humidity. *Mycobacterium tuberculosis* is intermediate between highly susceptible bacilli such as *Escherichia coli* and resistant fungi [35]. The higher the relative humidity, the less efficient the UV effect. In fact, with humidity above 70% the effect drops dramatically [36] and this can present a problem in tropical areas or during the warmer months in temperate climates in non-air conditioned areas.

Seminal studies by Riley *et al.* [37] have shown that UV light can protect guinea pigs from infection carried by air from rooms of individuals with TB. UV radiation parallels ventilation in decreasing airborne organisms in a logarithmic fashion [35] and can be expressed as air change equivalents (ACHE). One study involving AFB found that a single UV fixture could provide 10 ACHE, and two fixtures, 25 ACHE [38]. The amount of air flow in the room can modify this ACHE. Using a lower wattage, an air current pattern which may have lessened the exposure and a non-mycobacterial target cell, a 1992 study [39] found UV light to give 1.5–2 ACHE, one-tenth of the previous study. In an analysis of an outbreak of TB in a building, it was estimated that protection of overhead UV lighting exceeded what could have been produced by increased ventilation [35].

Despite this variability and concern over the potential health risks of UV radiation, Iseman [2] recommends UV lighting as perhaps the best available technology to confront nosocomial TB transmission. He estimates that such units could provide 12–15 ACHE in an average hospital room. It should not be used, however, as a substitute for HEPA filters, adequate exhaust ventilation or negative pressure. UV radiation has also been recommended as a supplement to other control measures by the American Thoracic Society/Centers for Disease Control (CDC) [40]. Providing adequate germicidal UV light without toxicity to health care deliverers from both short-term (keratoconjunctivitis and skin erythema) and long-term (cataracts and basal cell skin carcinoma) exposure dictates the importance of meeting proper safety guidelines in installation and maintenance [23]. This short wave length UV radiation is now classified as probably carcinogenic to humans by the International Agency for Research on Cancer [41]. Furthermore, UV can activate HIV gene promoters in tissue culture [42] but this observation is of unclear clinical significance.

### 9.3.4 Personal protective equipment

It had been commonplace for health care deliverers involved in the care of infectious TB patients to don a standard surgical mask. These masks (Figure 9.1) do not provide a tight facial seal or adequately filter particulate material of the droplet nucleus size [43]. They are now available in a molded form. Current recommendations from the US Public Health Service [5] suggest the use of a disposable particulate respirator (PR). Devices such as the dust-mist PR (Figure 9.2) provide a much better facial fit and particulate filtration. The PR may feel uncomfortable and this may limit its acceptability; the more efficient the seal, the greater the work of breathing and the higher the perceived discomfort [23]. When gaps occur in the seal, air will flow preferentially through the gap producing a PR working more like a funnel than a filter, providing minimal protection [44]. The degree of leak is related to the ability to obtain and maintain a proper fit and the non-availability of various sizes compared with a 'one size fits all' device.

Currently in the USA, disposable PRs are primarily certified by the National Institute for Occupational Safety and Health (NIOSH) for the industrial environment [45]. Minimal information has existed for their effectiveness against microorganisms [23]. A recent study [45a] found HEPA and dust-mist-fume PRs were more efficient in filtering *M. chelonae*. Even the least efficient mask had an efficiency of over 97%. These differences may only be relevant if the facial seal leakage is very low. In an effort to

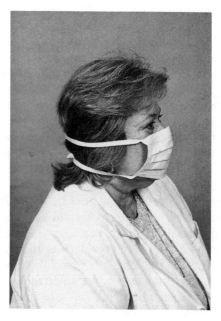

**Figure 9.1** Health care worker wearing a standard surgical mask. The lack of a seal is clearly shown.

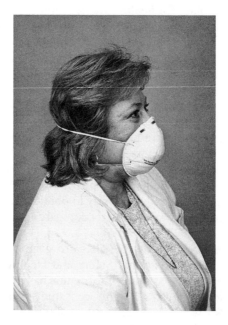

**Figure 9.2** Health care worker wearing a disposable particulate respirator. The improved seal of this device is evident compared with the standard surgical mask.

minimize the potential exposure to individuals providing care to the suspect TB patient or an individual who enters a room occupied by such a patient, Occupational Safety and Health Administration (OSHA) mandates the use of a HEPA PR. This seems in part due to the certification process not having been applied to the less costly PRs. Compared with the dust-mist or dust-mist-fume PR, the HEPA PR is more expensive, somewhat more uncomfortable to use and can contain latex which may be associated with allergy.

In the USA, NIOSH is required to develop criteria for the prevention of infectious diseases under the Occupational Safety and Health Act of 1970. The aim of the act is to create an environment where an exposure to potentially hazardous substances will be reduced well below levels determined to be safe. If no data are available to define the threshold for safety, it is assumed that any level of exposure is unsafe and should be avoided (zero risk) [45b]. Zero risk is not likely to be obtained in the TB arena even if the economic cost of more sophisticated respirators was within reach. Because of the inherent drawbacks of the disposable PR, NIOSH has recommended the use of a powered air purification respirator (PAPR) equipped with HEPA filters (Figure 9.3) for use when disposable PRs cannot be used effectively. The positive pressure produced inside the mask should minimize face seal leakage during the relatively low inhalation rate in the health care setting. Disadvantages include substantial cost, impaired voice communication, range of motion limitation and an intimidating appearance. Although the PAPR may afford greater protection than the disposable PR, the other standard methodologies are likely to be effective, except in very high risk situations (for example the bronchoscopy suite or the administration of inhalation pentamidine in TB patients) and measurable differences may not be appreciated. The standard CDC recommendations on TB control published in 1990 did not fail in the control of this disease. Rather, the increased spread of TB was related to the failure of the health care system. Iseman agrees [2], feeling that such devices cannot be a mainstay in TB control.

When personal respiratory protection devices are used a personal respiratory protection program should be in operation [44,46]. The program should include written standard operating procedures, training lectures and demonstrations, face seal testing and fit checking and inspections.

## 9.4 CHEMICAL AGENTS

There is no doubt that the use of TB case identification, antimycobacterial therapy, appropriate masks, adequate ventilation and UV light are all primary factors in the prevention of TB transmission. As reviewed succinctly by Rubin [47], however, chemical disinfection of inanimate surfaces could also play a role in prevention. The transmission of TB (and other

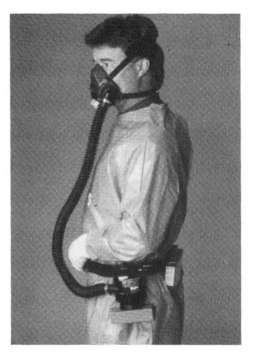

**Figure 9.3** A NIOSH approved battery powered air purifying respirator. Photograph used with permission of BioSafety Systems, San Diego, California.

pathogens) may occur from improperly disinfected bronchoscopes [48,49]. The gastroscope may also be a vehicle for transmission since sputum with tubercle bacilli is swallowed [50]. Fomites are very uncommon as a source of TB, however, several hospital workers have received compensation for allegedly acquiring TB from exposure to an inanimate object such as a suction apparatus or a hospital bed [51].

In addition to the cases of TB related to inadequate disinfection, many more infections and pseudo-infections have been reported related to non-tuberculous mycobacteria such as *M. chelonae* and *M. fortuitum* (Chapter 14). These AFB are commonly found in the environment, especially related to water. As examples, an outbreak of infection with *M. chelonae* from inadequately disinfected water used in hemodialysis has been reported [52] and our institution observed a pseudo-epidemic of *M. fortuitum* and *M. avium-intracellulare* associated with the cleaning of bronchoscopes with tap water subsequently found to have the same organisms [53].

The ability to kill mycobacteria is in part dependent on the environment in which the bacilli are maintained. Organic proteinaceous material, sputum in the case of the tubercle bacillus, adversely affects many disinfecting agents. Smith [54] reported that *M. tuberculosis* was cultured from a tuberculous cavity up to 1 year after embalming, demonstrating that formaldehyde could not be depended on to kill TB in the presence of substantial amounts of organic matter.

The choice of a specific disinfectant depends on a number of factors so that no single agent will be adequate for every circumstance (Table 9.4). Variables include the nature of the organism, the item to be disinfected, the amount of time needed, cost and the amount of toxicity and allergenicity to be tolerated.

**Table 9.4** Antimycobacterial disinfectants

| Agent | Antimycobacterial activity | Comment |
|-------|---------------------------|---------|
| Ethyl/isopropyl alcohol | ++ | Less effective in concentrations > 95% or in presence of organic debris |
| Phenolics | +++ | Effective in presence of organic debris. May have residual disinfectant effect |
| Formaldehyde | + | Infectivity of formalin-embalmed tissue brings out concern |
| Glutaraldehyde | ++ | Effective in presence of organic debris. Must be adequately maintained over time |
| Iodine/iodophors | + | Staining |
| Ethylene oxide | +++ | High cost of equipment. Lengthy exposure time needed |
| Peracetic acid | +++ | Useful for rapid turn round of fiberoptic equipment. Special sterilizer needed |

### 9.4.1 Alcohols

Both ethyl and isopropyl alcohol at concentrations of about 50% are useful mycobacteriocides and the effect is increased when added to other agents including iodine and formaldehyde [47]. Interestingly, ethanol concentrations about 95% are not as effective [55]. Alcohols are affected by organic debris so when using alcohol on skin, thermometers or metal instruments, care should be taken to wipe or wash off the organic debris prior to treatment.

### 9.4.2 Phenolics

Phenolic compounds have been used as highly effective disinfectants against *M. tuberculosis*. Rubin [47] has reviewed some of the older literature, finding great utility but disadvantages such as toxicity and odor. Ortho-phenyl phenol is, however, mostly odorless. Importantly, unlike the alcohols, phenolics are still effective in the presence of organic material. Additionally, o-phenyl phenol has a residual disinfectant effect for 30 days after application to dry surfaces [56]. Phenolics are useful in disinfecting glassware, metal instruments, linen, toilets, furniture and floors. They are, on the whole, more effectively tuberculocidal than most other disinfectants [57].

### 9.4.3 Formaldehyde

Although generally thought to have adequate antimycobacterial activity, it has been shown that viable *M. tuberculosis* could be obtained from formaldehyde (10% formalin) embalmed autopsy tissue. Certainly, reports such as that of Albert and Levinson regarding the infection of students related to embalmed cadavers [58] supports concern about this issue.

Used for disinfection of certain metal surfaces, formaldehyde is too corrosive and toxic for most circumstances. In a dialysis outbreak of *M. chelonae* [52], the organism survived exposure to 2% formaldehyde for 24 hours but was killed by a 4% solution.

### 9.4.4 Glutaraldehyde

Glutaraldehyde, used as an alkalinized 2% aqueous solution, is recognized to have considerable antimycobacterial activity [47,59]. It is noncorrosive and much less irritating than formaldehyde. This disinfectant has remained active in the presence of proteinaceous material such as serum [60]. It is still recommended to clean the surface to be disinfected thoroughly prior to treatment, particularly if prolonged treatment is not feasible. Even though it is an effective agent, a majority of centers in England were not using glutaraldehyde in an effective treatment protocol [61]. To remain effective, the product must be adequately maintained as it loses its potency over time. Although it is thought to be nontoxic and nonallergenic, irritated mucosal membranes and skin may occur.

### 9.4.5 Iodine and iodophors

Iodine (0.2–0.5%) combined with alcohol (70–80%) is considered to be the choice for thermometer disinfection. Although these agents stain fabrics and may be corrosive, they are relatively nontoxic and may be used in the disinfection of metal and glass instruments and as a skin preparation before surgery [47]. It has been reported [48] that certain strains of *M. tuberculosis* were not killed by iodophors at various strengths even after 30 minutes of exposure.

### 9.4.6 Ethylene oxide

This reasonably nontoxic, highly diffusible gas is not damaging to most materials and can be used in the disinfection of such surfaces as leather, paper, plastic, wood, metal and rubber. The disadvantages of ethylene oxide are the relatively high cost of the equipment needed for its use and the lengthy exposure time needed for appropriate treatment [47]. It remains one of the best agents for fiberoptic devices, which can be damaged by autoclaving [48,49].

### 9.4.7 Miscellaneous agents

Peracetic acid can be used to sterilize heat sensitive immersible instruments with a rapid turn round time. It is active against mycobacteria. Hexachlorophene may be active against Gram-positive cocci but is not antimycobacterial and the quaternary ammonium salts have no activity [47]. Mercurial compounds are also felt to be noneffective.

## 9.5 NONADHERENCE TO CHEMOTHERAPY

Noncompletion of TB treatment plays a key role in the prevalence and resistance patterns of this infection. Although not truly a chronic disease, the prevention or cure of TB necessitates administration of medication for months. Compliance, the term generally used to refer to the act of completing chemotherapy, can imply that the patient is docile and subservient to the care provider [62]. Sumartojo [62], therefore, has suggested that adherence be used, reflecting a more active patient role in the management of the therapy and the importance of cooperation between the health care recipient and deliverer.

In the USA, about 20% of TB patients do not complete chemotherapy [63]. A study from New York City reported that 83% of infected patients, in the setting of rampant homelessness, substance abuse and HIV infection, failed to complete even the initial 12 weeks of treatment [64]. Additionally, a third of those given preventive isoniazid (INH) did not complete the course [62].

### 9.5.1 Nonadherence measurements and correlates

How adherence to TB regimens should be measured is not well established. Methodology includes self reporting, estimates by the health care deliverer, appointments kept, medication counts, prescriptions filled, assays of medication in body fluid and electronic devices that record the removal of pills from a container [62]. No method is completely accurate as each is measuring different aspects of adherence. Indeed, multiple measurements for adherence seem to be needed to assess whether the patient is taking the prescribed medications.

Difficulties in interpreting these parameters are well described. In two studies, nonadherent patients were identified by health care deliverers only about 30% of the time [65,66] and 8% of adherent individuals were thought to be nonadherent [65]. These measurements are dependent on the techniques used to elicit responses and the relationship between the health care worker and the patient. Both INH and rifampin can be identified in the urine but positive results cannot measure whether the drug is ingested regularly. Likewise, electronically recording when and how often the medication bottle is opened does not measure if the drug is actually taken.

Many factors can be involved in nonadherence. These often reflect a lack of access to relevant information about health and illness, minimal financial resources for medical treatment, or mistrust of the health care system. Sumartojo [62] cites unpublished data from the US Public Health Service which includes homelessness, illicit substance abuse, emotional disturbance, poor access to transportation, lack of family and/or social support, migrant status, illiteracy, unemployment, low income and minority status as relevant variables. A 1993 Canadian study did not associate gender, age and immigration status with default of therapy but found adherence was associated with initial hospitalization compared with no hospitalization, a 6 month plan of therapy rather than a 12-month plan, a shorter interval before the first follow-up visit and a positive nursing assessment for patient understanding [67].

Cultural issues can also be very important in TB treatment. As an example, many Hispanics have believed that TB can be treated with over-the-counter medicines and that hospitalization for TB may subject the index case to familial rejection [68,69]. Some patients reported that they would prefer death to the social rejection associated with this disease [69].

### 9.5.2 Interventions to improve adherence

Some interventions that have been used to improve adherence are listed in Table 9.5.

*(a) Patient incentives*

Financial rewards such as money, bus or train tokens and food have been used to improve the default rate in therapeutic interventions. Minimal objective research, however, has been done to assess these effects [62]. One report, however, combining patient education with financial incentives

**Table 9.5** Methodology to improve adherence to chemotherapy

---

Patient incentives
- Money
- Bus or train tokens
- Food
- Enablers
    Travel to health care facilities
    Free medications

Social incentives (increased interpersonal contacts)

Education

Treatment strategies
- Injectable medications
- Blister calender packs
- Six-month regimens
- Directly observed therapy

Community health workers

Comprehensive services

---

found adherence improved in an INH preventive group (68% compared with 38%) but not in the treatment group [70].

Social incentives involving increased interpersonal contacts have been shown to affect adherence. As one example, a 'breakfast club' was set up which supplied nutrition and friendship [71]. Furthermore, an Indian study using the incentive of familial involvement by meeting with home public health visitors increased adherence [72]. Some incentives are enablers so that patients may attend a clinic or take their therapy rather than just be rewarded for doing so [62].

Each incentive should be combined with a variety of educational interventions. The delivery of such education and its location can also be a significant variable in adherence. A study from Spain showed that education delivered by a nurse visiting the patient's home produced better results than information delivered by telephone and both were more effective than education delivered by a physician in his or her office [73].

*(b) Treatment strategies*

A number of therapeutic interventions have been used to improve adherence. In some patients, the use of an injectable drug, such as an aminoglycoside or capreomycin, may enhance the significance of the infection to the patient, improving the chance of adherence to therapy [62]. Since this necessitates patient contact with a health care deliverer, part of the effect may be related to education or social interaction. In a study of over 250 000 TB patients in the Philippines, the use of blister calendar packs of medications increased adherence to over 80% compared with 41%

historically [74]. Fixed combination medications, such as isoniazid/rifampin can also improve adherence by lowering the number of pills that the patient has to take. As noted previously, the shorter 6 month course can improve compliance compared with 12–18 month courses.

Supervised or directly observed therapy (DOT) improves adherence to a therapeutic or preventive regimen in TB patients [62]. In response to the increase in total TB and drug-resistant TB in the USA, new recommendations suggest DOT should be considered in all TB patients [5]. DOT can vary from supervised therapy in the home to a clinic or even a designated street corner. Therapy can be administered by a health care worker or another person considered to be responsible, such as a family member, teacher or employer. Community-based volunteer health workers can be very useful in the success of these programs based on their respect in the area, reliability and close residence to the patient [62]. A study from the Philippines using church-based volunteers clearly underscores this resource [75]. Although DOT may be more labor intensive and costlier than other methods, when done appropriately and combined with other interventions, it can be effective enough to decrease secondary resistance and case spread and thus prove to be cost effective in TB control.

A CDC study involving patients in 10 cities quoted by Sumartojo [62] found a 50% decrease in nonadherence in DOT patients compared with those responsible for their own medication (5% failure compared with 10%). The positive effects of DOT do not necessarily continue if the supervision is discontinued prior to the end of therapy. In a study among Canadian Indians [76], daily DOT for preventive therapy resulted in only 19% nonadherence compared with 48% in an educational intervention group and 75% in a control group. Within 3 months after these interventions were stopped, there was no difference between the groups in the ingestion of INH. Even in a shelter for homeless men, a DOT program using biweekly INH produced a 49% adherence rate [77]. These increased adherence rates can translate into clinical responses as shown in a rural American study where 87% of DOT patients became sputum negative by 3 months, compared with 61% of standard therapy patients [78]. Furthermore, a Texas study published in 1994 found that the aggressive use of DOT could dramatically decrease acquired drug resistance and both overall and multi-drug-resistant relapse [78a].

Combining short course therapy with DOT has been successful even in situations where the risk of nonadherence is great. Miles and Maat [79] in an open refugee camp on the Thai–Cambodian border and Manalo et al. [75] in a population with a high prevalence of drug resistance reported success using these modalities.

## (c) Comprehensive services

TB treatment programs that incorporate multiple modalities to address the individual patient's needs can further improve adherence. Curry [80], in San

Francisco, was able to decrease the missed appointment rate from 34% to 6% using a neighborhood-based clinic system including a specialized, motivated medical team and greater convenience for the patients. The presence of motivated health care workers with a positive attitude towards their patients was an important aspect of the program. A comprehensive TB clinic in Chicago [81] combined this with easy accessibility and assistance with social and financial issues. Poor performance by the care deliverer, manifesting as inadequate record keeping, lost charts and non-recorded laboratory data, was partly responsible for poor patient adherence. Such comprehensive services have been shown to be effective in successful TB treatment even in previously nonadherent patients. As an example, Reichman's group in New Jersey [82] reported treatment success in 19 of 21 patients with long histories of past failures by the use of DOT and free comprehensive social and medical services.

Because of the importance of TB treatment adherence to public health overall, comprehensive programs can provide the motivation needed for the participation of potentially or previously nonadherent individuals. As stressed by Sumartojo [62], by tailoring treatment services to the specific needs of each patient and providing assistance for problems other than TB, such programs actively reach out to the patient. The diversity of problems in many patients is addressed by these services providing the patient with the additional assistance necessary which can facilitate the treatment and cure of TB.

*(d) Confinement*

Despite the use of adherence enhancing techniques, a small but significant number of individuals remain noncompliant. In such situations, the possibility of confining these patients in a hospital or other facility for treatment should be considered. The ability to do so will depend on legislation, co-operative court and law enforcement personnel and the presence of facilities for such confinement.

## 9.6 TUBERCULOSIS IN DEVELOPING COUNTRIES

Despite the achievements made in effective prophylaxis and therapy, TB continues to rank among the most serious of health problems throughout the world. Globally, 1.7 billion individuals, approximating to one third of the world's population, are or have been infected with the tubercle bacillus. The age distribution of the infection is dramatically different between the industrialized and developing worlds. In industrialized countries, 80% of people infected with TB are over the age of 50 whereas 75% of those in developing countries are less than 50 [83]. While the toll of TB in children in the developing world is substantial, the greatest attack rate is in the economically most productive age group (15–59 year olds) [83].

Estimates for 1990 were that 8 million new TB cases developed globally, with 95% in the developing world [84]. Of these cases, 50% are smear positive and therefore significantly infectious [85]. The largest number of cases occur in the World Health Organization's (WHO) Southeast Asian, Western Pacific and African regions. Because of poor distribution of health care services and difficulties accessing and using such facilities, especially in the rural areas, no more than half of these new cases are even diagnosed [86]. This presents a significant problem in source identification. Mortality from TB in 1990 was estimated to be 2.9 million, making it the largest single cause of death from a pathogen in the world [83]. Although 98% of the deaths are in the developing world, accounting for 25% of avoidable adult deaths, more than 40 000 deaths occurred in industrialized nations [84].

### 9.6.1 Problems in tuberculosis control in the developing world

Little, if any, of the decrease in TB seen in the industrialized countries through the second portion of the 20th century has been reflected in the developing nations. As an example, the annual decrease in TB in recent years was 14% in The Netherlands, 1.4% in Uganda and negligible in Lesotho [87]. Clearly, the advances that have occurred in developed countries have not been applied in the developing world. The methods for TB control are no different, but the quality of the control procedures and how they can be used are quite different between these areas. Examples of these differences are listed in Table 9.6.

**Table 9.6** Problems in tuberculosis control in developing nations

---

- Limited number and location of health care facilities
- Poor access to health care facilities
- Limited resources of the health care facility (cultures, X-rays)
- Different attitudes towards illness and medications produced by social and cultural backgrounds
- HIV infection and malnutrition increase risk of clinical infection
- Prolonged treatment regimens diminish adherence
- Increased antimycobacterial resistance patterns

---

Although treatment adherence rates in much of the developing world are poor, leading to low cure rates, countries that have built-in systems to monitor treatment outcomes can have cure rates of over 80%. These results are facilitated by financial and technical help from the International Union Against Tuberculosis and Lung Disease (IUATLD) [83]. The availability of medical services to treat TB is a substantial problem and contributes to difficulties in control of the disease. Kochi [83] estimated that only

46% of current TB cases in the developing world are in areas covered by TB services and that no significant change has occurred over the past 15 years. An in-depth study of the cost and impact of the treatment of smear positive TB in Malawi, Mozambique and Tanzania (all part of the IUATLD program) has shown that treating TB was less expensive than other cost effective interventions, such as measles immunization and oral rehydration therapy [88].

The HIV epidemic is having a severe effect on TB control programs in developing countries. Although only a small percentage of TB cases are HIV related, most of these dual infections are in the sub-Saharan area of Africa where TB service coverage is low [83]. In some areas, a 100% increase in reported TB cases has occurred, thought primarily to be related to HIV [89]. Complicating the situation are a number of factors (Table 9.7) which make the management of co-infection with *M. tuberculosis* and HIV more difficult.

**Table 9.7** Problems of co-infection with HIV and tuberculosis in the developing world

| |
|---|
| Increased demands |
| • Diagnostic services |
| • Hospital beds |
| • Medical supplies |
| Difficulties in diagnosis and treatment |
| • Drug reactions and intolerance |
| • Extrapulmonary tuberculosis |
| Social issues |
| • Increased stigma |
| Health care workers |
| • Fear of HIV acquisition |
| • Increased frustration regarding high mortality rates |
| • Decreased credibility of tuberculosis control |

Pio [90], in analyzing the impact of present control methods on the global TB problem, observed the slow or absent regression of the disease and the marked limitation of control measures. He felt it was unrealistic to expect a rapid reduction in global TB given the socio-economic conditions of many of the developing nations and the difficulties in applying the current methodology of case finding, treatment and prevention in these areas. Pio recommended the application of modern molecular biologic and immunologic technology to develop new methods and considered that without these applications, TB control was far away. Kochi [83] outlined the new WHO TB control strategy and felt that progress could be made by improvement of the cure rate with short course chemotherapy, combination medication tablets and expansion of TB service areas. WHO's proposed global target using this methodology included a decrease in the annual TB death rate by 40% (to 1.7 million), a decrease in global prevalence by 50% by the use of short course treatment and a decrease in incidence of the disease by 50% in 12 years by an increase in case finding coverage to 60–65%.

## 9.7 CONTROL THROUGH BCG VACCINATION

In the early 20th century, buoyed by success in the development of vaccines against smallpox and rabies, attempts were made to develop biological products to prevent TB. After a number of failures, Albert Calmette and Camille Guérin developed a weakened bacterial strain that was a good vaccine candidate. This work, at the Pasteur Institute in France, was done using *M. bovis*. After 13 years of *in vitro* subculturing, the organism was no longer able to produce progressive lesions in animals. The early work on the vaccine organism called Bacillus Calmette-Guérin (BCG) has been reviewed by several authors [91,92].

These investigations came to fruition in the spring of 1921 when Halle inoculated a child at high risk of acquisition of TB with the BCG vaccine. Soon after, the use of BCG spread across Europe. In 1930, a well publicized disaster occurred in Germany culminating in the death of 72 BCG vaccinated children. This was not due to a reversion of BCG to a more virulent form but rather to a laboratory error in which the vaccine was contaminated with the much more virulent *M. tuberculosis*. Despite this episode, by 1945, the use of BCG to prevent TB was well established.

BCG efficacy until then was mainly based on individual experiences, anecdotal observations or uncontrolled studies. Because of this, a dramatic dichotomy of BCG utilization developed which still exists in the world today. BCG is globally the most widely used vaccine with over 3 billion doses having been administered in the past four decades and more than 70% of the world's children now receiving BCG [93]. The recommended vaccine schedule may vary widely from country to country, however, including a single dose in infancy, a single dose in adolescence or repeated vaccination in childhood [94]. The USA has remained one of the few nations not to have used BCG on a national scale and its agencies issued an even more negative statement on BCG in 1988 [95]. The current recommendations no longer include the use of BCG for health care workers or other adults at high risk for TB acquisition. This policy change was developed with the assumption that prompt identification of the TB patient could be made and that INH therapy would minimize the effect of acquisition. This statement was issued before the full impact of the current wave of TB was appreciated. Newer suggestions from the Advisory Committee on Immunization Practices (ACIP) may be forthcoming.

### 9.7.1 BCG efficacy

It is paramount when regarding the use of BCG to analyze the studies designed to assess vaccine protectiveness. A critical review of eight controlled BCG trials was published in 1983 [96]. The trials had a range of observed efficacy from −56% to 80%. This review concluded that BCG can confer a high degree of protection against TB and that bias or inadequate statistical power may have contributed to the conflicting data.

More recently, TB morbidity in France was reported to be five times lower in BCG vaccinees compared with their nonvaccinated schoolmates [97]. Furthermore, a 1990 Brazilian case-control study [98] reported a more than 80% effectiveness against TB meningitis in children less than 5 years old. A study from Cameroon reported 66% protection by BCG against pulmonary TB in young adults [99].

On the negative side, several large studies have not demonstrated measurable efficacy in TB prevention. One, published in 1979, involved 260 000 individuals in Madras, India with a 7.5 year follow-up and no clear BCG protective effect [100]. Clemons [96] evaluated this study in his review and felt that it did not provide adequate protection against surveillance and diagnostic testing biases and did not examine the distribution of susceptibility factors. A study in Malawi involving more than 80 000 individuals also did not show protection against TB [101]. A meta-analysis of 14 prospective trials and 12 case-control studies of BCG [101a] found that BCG reduced the TB risk by 50%. The decrease occurred across many populations, study designs, forms of disease and age of vaccination.

### 9.7.2 Variability in BCG vaccines

Since 1948, the WHO has been involved in establishing and maintaining a quality control program for BCG. Milstien and Gibson [102] have reviewed data comparing different BCG strains. The number of culturable particles per dose varied from $3.7 \times 10^4$ to $3.2 \times 10^6$ between strains and as much as 10–15-fold between lots of the same strain. Even more dramatic, there was significant variability in the physicochemical characteristics of the BCG antigens produced by different strains. As an example, MPB7O, a unique BCG specific antigen is produced in variable quantities by some strains and not at all by others [102]. Much of this variability is related to each vaccine preparation being a mixture of different BCG mycobacteria, despite being referred to as a specific strain. Different production methods may influence the composition of the mixture (BCG hoard) and the composition of the mixture may differ between production lots of the same 'strain' [102]. Despite this, no clear BCG strain specific protective differences are described [101a].

### 9.7.3 Adverse reactions

BCG immunization is well tolerated with few serious complications. Side effects vary by strain and can change for the same strain over time [103]. The most common adverse effects are severe or prolonged ulceration at the vaccination site, lymphadenitis and osteitis. The incidence of regional suppurative adenitis depends on the type and concentration of vaccine used [102] and the technique of the vaccinator. For example, in Egypt, 10% of vaccinees in a public clinic developed adenitis needing treatment compared with 0.02% vaccinated in a clinic where immunization was given under stricter supervision [104]. Osteitis is also variable in incidence with rates of 0.01–300 per million vaccinations [102]. Disseminated BCG, at a rate of 1–10 cases per 10 million doses, is almost exclusively a problem of those with impaired immunity [103]. That BCG can persist in the body to cause symptoms later is shown by local infection 1 year after intravesical use [105] and BCG adenitis in a patient with AIDS 30 years after vaccination [106].

### 9.7.4 The future of BCG vaccination

TB prevention by BCG remains disparate throughout the world with explanations for the differences thought to be individual 'strain' potency differences, vaccination techniques and the age, genetics and nutrition of the vaccinees. The prevalence of environmental non-tuberculous AFB and the relative proportion of TB due to endogenous reactivation or new exogenous infection may also be relevant. It is surmised [107] that no single reason can explain all the disparity and multiple mechanisms are likely.

Citron [107] concluded in 1993, that BCG vaccination of the newborn should be continued in the developing world where TB is most prevalent. In developed countries with low TB prevalence, BCG could be given to high risk groups such as immigrants and their newborns and to the contacts of TB patients. Furthermore, in the midst of the epidemic of multi-drug-resistant TB in HIV patients in the USA, vaccination of health care workers at high risk may be increasingly important. This suggestion is made despite the variable results in efficacy of BCG in adolescents and adults. Nettleman [108] has estimated that even at 20% efficacy, BCG can be cost effective in TB prevention in health care workers and encourages further studies.

It is possible that further studies in analyzing vaccine components needed for protection [102] and more uniformity in different BCG preparations will produce some answers. Alternatively, improvements to BCG by adding other mycobacterial antigens [109] could potentially improve or confuse further efficacy data. Vaccines against the newly described *M. tuberculosis* gene product encoding for mammalian cell entry [110] or other specific bacterial products may also have future utility. Finally, Bretscher [111] has suggested that using lower BCG immunizing dosages rather than 'the largest acceptable dose' may produce a better cell mediated immune response.

## 9.8 CONCLUSIONS

The increased awareness of the resurgence of TB and recommendations from the WHO and the CDC to combat this problem are the first steps in the further control of this disease. Methods of tailoring control methodology to specific TB situations, such as the health care setting [23], long term care facilities for the elderly [112], migrant farm workers [113], the homeless [10], minority groups [11], foreign born immigrants [114], patients with multi-drug-resistant infection [115] and worldwide [83], have been published. No doubt these recommendations will affect the disease but most of the plans have some negative aspects. As quoted by the CDC in its 1989 plan for the elimination of TB in the USA [116], Samuel Johnson aptly summarized the problem:

> Nothing will ever be attempted if all possible objections must be first overcome.

## REFERENCES

1. Reichman, L.B. (1991) The U-shaped curve of concern. *Am Rev Respir Dis*, **144**, 741–2.
2. Iseman, M.D. (1992) A leap of faith. What can we do to curtail intrainstitutional transmission of tuberculosis. *Ann Intern Med*, **117**, 251–3.
3. Murray, J.F. (1989) The white plague: down and out, or up and coming? *Am Rev Respir Dis*, **140**, 1788–95.
4. World Health Organization (1992) Tuberculosis control and research strategies for the 1990s: Memorandum from a WHO Meeting. *Bull WHO*, **70**, 17–21.
5. American Thoracic Society (1992) Control of tuberculosis in the United States. *Am Rev Respir Dis*, **146**, 1623–33.
6. World Health Organization (1982) Tuberculosis control. Report of a Joint IUAT/WHO Study Group. *WHO Technical Report Series*, No. 671.
7. Craven, R.B., Wenzel, R.P. and Atuk, N.O. (1975) Minimizing tuberculosis risk to hospital personnel and students exposed to unsuspected disease. *Ann Intern Med*, **82**, 628–32.
8. Kantor, H.S., Poblete, R. and Pusateri, S.L. (1988) Nosocomial transmission of tuberculosis from unsuspected disease. *Am J Med*, **84**, 833–8.
9. Subcommittee of the Joint Tuberculosis Committee of the British Thoracic Society (1990) Control and prevention of tuberculosis in Britain: an updated code of practice. *Brit Med J*, **300**, 995–7.
10. Advisory Council for the Elimination of Tuberculosis (1992) Prevention and control of tuberculosis among homeless persons. *MMWR*, **41 (RR-5)**, 13–23.
11. Advisory Council for the Elimination of Tuberculosis (1992) Prevention and control of tuberculosis in U.S. communities with at-risk minority populations. *MMWR*, **41 (RR-5)**, 1–12.
12. Barnes, P.F., Verdegen, T.D., Vachon, L.A. *et al.* (1988) Chest roent-geno-grams in pulmonary tuberculosis. New data on an old test. *Chest*, **94**, 316–20.

13. Halperin, S.A. and Langley, J.M. (1992) Evaluation of a tuberculosis screening program at a children's hospital. *Am J Infect Cont*, **20**, 19–23.
14. Loudon, R.G. and Spohn, S.K. (1969) Cough frequency and infectivity in patients with pulmonary tuberculosis. *Am Rev Respir Dis*, **99**, 109–11.
15. Nakielna, E.M., Cragg, R. and Grzybowski, S. (1975) Lifelong follow-up of inactive tuberculosis: its value and limitation. *Am Rev Respir Dis*, **112**, 765–72.
16. Wells, W.F. (1934) On airborne infection. II. Droplets and droplet nuclei. *Am J Hyg*, **20**, 611–8.
17. Duguid, J.P. (1946) Expulsion of pathogenic organisms from the respiratory tract. *Brit Med J*, **1**, 265–8.
18. Chapman, J.S. and Dyerly, M.D. (1964) Presumably infected premises with respect to conversion of the tuberculin test. *Am Rev Respir Dis*, **89**, 197–9.
19. Riley, R.L. (1982) Disease transmission and contagion control. *Am Rev Respir Dis*, **125** (Supplement), 16–19.
20. Chan, J., Otten, J. and Cleary T. (1992) *Successful Control of an Outbreak of Multidrug-resistant Tuberculosis in an Urban Teaching Hospital.* Interscience Conference on Antimicrobial Agents and Chemotherapy, Anaheim, CA, American Society for Microbiology.
21. American Society of Heating, Refrigerating and Air Conditioning Engineers (1987) 1987 *ASHRAE Handbook: Heating, Ventilating and Air-conditioning Systems and Applications*, American Society of Heating, Refrigerating and Air Conditioning Engineers, Atlanta, GA, 23.1–23.12.
22. Health Resources and Services Administration (1984) *Guidelines for Construction and Equipment of Hospital and Medical Facilities.* U.S. Department of Health and Human Services, Public Health Service, Rockville, MD, PHS publication no. HRSA 84-14500.
23. Centers for Disease Control (1990) Guidelines for preventing the transmission of tuberculosis in health-care settings, with special focus on HIV-related issues. *MMWR*, **39 (RR-17)**, 1–29.
24. California Indoor Quality Program (1990) *Using Ultraviolet Radiation and Ventilation to Control Tuberculosis.* Air and Industrial Hygiene Laboratory and Tuberculosis Control and Refugee Health Programs Unit, Berkeley, CA, pp. 1–18.
25. Rudnick, J., Kroc, K., Manangan, L. *et al.* (1993) *How Prepared are U.S. Hospitals to Control Nosocomial Transmission of Tuberculosis?* Society of Hospital Epidemiologists of America, Chicago, IL.
26. Ehrenkranz, N.J. and Kicklighter, J.L. (1982) Tuberculosis outbreak in a general hospital: evidence for airborne spread of tuberculosis. *Ann Intern Med*, **77**, 377–82.
27. Haley, C.E., McDonald, R.C., Rossi, L. *et al.* (1989) Tuberculosis epidemic among hospital personnel. *Infect Control Hosp Epidemiol*, **10**, 204–10.
28. Hutton, M.D., Stead, W.W., Cauthen, G.M. *et al.* (1990) Nosocomial transmission of tuberculosis associated with a draining tuberculous abscess. *J Infect Dis*, **161**, 286–95.
29. Lundgren, R., Norrman, E. and Asberg, I. (1987) Tuberculosis infection transmitted at autopsy. *Tubercle*, **68**, 147–50.
30. Centers for Disease Control (1989) *Mycobacterium tuberculosis* transmission in a health clinic – Florida. *MMWR*, **38**, 256–64.

31. Adler, J.J. (1993) Hospital-acquired tuberculosis: addressing the challenge. *Hosp Pract*, **28**(9), 109–16, 120.

32. Sheretz, R.J., Belani, A., Kramer, B.S. *et al.* (1987) Impact of air filtration on nosocomial *Aspergillus* infection. *Am J Med*, **83**, 709–18.

33. Woods, J.E. and Rask, D.R. (1988) Heating, ventilation, air-conditioning systems: the engineering aproach to methods of control, in *Architectural Design and Indoor Microbial Pollution* (ed. R.B. Kundsin), Oxford University Press, New York, pp. 123–53.

34. Wells, W.F. and Fair, G.M. (1935) Viability of *E. coli* exposed to ultraviolet radiation in air. *Science*, **82**, 280–1.

35. Riley, R.L. and Nardell, E.A. (1989) Clearing the air. The theory and application of ultraviolet air disinfection. *Am Rev Respir Dis*, **139**, 1286–94.

36. Riley R.L. and Kaufman, J.E. (1972) Effect of relative humidity on the inactivation of airborne *Serratia marcescens* by ultraviolet radiation. *Appl Environ Microbiol*, **23**, 1113–20.

37. Riley, R.L., Mills, C.C., O'Grady, F. *et al.* (1962) Infectiousness of air from a tuberculosis ward. Ultraviolet irradiation of infected air: comparative infectiousness of different patients. *Am Rev Respir Dis*, **85**, 511–25.

38. Riley, R.L., Knight, M. and Middlebrook, G. (1976) Ultraviolet susceptibility of BCG and virulent tubercle bacilli. *Am Rev Respir Dis*, **113**, 413–18.

39. Macher, J.M., Alevantis, L.E., Chang, Y.-L. and Liu, K.-S. (1992) Effect of ultraviolet germicidal lamps on airborne microorganisms in an outpatient washing room. *Appl Occup Environ Hyg*, **7**, 505–13.

40. American Thoracic Society/Centers for Disease Control (1990) Diagnostic standards and classification of tuberculosis. *Am Rev Respir Dis*, **142**, 725–35.

41. International Agency for Research on Cancer (1992) *IARC Monographs on the Evaluation of Carcinogenic Risks for Humans: Solar and Ultraviolet Radiation*, Volume 55, World Health Organization, Lyons, France.

42. Valerie, K., Delers, A., Bruck, C. *et al.* (1988) Activation of human immunodeficiency virus type 1 by DNA damage in human cells. *Nature*, **333**, 78–81.

43. Pippin, D.J., Verderame, R.A. and Weber, K.K. (1987) Efficacy of face masks in preventing inhalation of airborne contaminants. *J Oral Maxillofac Surg*, **45**, 319–23.

44. National Institute for Occupational Safety and Health (1987) *Guide to Industrial Respiratory Protection,* U.S. Department of Health and Human Service (NIOSH) Publication, **70**, pp. 87–116.

45. Hutton, M.D. (1992) What is a disposable particulate respirator? *Am J Infect Cont*, **20**, 41.

45a. Chen, S.K., Vesley, D., Brosseau, L.M. and Vincent, J.H. (1994) Evaluation of single-use masks and respirators for protection of health care workers against mycobacterial aerosols. *Am J Infect Cont*, **22**, 65–74.

45b. Gerberding, J.L. (1993) Occupational infectious diseases or infectious occupational diseases? Bridging the views on tuberculosis control. *Infect Cont Hosp Epidemiol*, **14**, 686–8.

46. Occupational Safety and Health Administration 29CFR1910-134 (1994) *Occupational Safety and Health Standards: Personal Protective Equipment, Respiratory Protection*, Code of Federal Regulations, U.S. Government Printing Office, Washington, DC.

47. Rubin, J. (1991) Mycobacterial disinfection and control, in *Disinfection,*

*Sterilization and Preservation* (ed. S.S. Block), Lea and Febiger, Malvern, PA, pp. 374–84.

48. Nelson, K.E., Larson, P.A., Schraufnagel, D.E. and Jackson, J. (1983) Transmission of tuberculosis by flexible fiberbronchoscopes. *Am Rev Respir Dis*, **127**, 97–100.

49. Leers, W.D. (1980) Disinfecting bronchoscopes: how not to transmit *Mycobacterium tuberculosis* by bronchoscopy. *Can Med Assoc J*, **123**, 275–80.

50. Ayliffe, G.A.J. (1988) Equipment related infection risks. *J Hosp Infect*, **11**(Suppl A), 279–84.

51. Notlebart, H.C. (1980) Nosocomial infections acquired by hospital employees. *Infect Control*, **1**, 257–9.

52. Centers for Disease Control (1983) Nontuberculous mycobacterial infections in hemodialysis patients –Louisiana. *MMWR*, **32**, 244–6.

53. Chapnick, E.K., Lutwick, S.M. and Lutwick, L.I. (1993) Acid fast bacilli in bronchoalveolar lavage. *Infect Med*, **10**, 7, 39.

54. Smith, C.R. (1968) Mycobacteriocidal agents, in *Disinfection, Sterilization and Preservation* (eds C.A. Lawrence and S.S. Block), Lea and Febiger, Philadephia, PA, pp. 504–14.

55. Spaulding, E.H. (1964) Alcohol as a surgical disinfectant. *Assoc Oper Rm Nurse J*, **2**, 67–71.

56. Lester, W. and Dunkin, E.W. (1955) Residual surface disinfection. *J Infect Dis*, **96**, 40–53.

57. Bergan, T. and Lystad, A. (1971) Antitubercular action of disinfectants. *J Appl Bacteriol*, **34**, 751–6.

58. Albert, M.E. and Levison, M.E. (1964) An epidemic of tuberculosis in a medical school. *N Engl J Med*, **272**, 718–21.

59. Stonehill, A.A., Krop, S. and Borick, P.M. (1963) Buffered glutaraldehyde – a new chemical sterilizing solution. *Am J Hosp Pharm*, **20**, 458–65.

60. Borick, P.M., Dondershine, F.H. and Chandler, V.I. (1964) Alkalinized glutaraldehyde, a new antimicrobial agent. *J Pharm Sci*, **53**, 1273–5.

61. Ayon, A.T.R. and Cotton, P.B. (1983) Endoscopy and infection. *Gut*, **24**, 1064–6.

62. Sumartojo, E. (1993) When tuberculosis treatment fails. A social behavioral account of patient adherence. *Am Rev Respir Dis*, **147**, 1311–20.

63. Snider, D.E. and Roper, W.L. (1992) The new tuberculosis. *N Engl J Med*, **326**, 703–5.

64. Brudney, K. and Dobkin, J. (1991) Resurgent tuberculosis in New York City. *Am Rev Respir Dis*, **144**, 745–9.

65. Wardman, A.G., Knox, A.J., Muers, M.F. and Page, R.L. (1988) Profiles of non-compliance with anti-tuberculous therapy. *Brit J Dis Chest*, **82**, 285–9.

66. Preston, D.F. and Miller F.L. (1964) The tuberculosis outpatient's defection from therapy. *Am J Med Sci*, **247**, 55–8.

67. Menzies, R., Rocher, I. and Vissandjee, B. (1993) Factors associated with compliance in the treatment of tuberculosis. *Tubercle Lung Dis*, **74**, 32–7.

68. Rubel, A.J. and Garro, L.C. (1992) Social and cultural factors in the successful control of tuberculosis. *Pub Health Rep*, **107**, 626–36.

69. Mata, J.I. (1985) Integrating the client's perspective in planning a tuberculosis education and treatment program in Honduras. *Med Anthropol*, **Winter**, 57–64.

70. Morisky, D.E., Malotte, C.K., Choi, P. *et al.* (1990) A patient education program to improve adherence rates with antituberculous drug regimens. *Health Educ Quart*, **17**, 253–67.

71. Edwards, B.B. (1988) The breakfast club. *Florida Nurse*, **36**, 9.

72. Seetha, M.A., Srikantaramu, N., Aneja, K.S. and Singh, H. (1981) Influence of motivation of patients with their family members on the drug collection by patients. *Indian J Tuberc*, **28**, 182–90.

73. Sanmarti, L.S., Meigias, J.A., Gomez, J.C. *et al.* (1993) Evaluation of the efficacy of health education on the compliance with antituberculosis chemoprophylaxis in school children. A randomized clinical trial. *Tubercle Lung Dis*, **74**, 28–31.

74. Valeza, F.S. and McDougall, A.C. (1990) Blister calender packs for treatment of tuberculosis. *Lancet*, **335**, 473.

75. Manalo, F., Tan, F., Sbarbaro, J.A. and Iseman, M.D. (1990) Community-based short-course treatment of pulmonary tuberculosis in a developing nation. *Am Rev Respir Dis*, **142**, 1301–5.

76. Wobeser, W., To, T. and Hoeppner, V.H. (1989) The outcome of chemoprophylaxis on tuberculosis prevention in Canadian Plains Indians. *Clin Invest Med*, *12*, 149–53.

77. Nazar-Stewart, V. and Nolan, C.M. (1992) Results of a directly observed intermittent isoniazid preventive therapy program in a shelter for homeless men. *Am Rev Respir Dis*, **146**, 57–60.

78. Williamson, D.E., Hammack, C. and Burks, G. (1986) Effect of directly observed therapy with isoniazid and rifampin on 3 month sputum conversion in a Mississippi rural health district. *Am Rev Respir Dis*, **133**, A205.

78a. Weiss, S.E., Slocum, P.C., Blais, F.X. *et al.* (1994) The effect of directly observed therapy on the rates of drug resistance and relapse in tuberculosis. *N Engl J Med*, **330**, 1179–84.

79. Miles, S.H. and Maat, R.B. (1984) A successful supervised outpatient short-course tuberculosis treatment program in an open refugee camp on the Thai–Cambodian border. *Am Rev Respir Dis*, **130**, 827–30.

80. Curry, F.J. (1968) Neighborhood clinics for more effective outpatient treatment of tuberculosis. *N Engl J Med*, *279*, 1262–7.

81. Werhane, M.J., Snuket-Torbeck, G. and Schraufnagel, D.E. (1989) The tuberculosis clinic. *Chest*, **96**, 815–18.

82. McDonald, R.J., Memon, A.M. and Reichman, L.B. (1982) Successful supervised ambulatory management of tuberculosis treatment failures. *Ann Intern Med*, **96**, 297–302.

83. Kochi, A. (1991) The global tuberculosis situation and the new control strategy of the World Health Organization. *Tubercle*, **72**, 1–6.

84. Murray, G.D.L., Styblo, K. and Rouillon, A. (1990) Tuberculosis in developing countries: Burden, intervention and cost. *Bull Int Union Tuberc*, **65**, 6–24.

85. Snider, D.E. (1989) Research towards global control and prevention of tuberculosis with emphasis on vaccine development – introduction. *Rev Infect Dis*, **2**, S336–9.

86. Rubel, A.J. and Garro, L.C. (1992) Social and cultural factors in the successful control of tuberculosis. *Pub Health Rep*, **107**, 626–36.

87. Styblo, K. (1989) Overview and epidemiologic assessment of the current global tuberculosis situation with an emphasis on control in the developing countries. *Rev Infect Dis*, **11**, S339–46.

88. Murray, C.J.L., DeJonghe, E., Chum, H.J. *et al.* (1991) Cost effectiveness of chemotherapy for pulmonary tuberculosis in three sub-Saharan African countries. *Lancet*, **338**, 1305–8.

89. World Health Organization (1991) Proceedings of a WHO informal meeting. Development of guidelines for tuberculosis control in HIV epidemic countries/areas, 2–3 October 1989. *WHO TUB Unit Publication*, Geneva.

90. Pio, A. (1989) Impact of present control methods on the problem of tuberculosis. *Rev Infect Dis*, **11**, S360–S365.

91. Luelmo, F. (1982) BCG vaccination. *Am Rev Respir Dis*, **125**S, 70–2.

92. Gheorghiu, M. (1990) The present and future role of BCG vaccine tuberculosis control. *Biologicals*, **18**, 135–41.

93. Fine, P.E.M. and Rodrigues, L.C. (1990) Modern vaccines: mycobacterial diseases. *Lancet*, **335**, 1016–20.

94. Fine, P.E.M. (1989) The BCG story: lessons from the past and implications for the future. *Rev Infect Dis*, **11**, S353–59.

95. Centers for Disease Control (1988) Use of BCG vaccine in the control of tuberculosis. *MMWR*, **37**, 663–4, 669–75.

96. Clemons, J.D., Choung, J.J.H. and Feinstein, A.R. (1983) The BCG controversy. A methodological and statistical reappraisal. *JAMA*, **249**, 2362–9.

97. Schwoebel, V., Hubert, B. and Grosset, J. (1994) Tuberculous meningitis in France in 1990: characteristics and impact of BCG vaccination. *Tubercle Lung Dis*, **75**, 44–8.

98. Filho, V.W., deCastilho, E.A., Rodrigues, L.C. and Huttly, S.R.A. (1990) Effectiveness of BCG vaccination against tuberculosis meningitis: a case-control study in São Paulo, Brazil. *Bull WHO*, **68**, 69–74.

99. Blin, P., Delolme, H.G., Heyraud, J.D. *et al.* (1986) Evaluation of the protective effect of BCG vaccination by a case-control study in Yaounde, Cameroon. *Tubercle*, **67**, 283–8.

100. Tuberculosis Prevention Trial (1979) Trial of BCG vaccines in South India for tuberculosis prevention. *Indian J Med Res*, **70**, 349–63.

101. Pönnighaus, J.M., Fine, P.E.M., Sterne, J.A.C. *et al.* (1992) Efficacy of BCG vaccine against leprosy and tuberculosis in northern Malawi. *Lancet*, **339**, 636–9.

101a. Colditz, G.A., Brewer, T.F., Berkey. C.S. *et al.* (1994) Efficacy of BCG vaccine in the prevention of tuberculosis. Meta-analysis of the published literature. *JAMA*, **271**, 698–702.

102. Milstien, J.B. and Gibson, J.J. (1990) Quality control of BCG vaccine by WHO: a review of factors that may influence vaccine effectiveness and safety. *Bull WHO*, **58**, 93–108.

103. Centers for Disease Control (1988) Use of BCG vaccines in the control of tuberculosis. *MMWR*, **37**, 663–4, 669–74.

104. Megahed, G.M. and Mahmoud, M.E. (1986) Axillary lymphadenitis after BCG vaccination. *Dev Biol Stand*, **58**, 337.

105. Linn, R., Klimberg, I.W. and Wajsman, Z. (1989) Persistent acid-fast bacilli following intravesical Bacillus Calmette-Guérin. *J Urol*, **141**, 1197–8.

106. Reynes, J., Perez, C., Lamaury, I. *et al.* (1989) Bacille Calmette-Guérin adenitis 30 years after immunization in a patient with AIDS. *J Infect Dis*, **160**, 727.

107. Citron, J.M. (1993) BCG vaccination against tuberculosis: international perspectives. *Brit Med J*, **306**, 222–3.

108. Nettleman, M.D. (1993) *Use of BCG Vaccine in Healthcare Workers: a Decision Analysis*. Interscience Conference on Antimicrobial Agents and Chemotherapy, New Orleans, LA, American Society for Microbiology.

109. Bahr, G.M., Stanford, J.L., Rook, G.A.W. *et al.* (1986) Two potential improvements to BCG and their effect on skin test reactivity in the Lebanon. *Tubercle*, **67**, 205–18.

110. Arruda, S., Bomfim, G., Knights, R. *et al.* (1993) Cloning of an *M. tuberculosis* DNA fragment associated with entry and survival inside cells. *Science*, **261**, 1454–7.

111. Bretscher, P.A. (1992) A strategy to improve the efficacy of vaccination against tuberculosis and leprosy. *Immunol Today*, **13**, 342–5.

112. Centers for Disease Control (1990) Prevention and control of tuberculosis in facilities providing long-term care to the elderly. *MMWR*, **39 (RR-10)**, 7–20.

113. Centers for Disease Control (1992) Prevention and control of tuberculosis in migrant farm workers. *MMWR*, **41 (RR-10)**, 1–15.

114. Centers for Disease Control (1990) Tuberculosis among foreign-born persons entering the United States. *MMWR*, **39 (RR-18)**, 1–21.

115. Centers for Disease Control (1992) National action plan to combat multi-drug resistant tuberculosis. *MMWR*, **41 (RR-11)**, 5–48.

116. Centers for Disease Control (1989) A strategic plan for the elimination of tuberculosis in the United States. *MMWR*, **38 (S–3)**, 1–25.

# 10 Ethical and legal aspects of tuberculosis control

Sheldon H. Landesman

## 10.1 BACKGROUND

Tuberculosis (TB) rose sharply in incidence and prevalence during the 18th century and by the 1900s it had become one of the great killers of mankind [1]. First steps at controlling this infection were initiated after the discovery of tubercle bacillus by Koch and the subsequent understanding of transmission of the disease. Once it was understood that TB was transmissible via airborne droplets, educational campaigns and laws that restricted TB patients from certain types of work and penalized personal habits (e.g. spitting) were adopted.

Laws mandating isolation of TB patients were passed by many states and localities. In the USA, the policies and perceptions of the New York City Department of Health under Herman Biggs, led to New York City and eventually the rest of the country establishing extensive programs which combined rest cures for patients and detailed, although questionable, prevention efforts [2–4]. Many of the elements of these programs still exist today, including mandated physician reporting and treatment of cases, and voluntary or involuntary confinement of patients with active disease who cannot or will not complete therapy.

During the 19th century, TB was epidemic throughout society and affected all social levels. The rich, the poor, the high born and the immigrant suffered equally from what became known as the 'White Plague'. In the 1830s, TB accounted for nearly 25% of all deaths in the USA with a mortality rate of 400 per 100 000/year. After 1830, the mortality rate steadily dropped reaching 200 per 100 000/year by 1920 and 10 per 100 000/year at the onset of the chemotherapeutic era in 1948 [1]. The decline in TB occurred long before the germ theory of the disease was accepted. It continued a steady decline through the 20th century in a manner seemingly unaffected by the policies of isolating patients and using sanatoria. Improved social conditions presumably account for much of the improvement.

After the introduction of therapy, case rates and mortality continued to decrease to a point where the Centers for Disease Control (CDC) developed a campaign for the elimination of TB by the beginning of the second millennium [5]. The optimism of CDC in drafting a plan to eliminate TB was somewhat premature. Starting in 1978, TB case rates at first ceased their decline and then slowly started to increase through the 1980s and early 1990s [6].

In part, the rise in TB cases can be attributed to the marked propensity of HIV-infected individuals to re-activate TB if they have latent infection or the rapid development of active disease in the same population after primary exposure to the tubercle bacillus [7,8]. Concurrent with the rise in cases of active TB, the USA also experienced a marked, and almost frightening, increase in the incidence of multi-drug-resistant (MDR) TB (Chapters 3 and 13) and the occurrence of multiple outbreaks in congregate settings [8,9].

The increase in cases of MDR TB is a result of declining public health resources with the subsequent production of inadequate control programs. As a consequence, TB treatment completion rates diminished, especially in high prevalence areas. In cities like New York, less than 60% of patients completed their treatment [10]. Lower completion rates invariably result in an increase in MDR TB [9,11].

## 10.2 ELEMENTS OF TUBERCULOSIS

The modern landscape of TB can be said to contain a combination of new and old elements, each requiring careful re-examination and reorganization if this infection is to be brought under control in a manner consistent with modern law and 20th century medical ethics. These elements are summarized in Table 10.1.

Against this background, we must place recent changes in law and medical ethics. The changes in modern constitutional law, the passage of the Americans With Disabilities Act, and the voluntary noncoercive nature

**Table 10.1** Tuberculosis control elements, factors causing problems

- Increasing numbers of cases
- Propensity of latent tuberculosis-infected HIV patients to develop active infection
- Appearance of multi-drug-resistant tuberculosis
- Outbreaks of multi-drug resistance in congregate settings
- Antiquated laws for control

of public policy and law as it relates to HIV, will require us to revise current TB control strategies so as to make them consistent with the law, useful from a public health standpoint and ethically permissible.

As a background to the specifics of our current medical and ethical re-evaluation of TB control strategies, it is useful to review the relevant ethical and legal principles that will be referred to.

## 10.3 ETHICAL PRINCIPLES

Ethical principles include respect for persons, the harm principle, benificence and justice [12].

Respect for persons requires that individuals be treated as autonomous agents having the right to control their destinies. Respect for persons requires that people will be given the opportunity to decide what will or will not happen to them. From this concept flow the principles of informed consent and the right of privacy.

The harm principle permits limitations on a person's individual decisions and actions when these may injure or place at risk of injury another person (e.g. shouting fire in a crowded theater).

Beneficence requires that we act on behalf of the interest and welfare of others. The obligation of beneficence applies to communities as well as individuals. Actions must be weighed on an overall risk-to-benefit ratio prior to adoption. Public health policy decisions are often based on a balance between the harm principle and beneficence.

Justice is a principle that requires the burdens and benefits of society to be equally distributed. The principle of justice prescribes invidious discrimination.

These principles are not rigid classifications or laws. Rather, they provide a framework in which governmental and individual actions can be judged. These principles may also be in conflict with one another. As an example, the right of an individual not to take TB medication and the effect of that on TB transmission to others is an example where the respect for persons and the harm principle are in conflict with one another.

In the subsequent sections of this chapter we will examine the social, legal and ethical aspects of mandatory TB reporting and screening; mandated treatment; the use of directly observed therapy and its infringement on liberty; retention of patients for mandated treatment; and the differing public health responses to the TB and HIV epidemics.

## 10.4 MANDATORY TUBERCULOSIS REPORTING

Henry Biggs, New York City Commissioner of Health, was the first to require mandatory reporting of active TB cases [2–4,13]. This requirement, now commonplace, was initially resisted by physicians who viewed it as an unwanted intrusion of public health into their private clinical practice. Additionally, they perceived it as a burden that would add hardship to the lives of their unfortunate patients, branding them as outcasts of society. Nonetheless, Biggs prevailed and patients with TB and many other diseases are now reportable by name to public health authorities.

Biggs' purpose, developed in the prechemotherapy era of TB, was to identify, track and, if necessary, isolate infectious individuals. In this manner, he hoped to contain the disease. The utility of this effort and the entire sanatorium movement that sought to isolate patients with TB, has, however, been open to question [2–4]. With the advent of effective chemotherapy, mandatory reporting can more easily be justified than it was 90 years ago. Mandatory physician reporting followed by case management and treatment until cure, benefits both the patient and society.

## 10.5 TUBERCULOSIS SCREENING

TB screening using tuberculin skin testing is commonplace for persons admitted to hospitals. It is also a common part of pre-employment examinations. No express written consent is required as consent is presumed to exist in the absence of an explicit objection. TB screening is mandatory for persons working in health care settings, prisoners and other congregate settings. Mandatory testing does represent an infringement on individual liberty. Such screening is justified because it makes possible the identification and treatment of a disease that represents a public health threat. By comparison, there is no law or statute requiring a mammogram or electrocardiogram as a condition for employment: breast cancer and heart attacks are not communicable.

The state's ability to mandate TB screening appears to violate the principle of informed consent and autonomy or respect for persons. The legal principle for self determination and the ethical principle of respect for persons normally provide the basis for the right of informed consent. This right was enunciated in 1914 when it was stated 'every human being of adult years and sound mind shall have the right to determine what shall be done with his own body' [14]. This principle can be overridden when the public health is threatened [15]. To the extent that screening programs for patients, children, or employees are carried out without explicit informed consent or are required as prior condition of employment, the Supreme Court has ruled that the public health benefit overrides the minimal curtailment of individual liberty and autonomy that is incurred by the procedure.

Mandated screening for TB thus receives little resistance from a legal perspective and appears justifiable from an ethical perspective. It is interesting to note how different the perspective is for HIV disease, where HIV testing requires informed consent and there is an absence of mandatory HIV testing except for specific settings such as blood and organ donation.

## 10.6 MANDATED TUBERCULOSIS TREATMENT

TB is one of the few diseases where treatment can and has been required by the state. Given the infectious and transmissible nature of TB, many states have legislation that mandates treatment. This form of legal coercion is not unrestricted since a court order is often required. The public threat posed by TB provides the legal and ethical justification for mandated treatment [15]. The laws on imposed or mandated treatment are, however, highly variable. Moving across state lines can obviate a court ordered treatment without changing the risk of transmission [16].

The state also has an obligation towards the TB patient prior to issuance of any mandated treatment. State or municipalities supplying care for patients with active TB must make available those medical services and related amenities that will enhance compliance with therapy. Generally speaking, the minimum requirements for an adequate TB program include ready and easy access to standard TB outpatient care, minimal waiting time for evaluation and receipt of free medicines and neighborhood outreach programs for the more difficult patients.

Completion of TB therapy is in the community's as well as the patient's best interest. Therefore, it behooves the community to provide the additional amenities or assistance that will encourage completion of TB treatment (Chapter 9). This includes the availability of drug treatment slots (for the addicted TB patient), mental health referrals or assistance, and a user friendly TB clinic. These amenities are not required by law. Having them in place is, however, good medicine and good public health [17]. The ethical principle of beneficence impels governments to offer those inducements that will make the taking of medication an easier task. In this manner, the government offers additional benefits to a subset of its citizens in order to benefit all citizens.

## 10.7 DIRECTLY OBSERVED ANTITUBERCULOUS THERAPY

Mandating treatment does not produce a guarantee that the TB medications will be taken. The next step, a less restrictive alternative to confinement of the noncompliant patient, is the use of directly observed therapy (DOT) (Chapter 9). A recent report by a group of physicians, lawyers, public health officials and ethicists, published by the United Hospital Fund, recommended universal DOT as the initial therapeutic regimen for all TB patients regardless of their past history of compliance (or noncompliance) [18]. This recommendation is based on the high rate of noncompliance for nearly all therapies and the knowledge that noncompliance is characteristic of all social classes and education levels [19–21]. The United Hospital Fund working group recommended DOT to begin with, assuming that after the initial phase of therapy the physician or public health advisor can then make a reasonable judgement to decide whether the patient should continue on DOT or be followed in a clinic or doctor's office every month until completion of therapy.

This recommendation, although currently promoted by the CDC as a standard of care, has met with considerable opposition from civil libertarians. Their view is that DOT is an infringement on the liberty and autonomy of the individual and should be imposed only after evidence of a non-compliance hearing. They also believe that a judicial or administrative hearing is required before mandating this therapy [18,22].

## 10.8 CONFINEMENT OF PATIENTS WITH TUBERCULOSIS FOR COMPLETION OF THERAPY

The state has the power, when the community is endangered by a transmissible disease, to protect itself. As long as the state's action is not unreasonable or arbitrary, it can mandate treatment and/or confinement of a patient deemed a threat to the community. The principle is embodied in the Supreme Court decision mandating vaccination against smallpox. The court ruled that 'upon the principle of self defense a community has the right to protect itself against a disease which threatens the safety of its members' [15,22].

Civil commitment of a patient who is a danger to others, although sanctioned by the Jacobson decision [15], is not an unrestricted right. Generally speaking, health authorities must provide 'clear and convincing evidence' of the danger of the patient [22,23]. The state must also guarantee the right to counsel and the right to cross examine witnesses and provide counsel if the patient cannot afford a lawyer. However, it should be stressed that the individual laws in the 50 US states are extremely variable and the due process protection required prior to confinement range from almost nonexistent to so stringent as to make confinement nearly impossible.

Federal law has little direct impact on individual cases of mandated civil commitment of noncompliant patients with active TB. Protection of the public health is largely a state function. A federal presence exists largely in the decisional law of the Supreme Court which has, over the years, defined the requirements and burden of proof needed to control a person's liberty. The requirements listed above, taken from a West Virginia court ordered confinement, probably constitute the minimal requirements for constitutionally correct deprivation of liberty [23].

The CDC is drafting model legal guidelines for TB control. It has reviewed the state laws and has made recommendations to achieve some uniformity of law from state to state [24]. Gostin [16] has also recently published a review of TB laws in all 50 US states and has put forth proposals for revisions and uniformity of these laws. Tables 10.2–10.4 summarize some of the variables in state laws regarding TB as reported by the CDC.

**Table 10.2** Populations subject to tuberculosis screening by state 1993 [24]

| State | Medical facility employees | School employees | Foster home residents | School children | School bus drivers | Incarcerated persons | Food handlers | Park employees | Child or day care employees | Long-term care facility residents | Barbers/ beauticians | Correctional facility employees | Nursing home employees |
|---|---|---|---|---|---|---|---|---|---|---|---|---|---|
| AL |   |   |   |   |   |   |   |   |   |   |   |   |   |
| AK | X | X | X | X | X |   |   |   |   |   |   |   | X |
| AZ |   |   |   |   |   |   |   |   |   |   |   |   |   |
| AR | X | X |   |   |   |   |   |   |   |   |   |   | X |
| CA | X | X |   | X |   | X | X |   |   | X |   | X | X |
| CO | X |   |   |   |   |   | X | X | X |   |   | X |   |
| CT |   |   |   |   |   |   |   |   |   |   |   |   |   |
| DE | X | X |   | X |   | X | X |   |   |   |   |   | X |
| FL | X |   |   |   |   | X |   |   | X | X |   | X | X |
| GA |   |   |   |   |   | X |   |   | X | X |   | X | X |
| HI |   |   |   |   |   |   |   |   |   |   |   |   |   |
| ID |   |   |   |   |   |   |   |   |   |   |   |   |   |
| IL | X | X | X |   |   | X |   |   | X | X |   |   | X |
| IN | X | X |   |   |   |   |   |   |   | X |   |   | X |
| IA | X | X |   |   | X |   |   |   |   | X |   | X | X |
| KS |   | X |   | X |   |   |   |   |   |   |   |   | X |
| KY |   |   |   |   |   |   |   |   |   |   | X |   |   |
| LA | X |   |   |   |   |   | X |   |   |   |   |   |   |
| ME |   |   |   |   |   |   |   |   | X | X |   |   |   |
| MD |   | X |   |   |   |   |   |   | X |   |   |   | X |
| MA |   | X |   |   | X | X |   |   |   |   | X |   | X |
| MI |   | X |   |   |   | X |   |   |   |   |   |   |   |

| State | 1 | 2 | 3 | 4 | 5 | 6 | 7 |
|---|---|---|---|---|---|---|---|
| MN | X |   | X | X | X | X | X |
| MS | X | X |   |   | X |   | X |
| MO | X | X | X |   | X | X |   |
| MT |   | X |   |   |   |   |   |
| NE |   |   |   |   |   |   |   |
| NV |   |   |   |   |   |   |   |
| NJ | X | X | X |   | X |   | X |
| NH | X | X |   | X |   | X | X |
| NM | X | X | X | X |   | X | X |
| NY |   | X | X |   |   |   |   |
| NC |   |   |   |   |   |   |   |
| ND |   |   |   |   |   |   |   |
| OH | X | X |   | X | X |   | X |
| OK | X |   |   |   |   |   | X |
| OR | X |   | X |   |   |   | X |
| PA |   |   |   |   |   |   |   |
| RI |   |   |   |   |   |   |   |
| SC |   | X |   |   | X |   |   |
| SD |   |   |   |   | X |   |   |
| TN |   |   |   |   |   |   |   |
| TX | X | X | X | X | X |   | X |
| UT | X |   |   |   | X |   | X |
| VT |   |   |   |   |   |   |   |
| VA |   | X | X |   |   |   |   |
| WA | X |   |   |   | X | X |   |
| WV | X | X |   |   | X | X | X |
| WI | X | X |   |   |   | X | X |
| WY |   |   |   |   | X |   | X |

**Table 10.3** Tuberculosis control programs by state 1993 [24]

| State | Voluntary treatment | Outpatient treatment | Home quarantine | Commitment | Commitment until no longer a threat | Commitment until cured | Commitment for unspecified time | Consideration of carrier's religious belief | Penalty for nonadherent patients |
|---|---|---|---|---|---|---|---|---|---|
| AL | X | X | X | X | X | X | | X | |
| AK | X | X | | | | X | | | X |
| AZ | X | | X | X | | | | | |
| AR | X | | X | X | X | | | | |
| CA | X | | X | X | | | | X | X |
| CO | | X | X | X | X | X | | X | X |
| CT | | | X | X | X | | | | |
| DE | | X | X | X | | | X | | |
| FL | X | X | X | X | X | | | | X |
| GA | X | X | X | X | X | | | | X |
| HI | X | | X | X | X | X | | | |
| ID | | | X | X | | | | | |
| IL | | X | X | X | | | X | | |
| IN | X | | X | X | | | | | |
| IA | X | | X | X | | | | | X |
| KS | X | X | X | X | X | | | | X |
| KY | | | X | X | | | | | |
| LA | | | X | X | | | | | X |
| ME | | | X | X | X | | | | |
| MD | X | X | X | X | X | | | X | X |
| MA | | | | X | | | X | | |
| MI | | X | X | X | X | | | X | X |

| State | 1 | 2 | 3 | 4 | 5 | 6 | 7 | 8 | 9 |
|-------|---|---|---|---|---|---|---|---|---|
| MN |   |   |   | x | x |   |   |   |   |
| MS | x |   | x | x | x |   |   |   | x |
| MT | x |   | x | x | x | x |   |   |   |
| MO | x | x |   | x | x | x |   |   |   |
| NE | x | x |   | x |   |   |   | x | x |
| NV | x |   |   | x | x |   |   |   |   |
| NJ | x |   |   | x | x | x |   |   |   |
| NH |   |   |   | x | x |   |   |   |   |
| NM | x |   |   |   |   |   |   |   | x |
| NY | x | x |   | x | x | x |   |   |   |
| NC | x |   |   | x | x |   |   |   |   |
| ND | x |   |   | x | x |   |   |   |   |
| OH |   | x |   | x | x | x |   |   | x |
| OK | x |   |   | x | x |   |   |   | x |
| OR |   |   |   | x | x |   |   |   | x |
| PA | x |   |   | x | x |   |   |   |   |
| RI |   |   |   | x | x |   |   |   |   |
| SC | x |   |   | x | x |   |   |   | x |
| SD | x |   |   | x | x | x |   |   | x |
| TN | x | x |   | x | x | x |   |   |   |
| TX | x | x |   | x | x |   | x |   |   |
| UT | x | x |   | x | x | x |   | x | x |
| VT |   | x |   | x | x | x |   |   | x |
| VA |   |   |   | x | x |   |   |   |   |
| WA | x | x |   | x | x | x |   | x | x |
| WV |   |   |   | x | x |   |   |   |   |
| WI | x | x |   | x | x |   |   |   | x |
| WY |   | x |   | x | x |   |   |   | x |

**Table 10.4** Persons restricted from activities and/or employment if infected with tuberculosis by state 1993 [24]

| State | Food handlers | School children | School employees | Care providers[a] | Household contacts |
|-------|---------------|-----------------|------------------|-------------------|--------------------|
| AL | | | | | |
| AK | | | | | |
| AZ | | | | | |
| AR | X | X | X | | |
| CA | | | | | |
| CO | | | | | |
| CT | | | | | |
| DE | | | | | |
| FL | | | | X | |
| GA | | | | | |
| HI | X | X | X | | |
| ID | X | X | X | X | X |
| IL | | X | | | |
| IN | | | | | |
| IA | | | | | |
| KS | | X | X | | |
| KY | | | | | X |
| LA | | | | | |
| ME | | X | X | | |
| MD | | | X | | |
| MA | | | | | |
| MI | | X | | | |
| MN | | | | | |
| MS | | X | X | | |
| MO | X | X | | | |
| MT | X | X | | X | |
| NE | | | | | |
| NV | | | | | |
| NJ | X | | | | |
| NH | | | | | |
| NM | | | X | | |
| NY | | | | | |
| NC | | | | | |
| ND | X | X | X | X | |
| OH | | | | | |
| OK | | X | | | |
| OR | | X | X | X | |
| PA | | | | | X |
| RI | | | | | |
| SC | X | X | | | X |
| SD | | | | | |
| TN | | X | X | X | |
| TX | | | | | |
| UT | | | | | |
| VT | | | | | |
| VA | | | | | |
| WA | | | | | |
| WV | | | X | | |
| WI | | X | X | X | |
| WY | | | | | |

[a] Includes day care providers, nursing-home employees, and home health-care workers.

Recently, New York City revised its legal statute for determining noncompliant patients. This revision was designed to bring current laws up to modern day standards of due process as well as providing a useable mechanism for confining persistently noncompliant patients. California recently based its revised state law on the New York City statute. The basic elements of the revision are:

- guaranteed right to counsel for any person subject to civil commitment for noncompliance
- individualized assessment of the person's circumstances and/or behavior constituting the basis for issuance of the order
- rapid judicial action on a commitment order (5 days between detention and a hearing)
- periodic court review on any civil commitment order (60 days)
- a clear and convincing standard with regard to the danger the patient poses to the community
- a provision for Commissioner ordered DOT, often as a prelude to commitment
- the presence of evidence that there exists 'substantial likelihood' that the patient cannot, will not, or has not previously complied with the TB medication regimen.

This revision has, so far, stood up to legal challenge. Currently, 25 persistently noncompliant persons have been committed to a long-term hospital facility in order to ensure completion of therapy.

## 10.9 TUBERCULOSIS–HIV CONNECTION

The coercive nature of TB control laws with mandated testing, reporting, treatment and, if needed, confinement, are in sharp contrast to the public health strategy with regard to HIV infection. In the latter, individual consent, often written, is required prior to HIV testing and there are only patchy requirements for mandatory reporting of HIV-infected individuals. Although many states require mandated reporting of any HIV-positive persons, in the states where HIV disease is most common (New York, Florida, California and New Jersey), only AIDS cases are reportable. In addition, there is no mandated treatment and no confinement of sexually active HIV-infected people who may be infecting others.

The contrast between the coercive nature of TB control laws and the voluntary strategy of HIV-related laws may be due to the differences in perceived effectiveness of control measures. Identification of TB patients followed by isolation and removal from an environment where transmission occurs with subsequent treatment until cure, results in protection of individuals and society. TB programs curtail, to some extent, the liberty of the individual. This infringement on liberty is justified by the benefits obtained by the patient and the community. For HIV disease, the long duration of an asymptomatic infectious disease, the pleasurable and instinctual behaviors by which the disease is transmitted, the lack of effective treatment and the discrimination attendant with identification, have combined to make coercive control measures less effective. If coercive measures that deprive a person of autonomy and liberty do not accomplish their communal goal, they can rarely be justified, either on ethical or legal grounds. There appears to be a societal and public health consensus that voluntary rather than coercive measure are the best way to control HIV. These differing public health strategies may need to be reconciled if the rise in TB cases, largely related to HIV disease, is to be controlled.

As we try to control TB among HIV-infected persons, suggestions for the use of coercive TB-type control measures have been put forward. For example, the question of whether mandatory HIV testing in the work place ought to be initiated so as to identify potentially dual infected (HIV and *Mycobacterium tuberculosis*) people has been raised [25]. The purpose of the HIV testing would be the identification of individuals at high risk for developing active TB and their consequent exclusion from the workplace. Careful review of this question and similar questions by the United Hospital Fund panel concluded that mandatory HIV testing and exclusion of HIV-positive persons would not result in enhanced control of TB in the workplace. Less restrictive measures, with less infringement on an individual's liberty and autonomy could accomplish the same goal. Employee education, mandated TB testing and voluntary HIV testing would be adequate for creating a safe work environment.

## REFERENCES

1. Dubos, R. and Dubos, J. (1987) *The White Plague: Man and Society*, Rutgers University Press, New Brunswick, NJ.
2. Rothman, S. (1992) The sanatorium experience: myths and realities, in *The Tuberculosis Revival: Individual Rights and Societal Obligations in a Time of AIDS*, United Hospital Fund, New York, pp. 67–75.
3. Rothman, S. (1993) Seek and hide: public health departments and persons with tuberculosis, 1890–1940. *Law Med Ethics*, **21**, 289–95.
4. Winslow, C.E.A. (1929) *The Life of Herman Biggs*, Lea and Febiger, Philadelphia, PA.
5. Centers for Disease Control (1989) Strategic plan for the elimination of tuberculosis in the United States. Recommendations of the Advisory Committee for the Elimination of Tuberculosis. *MMWR*, **39 (S–3)**, 1–26.
6. Centers for Disease Control (1992) National action plan to combat multidrug resistant tuberculosis. *MMWR*, **41 (RR–11)**, 6–8.
7. Selwyn, P.A., Hartel, D., Lewis, V.A. *et al.* (1989) A prospective study of the risk of tuberculosis among intravenous drug users with human immunodeficiency virus infection. *N Engl J Med*, **320**, 545–50.
8. Daley, C.L., Small, P.M., Schecter, G.F. *et al.* (1992) An outbreak of tuberculosis with accelerated progression among persons infected with human immuno-

deficiency virus: an analysis using restriction-fragment-length polymorphisms. *N Engl J Med*, **326**, 231–5.

9. Frieden, T.R., Sterling, T., Pablos-Mendez, A. *et al.* (1993) The emergence of drug resistant tuberculosis in New York City. *N Engl J Med*, **328**, 521–6.

10. Bloom, B.R. and Murray, C.J.L. (1992) Tuberculosis: commentary on a re-emergent killer, *Science*, **257**, 1055–64.

11. Brudney, K. and Dobkin, J. (1991) Resurgent tuberculosis in New York City. *Am Rev Respir Dis*, **141**, 347–51.

12. Bayer, R., Levine, C. and Wolf, S.M. (1986) HIV antibody screening: an ethical framework for evaluating proposed programs. *JAMA*, **256**, 1768–74.

13. Fox, D.M. (1945) Social policy and city politics. *Bull Hosp Med*, **42**, 169–75.

14. Schloendorff v. Society of New York Hospital, 105 N.E. (NY 1914): Overruled on other grounds by Bing v. Thunig: 143 N.E. 2d 3 (1957).

15. Jacobson v. Massachusetts, 197 U.S. 11 (1904).

16. Gostin, L.O. (1993) Controlling the resurgent tuberculosis epidemic: A 50-state survey of TB statutes and proposals for reform. *JAMA*, **269**, 255–61.

17. Bayer, R., Dubler, N. and Landesman, S.H. (1993) The dual epidemics of tuberculosis and AIDS: ethical and policy issues in screening and treatment. *Am J Pub Health*, **83**, 649–54.

18. Dubler, N.N., Bayer, R., Landesman, S.H. and White, A. (1992) Tuberculosis in the 1990s: ethical, legal and public issues of screening, treatment and the protection of those in congregate facilities, in *The Tuberculosis Revival: Individual Rights and Societal Obligations in a Time of AIDS*, United Hospital Fund, New York, pp. 1–45.

19. Sbarbaro, J.A. (1979) Compliance inducements and enforcements. *Chest*, **76**, 750–66.

20. Addington, W.W. (1985) Patient compliance: The most serious remaining problem in control of tuberculosis in the U.S. *Clin Chest Med*, **76**(Suppl), 741–3.

21. Mohler, D.N., Wallin, D.C. and Dreyfus, E.G. (1955) Studies in home treatment of streptococcal disease. I. Failure of patient to take penicillin by mouth as prescribed. *N Engl J Med*, **252**, 1116–18.

22. Annas, G.J. (1993) Control of tuberculosis: the law and the public's health. *N Engl J Med*, **328**, 585–8.

23. Greene v. Edwards, 263 S.E. 2d 661 (W. Va. 1980).

24. Centers for Disease Control and Prevention (1993) Tuberculosis control laws – United States, 1993. *MMWR*, **42 (RR–1)**, 1–28.

25. Kuvin, S.F. (1992) Control of tuberculosis depends on AIDS testing. *New York Times*, 1 April, p. A24.

| 11 | # Antitubercular drugs |
|----|------------------------|

Peter G. Barber, William M. Goldman, Annette J. Stahl
Avicolli, Rosemary Smith, Neal Rairden, Octavio Maragni,
Jeneane Chirico, Constance Mangone

## 11.1 ISONIAZID

Isoniazid (isonicotinic acid hydrazine, INH) was first found to have *in vitro* activity against *Mycobacterium* sp. in 1945. In 1952, INH was reported to be a useful agent when two groups independently showed that it was a potent anti-TB drug in animal and human studies [1]. INH (Figure 11.1) remains an inexpensive, well tolerated and very valuable agent for the treatment of tuberculosis (TB).

### 11.1.1 Mechanism of action and activity

INH is bacteriocidal for TB. Its mechanism of action, however, remains unclear. One step inhibited [2] is the desaturation of the $C_{24}$ and $C_{26}$ long chain fatty acid precursors of mycolic acid, a unique part of the mycobacterial cell wall [3]. This effect may explain the narrow spectrum of INH. The drug also affects $NAD^+$ and pyridoxal phosphate metabolism [4] and produces a cuprous complex toxic to the bacillus [5]. INH appears to be inhibitory to resting bacilli and bacteriocidal to actively replicating ones [6]. It has been found to be more active than other first line agents in early bacteriocidal activity against TB [6a].

The minimal inhibitory concentration for INH is 0.025–0.5 µg/ml for the tubercle bacillus [7]. Resistance can develop when therapy is inadequate [8,9]. Recent work has suggested that the mechanism of resistance, for at least a subgroup of organisms, is deletion [4] or mutation [9a] of the catalase-peroxidase gene. A second gene, involved with mycolic acid synthesis,

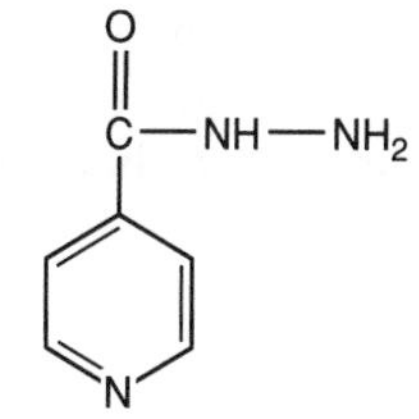

**Figure 11.1** Isoniazid.

has also been found which encodes a target for both INH and ethionamide [9b]. *Mycobacterium kansasii* is the most sensitive of the non-TB mycobacteria.

### 11.1.2 Pharmacokinetics

Isoniazid is readily absorbed from the gut with peak levels of 3–7 µg/ml 1–2 hours after an oral 300 mg dose [10]. Intramuscular (IM) therapy achieves similar levels [11]. Levels will be lower if INH is given with food or aluminum-containing antacids [12]. Not protein bound, INH distributes widely into all fluids and tissues, including cerebrospinal, pleural and ascitic fluids, sputum and caseous tissue [10]. Spinal fluid levels are about 20% of the blood in normal meninges [13] and almost 100% in inflamed meninges. It diffuses across the placenta, and breast milk concentrations are similar to serum.

The major pathway for INH metabolism is acetylation to acetylisoniazid by a noninducible hepatic enzyme. Sulfamethazine and dapsone are other drugs acetylated by the same mechanism [14]. The rate of acetylation is constant in any individual but varies in different patients. People are characterized as rapid or slow acetylators with slow acetylation inherited as an autosomal recessive [14]. Heterozygotes have intermediate acetylation rates. Acetylation phenotype frequencies vary in different ethnic groups. Most patients of Asian descent, such as Eskimos, Japanese and Chinese are rapid acetylators while Scandinavians, North African Caucasians (i.e. Moroccans and Egyptians) and Jews tend to be slow acetylators. In the USA, 50–60% of Caucasians are slow acetylators [9,15]. Rapid acetylators have an INH serum half life of 0.5–1.6 hours and slow acetylators 2–5 hours. Serum levels are 30–50% lower in rapid acetylators [16]. Levels are increased by the concurrent administration of para-aminosalicylic acid due to interference with acetylation.

INH is excreted by the kidneys as either parent drug or metabolite with slow acetylators excreting more unchanged INH [17]. Prednisolone will decrease INH concentrations in both rapid and slow acetylators by enhancing renal clearance [18] and enhancing acetylation in slow acetylators. Although the elimination of INH is primarily dependent on the rate of acetylation, with levels higher with liver disease [19], retention of the drug will occur in those individuals with renal failure. The half life of INH in patients with kidney failure is 8–11 hours [10].

### 11.1.3 Adverse effects

INH inhibits the microsomal mixed function oxidase system [20] decreasing clearance and prolonging the effects of drugs such as phenytoin which are metabolized by this system. Such interactions are more significant in slow acetylators [21].

The significance of INH hepatotoxicity was not well recognized until the report of Garibaldi *et al.* in 1970 [22], nearly 20 years after the drug's introduction. In this study, 19 cases of clinical liver disease (0.82%) among 2321 Washington, DC federal employees receiving INH (with two deaths) were found over a 9 month period. A multicenter trial conducted among nearly 14 000 persons receiving INH found a 1.04% rate of probable hepatotoxicity and an additional 1.03% incidence possibly related to INH [23]. This study found advancing age to be associated with increasing risk and the rate of toxicity more than four times greater for daily drinkers than for nondrinkers. A striking difference in hepatotoxicity in males was noted, with Orientals having a rate almost double that of Whites and nearly 14 times that of Blacks.

Subclinical liver injury, as indicated by elevated aminotransferases, occurs in 12–18% of those receiving INH [24–26]. While most elevated hepatic enzymes will normalize during continued use of INH, a few patients progress to overt disease with hepatic necrosis. Progression is associated with the symptoms of anorexia, vomiting, abdominal discomfort, weakness and fatigue [27]. Although clinical hepatotoxicity is clearly age dependent, anecdotal case reports have appeared in adolescents and children [28,29]. Chronic infection with hepatitis B does not clearly increase the incidence of INH hepatotoxicity [30].

Although some symptoms of INH liver disease suggest an idiosyncratic reaction [31], the hepatic toxicity is likely related to a metabolite, perhaps monoacetylhydrazine [25]. The age related risk may relate to a decreased ability to repair the liver damage with advancing age. Although initial observations suggested that rapid acetylators have a higher incidence of hepatoxicity [27,32], this is apparently not the case [33,34]. In fact, in one controlled study, slow acetylators had a higher rate of hepatotoxicity [35]. Since rapid acetylators produced more acetylisoniazid, precursor of monoacetylhydrazine, this group would be likely to have a higher rate of toxicity. The same N-acetyltransferase, however, converts more monoacetylhydrazine to a nontoxic diacetyl form in the rapid acetylator. Because of this, similar amounts of the hepatotoxic intermediates are present in both acetylator phenotypes [36]. It has been postulated that enzyme induction by rifampin may be responsible for the enhancement of hepatotoxicity [37] and INH hydrolase induced by rifampin seems to increase hepatotoxic metabolites in slow acetylators [38].

Neurotoxicity can be associated with INH. Dose related peripheral neuropathy occurs in about 1% of patients on 3–5 mg/kg/day and is more common with higher doses [16]. The neuropathy is rapidly reversible if INH is withdrawn promptly after symptom onset, but may persist if therapy continues [16]. The neuropathy is caused by pyridoxine deficiency caused by inactivation of the coenzyme function of pyridoxal phosphate by INH metabolites. It is more likely to occur in malnourished individuals, alcoholics, the elderly, pregnant women and slow acetylators and can be prevented by the supplemental use of pyridoxine. Pyridoxine does not counteract the anti-TB properties of INH [39].

Central nervous system effects of INH are symptoms of increased excitability, ranging from irritability to overt seizures. Seizures may be more common in slow acetylators [16]. Caution must be used when administering INH to patients receiving phenytoin as toxicity from this anticonvulsant is more likely to occur in slow acetylators receiving both drugs. The INH related seizure activity is reversed by pyridoxine. Large doses of pyridoxine (equivalent to the gram amount of INH ingested) can be used in patients with INH overdose [40], in which metabolic acidosis and coma can occur. Memory impairment, depression, optic neuritis and toxic encephalopathy have been rarely reported [41].

INH may cause a syndrome reminiscent of lupus erythematosus [42]. The symptoms are associated with a reactive antinuclear antibody (ANA), but 20% of TB patients receiving INH will develop an ANA without lupus symptoms [43]. The lupus-like syndrome usually resolves promptly when INH is discontinued. Isolated febrile reactions from INH are uncommon, but can simulate a septic process with rigors [44].

INH can affect the metabolism of and reactions to certain foods or nutrients. It can, at usual doses, lower serum calcium and phosphate levels [45]. This effect is related to the inhibition of the production of dihydroxy-vitamin D. Additionally, similarity in structure to some monoamine oxidase inhibitors might suggest that INH users may have dietary intolerances to food rich in tyramine, such as cheese and red wine. This may occur but is very rare [46]. Pyridoxine deficiency from INH can produce a pellagra-like syndrome related to effects on tryptophan metabolism.

The drug remains part of the standard of treatment in the pregnant female with active TB. INH chemoprophylaxis may also be used during pregnancy.

### 11.1.4 Monitoring parameters

It has been stated that, in the absence of clinical symptoms of an influenza-like illness, anorexia, or abdominal discomfort, periodic monitoring of aminotransferase levels is not useful in detecting significant hepatotoxicity

[47]. Byrd *et al.* [25] found, however, that there was no statistical difference in the development of such symptoms between an INH and a placebo group and no relationship between symptoms and elevated aminotransferases. These authors later reported that monthly biochemical and clinical monitoring could be used to avoid irreversible hepatic damage [48]. Although the height at which asymptomatic elevations of aminotransferase enzymes should necessitate discontinuance of INH is arbitrary, five times normal baseline level is a reasonable cutoff.

Careful clinical monitoring of neuropathic symptoms is adequate in preventing toxicity when normal doses are given to low risk groups. Individuals at higher risk for INH neuropathy, such as the elderly, pregnant and malnourished patients, should receive supplemental pyridoxine. Those concomitantly receiving ethionamide, para-aminosalicylic acid (PAS) or cycloserine should also be given pyridoxine.

### 11.1.5 Dosage

INH is given at a dose of 5 mg/kg (300 mg in the adult) as a single daily dose. Divided doses can result in low blood levels, especially in rapid acetylators. Twice weekly doses of 15 mg/kg (900 mg) can be used in directly observed therapy regimens or as self administered therapy in reliable patients. The dosage can be given intramuscularly as a 100 mg/ml solution and although not recommended for intravenous use, INH has been given by this route.

Dosages reduced by half have been used in severe hepatic insufficiency and a dose of 150–200 mg/day has been used in severe renal failure, especially in slow acetylators [49].

### 11.2 RIFAMPIN

Rifampin (rifampicin in the UK) is a semisynthetic derivative of rifamycin B (Figure 11.2). It is a water-soluble, reddish-brown crystalline powder [50]. The drug is a first line anti-TB agent which, in combination with INH, has made TB therapy much more effective.

### 11.2.1 Mechanism of action and activity

Rifampin can be inhibitory against *M. tuberculosis* at levels as low as 0.005 µg/ml. The drug achieves its antibacterial effect by binding, with high affinity, to DNA-dependent RNA polymerase. The binding inhibits the initiation of RNA chain formation. It does not have this effect on mammalian cells [51].

This commonly used agent is active *in vitro* and *in vivo* against *M. tuberculosis, M. bovis, M. kansasii, M. marinum, M. leprae* and some strains of

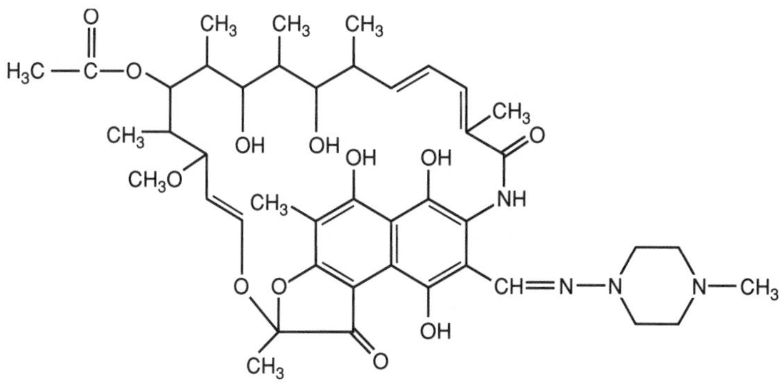

**Figure 11.2** Rifampin.

*M. avium-intracellulare* complex [52]. Its cidal effect against the tubercle bacillus is more efficient than INH because it is better at killing bacilli that are predominantly metabolically dormant [53]. It is also effective *in vivo* and *in vitro* against *Staphylococcus aureus, Neisseria meningitidis, Haemophilus influenzae* and *Legionella pneumophila* [52]. Widespread use of rifampin for bacterial infections could result in increasing amounts of resistance in TB. The more broad spectrum nature of rifampin compared with most other agents makes a clinical response to an empiric regimen containing rifampin less diagnostic for TB.

Resistance development has been seen *in vitro* and *in vivo*. *In vitro*, it is a one step process, which is likely related to a modification in the beta subunit of the RNA polymerase. Resistant clones can be easily selected for and produce a predominantly rifampin resistant population [51].

### 11.2.2 Pharmacokinetics

A 600 mg oral dose of rifampin will achieve a peak level of about 7 µg/ml, with a range of 4–32 µg/ml. In children, levels are somewhat lower [54]. Peak concentrations may be slightly reduced or delayed if taken with food. An intravenous administration of rifampin produces levels of about 9 µg/ml after 300 mg and 17.5 µg/ml following 600 mg [55–57].

Rifampin is widely distributed into many body tissues and fluids including ascitic fluid, pleural fluid, liver, lungs, bile, prostate and CSF. The drug is 80–90% protein bound and will cross the placenta and distribute into breast milk [56]. When the meninges are inflamed, rifampin levels may reach 10–20% of the serum. The drug penetrates well intracellularly into leukocytes and nerve cells and is effective in nerve involvement in lepromatous leprosy [58].

Rifampin is metabolized by the liver by deacetylation into an active metabolite and undergoes significant enterohepatic circulation. The plasma half life is approximately three hours after a single 600 mg dose. After repeated doses, however, it is 1.5–2 hours, related to the induction of hepatic microsomal enzymes [56]. Up to one-third of a rifampin dose is excreted in the urine. About 60% of rifampin is excreted in the feces, primarily in the deacetylated form [56]. Both serum levels and urinary excretion increase in hepatic failure which necessitates dosage reduction [56]. No dose reduction is needed in renal failure.

Drug absorption is reduced in the presence of PAS or clofazimine. Therefore, these drugs should be given separately from rifampin. The hepatic uptake and elimination of rifampin is inhibited by probenecid and serum levels may rise substantially [59]. Trimethoprim/sulfamethoxazole may also increase rifampin levels.

### 11.2.3 Adverse effects

Rifampin has been shown to induce the hepatic microsomal enzymes involved in drug metabolism, resulting in decreased blood levels and pharmacologic effects of a variety of medications many of which are listed in Table 11.1 [60]. When the rifampin is withdrawn, drug levels will rise and may be associated with toxicity.

The most common adverse effects associated with rifampin are gastro-intestinal and include epigastric distress, nausea, vomiting, anorexia and diarrhea. These side effects may be reduced if the drug is taken with food

**Table 11.1** Drugs which have decreased effect in the presence of rifampin[a]

| | |
|---|---|
| Acetaminophen | Haloperidol |
| Anticoagulants, oral | Itraconazole |
| Barbiturates | Ketoconazole |
| Benzodiazepines | Methadone (and other |
| Chloramphenicol | narcotics) |
| Ciprofloxacin | Metoprolol |
| Clofibrate | Mexilitine |
| Contraceptives, oral | Nifedipine |
| Corticosteroids | Nortriptyline |
| Cyclosporine | Propranolol |
| Dapsone | Quinidine |
| Diazepam | Sulfones |
| Digitalis derivatives | Sulfonylureas |
| Diltiazem | Theophyllines |
| Disopyramide | Tocainide |
| Estrogens | Verapamil |
| Fluconazole | |

[a] Before adding rifampin to a patient's drug regimen or adding an additional drug to rifampin, it is important to check its interaction with rifampin even if it is not listed above.

[64]. Transient elevations of liver function tests occur in about 14% of patients who receive rifampin. Low level elevations may normalize even if the drug is continued. Prolonged use or overdose may cause clinical

hepatotoxicity. Sixteen deaths from hepatotoxicity were reported among 500 000 rifampin recipients [50]. Liver function abnormalities are also more likely to occur in alcohol abusers, patients receiving other hepatotoxic drugs, such as INH and halothane, and patients with hepatitis or cirrhosis [38,61–63].

Another common effect is an orange discoloration of urine, feces, sweat, tears and sputum [64,65]. Soft contact lenses may be stained permanently if worn during rifampin therapy. An influenza-like syndrome with fever, chills and malaise is associated with high dose intermittent rifampin therapy (900–1200 mg twice weekly) [65], but not with lower dose intermittent treatment. Oral desensitization to rifampin has been used in patients with cutaneous hypersensitivity reactions, such as urticaria, so that the patient may continue to use this agent [65a]. A variety of uncommon adverse effects involving the CNS, skin and bone marrow are described [64,65].

Although animal studies find adverse fetal effects from rifampin, there are no controlled studies in pregnant women. In rodents, increased spina bifida and cleft palate were seen when 15–20 times the usual human dose was used. The incidence of congenital malformations in pregnant women who received rifampin was similar to that expected in nonexposed patients [66]. The drug has been implicated, however, in the development of hemorrhagic disease of the newborn [67]. It is generally accepted, however, that rifampin is not a proven human teratogen and its use in pregnancy is recommended [68–70] if the benefit outweighs the risk. Although rifampin is excreted in breast milk, it is not thought to represent a significant risk to the infant. Rifampin therapy is considered to be compatible with breast feeding by the American Academy of Pediatrics [71], along with INH and ethambutol.

Rifampin has been demonstrated to have immunosuppressive properties. Overall, however, if it occurs at the doses used to treat TB, the effect appears not to modify treatment adversely or enhance susceptibility to other infections [16].

### 11.2.4 Monitoring parameters

A complete blood count (CBC), serum aminotransferase and bilirubin levels should be measured prior to rifampin use and monitored during therapy. Liver function tests are often monitored monthly. Serum levels of drugs such as warfarin, phenobarbital and dilantin should be monitored.

### 11.2.5 Dosage

For the initial treatment of TB, rifampin is always used in combination with other agents. The dose for adults is 600 mg orally or intravenously once daily. Children may be given 10–20 mg/kg, not to exceed 600 mg daily. For

INH-resistant, rifampin-sensitive organisms, rifampin can be used for preventive therapy. In a mouse model, rifampin was effective and the rifamycin derivatives, rifabutin and rifapentine, could also be used [72].

## 11.3 PYRAZINAMIDE

Pyrazinamide (PZA) (Figure 11.3) is a synthetic pyrazine analog of nicotinamide. It was synthesized and found to be active for TB in 1952. PZA has a unique ability to act within the macrophage and in acidic environments. PZA is an integral part of short course therapy, reducing the time to sterilize the sputum. It appears to be most effective in the first 2 months of therapy with much less effect afterward. Therefore, it is often discontinued after 2 months of therapy while continuing other agents [73–75].

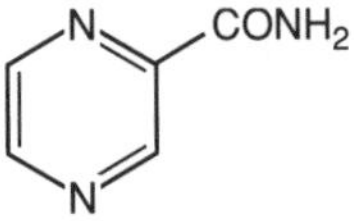

**Figure 11.3** Pyrazinamide.

### 11.3.1 Mechanism of action and activity

The exact mechanism of action of PZA is not known. The drug is bactericidal at acid pH (5.0–5.5) but has little, if any, activity at higher pH. PZA is therefore active in the acidic pH of the intracellular environment of macrophages. PZA is hydrolyzed to pyrazinoic acid by enzymes produced by *M. tuberculosis*. Pyrazinoic acid also has anti-TB effects and lowers intracellular pH, inhibiting mycobacterial growth [76]. The drug has little *in vitro* activity [77] but is very active in animal models [78].

PZA is a highly specific agent which is not active against most of the non-TB mycobacteria as well as *M. bovis*. The MIC for PZA is less than 20 µg/ml in susceptible organisms and resistance may be related to the absence of the hydrolyzing enzyme. As with other drugs, resistance occurs rapidly when it is used alone. When in combination with other active agents, resistance develops slowly.

### 11.3.2 Pharmacokinetics

PZA is well absorbed from the gut and attains peak levels within 2 hours. Concentrations of 30–50 µg/ml are attained with a dose of 20–25 mg/kg (1.5 g adult dose) [76]. Pyrazinoic acid has higher plasma concentrations than PZA, peaks 4–8 hours after an oral dose [76,79] and is metabolized by xanthine oxidase.

PZA is widely distributed into body tissues and fluids including the liver, lungs and CSF [79,80]. CSF concentrations may equal that of the plasma. It penetrates well intracellularly and its activity at acid pH makes the drug uniquely qualified in the treatment of intracellular tubercle bacilli.

The serum half life of PZA is 9–10 hours with normal renal and hepatic function [76] and is prolonged in patients with impaired renal or hepatic function.

### 11.3.3 Adverse effects

Drug-induced hepatotoxicity is a dose-related phenomenon. With doses of 40–50 mg/kg/day, 15% develop drug-induced hepatitis with fever, malaise and splenomegaly. Jaundice is seen in 2–3% of patients. Doses of 20–35 mg/kg/day or 90 mg/kg/week have a much lower incidence of severe hepatic reactions, although transient elevations in serum aminotransferases are common [81–83].

PZA inhibits renal excretion of uric acid and may cause hyperuricemia with episodes of gout. The hyperuricemia results from competition for renal excretion of uric acid by PZA metabolites. The effect of probenecid on PZA related hyperuricemia varies with the relative doses [84]. Arthralgias unrelated to hyperuricemia may also occur and are more common with daily than with intermittent dosing [82,83,85]. The arthralgias appear in the first few months and are usually self limited.

While anorexia, nausea and vomiting may occur without liver toxicity, liver function tests should be performed in any patient with these complaints. PZA has rarely caused cutaneous reactions but facial flushing similar to that seen with nicotinic acid is relatively common [82,85].

There is little information on the use of PZA in pregnancy. Pregnant women with drug susceptible organisms can be treated with INH, rifampin and ethambutol, and the use of PZA should be considered if resistance to these drugs is likely [86].

### 11.3.4 Monitoring parameters

Prior to initiation of therapy CBC, serum creatinine, blood urea nitrogen (BUN), uric acid, bilirubin, lactate dehydrogenase (LDH) and aminotransferases should be evaluated. Liver function tests should be evaluated monthly. If serum aminotransferases are found to be greater than five times baseline levels or the patient has complaints consistent with hepatic damage, discontinuation of all hepatotoxic drugs should be considered.

Uric acid levels should also be evaluated on a monthly basis, especially in patients with pre-existing hyperuricemia. Patients complaining of arthralgia or myalgia should have their uric acid levels re-evaluated, especially if the patient is predisposed to gouty arthritis.

### 11.3.5 Dosage

While the manufacturer recommends 20–30 mg/kg/day in three to four divided doses, the American Thoracic Society (ATS) and the Centers for Disease Control (CDC) recommend a dose of 15–30 mg/kg (up to 2 g/day) given once daily. For patients with HIV at least 20 mg/kg/day should be used. Doses as high as 60 mg/kg/day have been used in the treatment of INH-resistant TB, but these doses are generally not recommended [87].

In order to increase compliance, PZA has been given in doses of 50–70 mg/kg twice weekly along with other agents. Although the safe use of PZA has not been definitely established in children, a twice weekly PZA dose of 50–70 mg/kg (up to 2 g) is recommended for children less than 18 years of age [87].

PZA should be used cautiously in those with creatinine clearances of less than 50 ml/min. In such patients, the lower end of the recommended dosage range (i.e. 15–20 mg/kg/day or 50 mg/kg twice a week) should be used. It is generally not recommended to use PZA in patients with active liver disease or severe renal insufficiency [87].

## 11.4 ETHAMBUTOL

Ethambutol (EMB) is a bacteriostatic, synthetic agent (Figure 11.4) discovered among compounds screened for activity against the tubercle bacillus in 1961. EMB is considered to be first line therapy in patients with TB along with INH, rifampin and PZA.

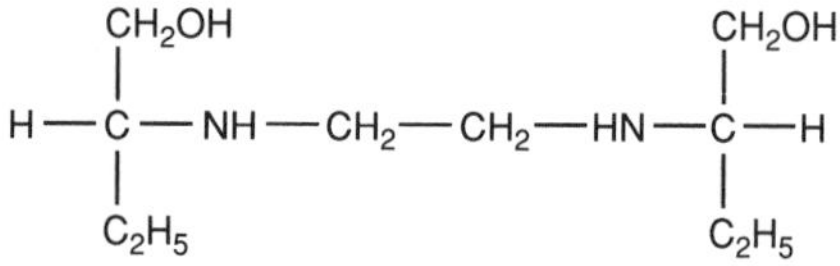

**Figure 11.4** Ethambutol.

### 11.4.1 Mechanism of action and activity

Although the mechanism of action is not known, it appears to have effects on RNA synthesis [88]. EMB also inhibits the incorporation of mycolic acid into the cell wall [89]. The drug diffuses only into actively growing mycobacterial cells. EMB is a highly specific agent with activity only against mycobacteria. As many as 90% of strains of *M. tuberculosis* are inhibited by 2 μg/ml or less [90]. Most strains of *M. kansasii* and *M. marinum* are also susceptible but *M. avium-intracellulare*, *M. scrofulaceum* and *M. fortuitum* are resistant [90,91]. Primary resistance can occur, but cross resistance with other anti-TB drugs is unusual.

## 11.4.2 Pharmacokinetics

From a dose of EMB, 75–80% is absorbed from the gut and the rate is not affected by food. Aluminum-containing salts, however, can reduce the absorption. Following an oral dose of 15–25 mg/kg, a peak level of 2–5 µg/ml occurs. The drug is widely distributed with the highest concentrations found in erythrocytes, kidney and lung (including caseous lesions). Lower concentrations are found in ascitic and pleural fluid. Although little drug crosses into the CSF with normal meninges, 10–15% of serum levels appear in the CSF in patients with inflamed meninges. EMB crosses the placenta and achieves levels in milk which are similar to the serum [10,92].

The drug is metabolized in the liver to two inactive forms. In the feces, 20% is found as unmetabolized, nonabsorbed drug. The remaining 80% is excreted by the kidney, 50% as EMB and 50% as inactive metabolites [10,92]. The serum half life is 3–4 hours in individuals with normal renal function and is prolonged with impaired renal function [10,93].

## 11.4.3 Adverse effects

The major adverse effect of EMB is optic neuritis, with a decrease in visual acuity, constriction of visual fields, central and peripheral scotomas and loss of red–green color discrimination. Like PZA, hyperuricemia can occur, is related to decreased urinary uric acid excretion and can precipitate gouty arthritis. Other adverse effects are quite uncommon. Gastrointestinal intolerance is infrequent [47].

Concern has been voiced that an overemphasis on the ocular effects of this drug could minimize usage. A lower percentage of adverse reactions from EMB culminating in death have been noted compared with other anti-TB drugs [94]. In another report, ocular toxicity was found in only 10 of 2184 individuals receiving EMB (0.04%). In nine of the ten individuals, it was noted after 8 weeks or more of treatment; only two had visual complaints [95]. Other sources [47] have reported a 1% incidence of ocular toxicity.

The drug has been used safely in children 6 years of age and older. Caution is advised, however, when using it in those under 13 years old owing to inaccuracies in monitoring visual acuity in this population [96,97]. For this reason, some physicians do not use EMB in children.

In patients with visual defects such as cataracts, recurrent inflammatory conditions of the eye, optic neuritis and diabetic neuropathy, the evaluation of visual acuity is more difficult. Consideration should be given as to whether the benefits of EMB justify the possible additive ocular effects.

EMB has been used to treat TB in pregnant women without any adverse effects on the fetus. The drug can be shown, however, to be teratogenic in animal studies when used in high doses [98]. It should, therefore, be used when potential benefits outweigh any possible risk to the fetus [98,99].

### 11.4.4 Monitoring parameters

Visual testing should be performed prior to initiation of therapy and periodically during therapy. Testing should be done monthly in patients receiving more than 15 mg/kg/day EMB. Examination should include Snellen eye chart, ophthalmoscopy, finger perimetry and testing of color discrimination. All patients should be questioned periodically about subjective visual symptoms and should be instructed to report any such changes as soon as they are noticed. If substantial changes in visual acuity occur, EMB should be discontinued immediately [47,96,97]. In most cases of optic neuritis associated with high dose or prolonged use, the ocular effects are reversible on stopping the drug.

Periodic tests of the renal, hepatic and hematopoietic systems during long term therapy should also be performed [47,96,97]. Serum uric acid levels should be evaluated at baseline and intermittently in patients who are predisposed to gout [100].

### 11.4.5 Dosage

Dosing is usually 15 mg/kg/day as a single oral dose. Initially, particularly in patients who have been previously treated for TB, the dose may be increased to 25 mg/kg/day for the first 60 days or until acid-fast bacillus (AFB) cultures are negative, with the dose is then decreased to 15 mg/kg/day [96,97].

Dosage should be modified in patients with renal impairment. Patients with creatinine clearances greater than 50 ml/min may receive the normal dosage. Patients with clearances of 10–50 ml/min should receive 7.5 mg/kg/day and a dose of 5 mg/kg/day should be used if the clearance is less than 10 ml/min [10,92,93]. It is recommended that patients receiving hemodialysis be given 15 mg/kg on the day of dialysis. Patients receiving peritoneal dialysis should receive 15 mg/kg/day on days when peritoneal dialysis is being administered [10,93,101].

### 11.5 ETHIONAMIDE

Soon after the discovery of INH, several independent groups discovered the anti-TB activity of thioisonicotinamide. The compound's α-ethyl derivative, ethionamide, synthesized in France in 1956 (Figure 11.5) was

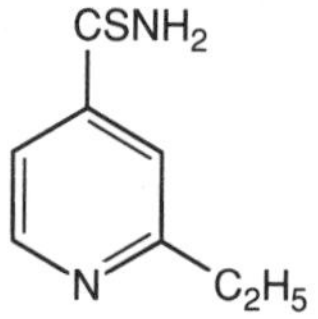

Figure 11.5 Ethionamide.

found to be more effective than the parent drug [13,102]. It is a bright yellow powder with a sulfide odor. Ethionamide is a second line agent that is not recommended for treatment regimens in previously untreated patients because of its frequent and potentially serious toxicities [103].

### 11.5.1 Mechanism of action and activity

While the drug is thought to inhibit peptide synthesis, the precise mode of action is unclear [104,105]. The similarity in structure to INH could offer some answers about ethionamide's activity, but the lack of cross resistance between INH and ethionamide [106] suggests that this may not be the case. The report of a gene encoding for a target for both INH and ethionamide, however, suggests cross resistance can occur [9a].

Active only against some mycobacteria, ethionamide inhibits the TB bacillus *in vitro* at 0.6–1.2 µg/ml [106]. Three-quarters of photochromogenic mycobacteria are inhibited *in vitro* by 10 µg/ml or less [13,102]. Ethionamide is reported to be equally effective *in vitro* against intracellular and extracellular TB bacilli [13].

### 11.5.2 Pharmacokinetics

Administered orally, ethionamide is rapidly absorbed with a bioavailability approaching 100%. Following a dose of 1 g, a serum level as high as 20 µg/ml may be attained, falling to 3 µg/ml at 9 hours and less than 1 µg/ml at 24 hours [13]. The drug is widely distributed in most body tissues and fluids with tissue concentrations approximating blood levels. Levels of drug in lung tissue were found to be 85–90% of those in the serum [107]. CSF levels are similar to serum levels in both inflamed and normal meninges. Although the risk in pregnancy is not well defined, the drug crosses the placenta and its use in pregnancy should be avoided if possible. The concentration in breast milk is unknown.

Ethionamide has a serum half life of 2 hours, and is extensively metabolized. The sulfoxide derivative retains activity and may be converted back to the parent drug *in vivo* [108]. Most elimination is via the renal route, with 1% being unchanged drug, 5% active metabolites and the remainder inactive metabolites [105].

### 11.5.3 Adverse effects

There is an increased rate of CNS side effects from cycloserine (altered mental status and seizures) and from INH (dizziness and drowsiness) with the concomitant use of ethionamide. Likewise, other neurological effects, such as optic and peripheral neuritis from aminoglycosides, capreomycin and ethambutol may be increased with concurrent use of ethionamide [105]. Like INH, ethionamide can cause a peripheral neuropathy related to an increased pyridoxine requirement. Since pyridoxine is needed as a cofactor in synthesizing nicotinamide, a pellagra-like encephalopathy and neuropathy can occur during drug treatment [109].

Hepatotoxicity occurs during ethionamide therapy in 5% of cases. One report, however, found 37% of those on ethionamide-containing regimens developed hepatotoxicity compared with 12% not on ethionamide [110]. Aminotransferase elevations are generally reversed when the drug is stopped [102,105]. Hepatitis appears to be more common in diabetic patients [103,111], and diabetes may be more difficult to control while taking ethionamide [102].

The most common side effects are gastrointestinal and include nausea, vomiting and anorexia [102]. Additionally, CNS effects of headache, giddiness, optic neuritis and depression can occur [102,112]. Vitamin B complex supplementation does not reduce the incidence of these events [113]. The drug can also be associated with the development of hypothyroidism with goiter [114,115].

Ethionamide is teratogenic in animals in high doses and cannot be recommended during pregnancy.

### 11.5.4 Monitoring parameters

Although mild serum aminotransferase elevations can return to normal despite continued ethionamide use, close observation of hepatic function is recommended, particularly in diabetic patients. Periodic eye and neuropsychiatric evaluations are also indicated. Visual symptoms should prompt discontinuation of the drug.

### 11.5.5 Dosage

The initial dosage of ethionamide is usually 125 mg twice daily. The dose is then increased by 125 mg every 5 days until 1 g/day is reached. A single daily dose of 1 g/day taken after dinner may be given with possible increased efficacy but divided daily doses are better tolerated with fewer gastrointestinal side effects. To minimize peripheral neuropathy, especially for patients also taking INH, pyridoxine supplementation is recommended.

### 11.6 AMINOGLYCOSIDES

Aminoglycosides are made up of two or more amino sugars attached to a hexose nucleus via glycosidic linkages [116]. They are best classified as aminoglycosidic aminocyclitols. Of the group, streptomycin and kanamycin (Figure 11.6) are most often used in TB treatment. Amikacin, a semisynthetic aminoglycoside, is used primarily for non-TB mycobacteria and is discussed later.

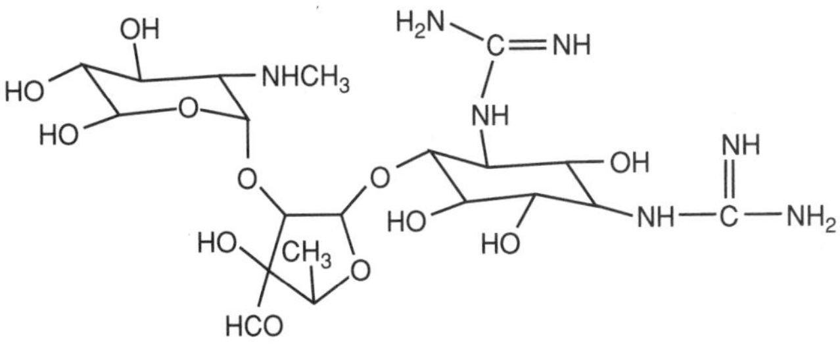

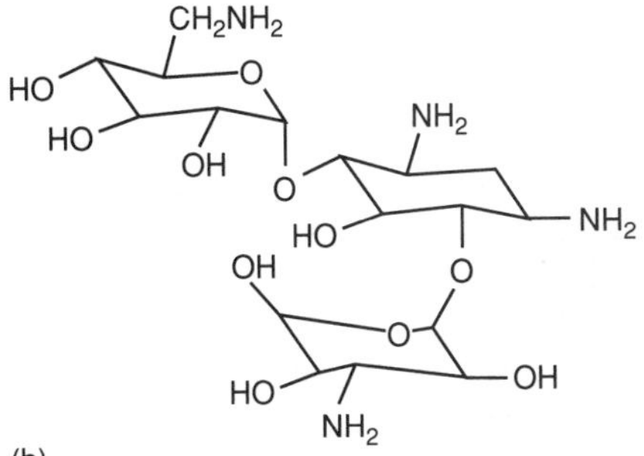

**Figure 11.6** Streptomycin (a) and kanamycin (b).

Streptomycin was the first effective anti-TB agent when it was introduced by Waksman *et al.* in 1944 [117]. Kanamycin was first described in Japan in 1957. Kanamycin is composed of two isomers, but only kanamycin A has anti-TB activity [118]. The biological activity is pH dependent, with more effect at higher pH values. *In vitro* susceptibility testing should be carried out in test medium at a pH in the range of 7.3–7.5. Calcium and magnesium concentrations in the sensitivity media should be controlled as high levels can lead to apparent decreased activity [119].

### 11.6.1 Mechanism of action and activity

Aminoglycosides are bacteriocidal to tubercle bacilli [120]. Streptomycin binds to a single site on the bacterial ribosome, blocking the initiation stage in translocation and preventing polypeptide elongation. Kanamycin binds to multiple sites on the ribosome. Single step mutations involving the streptomycin ribosomal protein do not result in high level resistance to kanamycin [119]. Resistance to aminoglycosides may arise through mechanisms including alteration of the ribosomal binding site, interference with drug transport and production of inactivation enzymes [121]. Most strains of *M. tuberculosis*, *M. kansasii* and *M. marinum* are sensitive *in vitro* to streptomycin at 10 μg/ml. Similarly, most strains of TB are inhibited by

10 µg/ml or less of kanamycin. Although the drugs are bacteriocidal at concentrations significantly less than blood levels, *in vivo* activities are relatively low. This relates to poor intracellular penetration [122]. These agents also have broad facultative Gram-negative bacilli activity.

### 11.6.2 Pharmacokinetics

The aminoglycosides are poorly absorbed when given orally, requiring the parenteral route to produce adequate levels. After a 0.5–1 g intramuscular dose of streptomycin or kanamycin, peak levels are 10–55 µg/ml and 10–30 µg/ml, respectively [121]. An adequate level for treatment is considered to be 10 µg/ml although streptomycin levels as low as 0.4 µg/ml may inhibit *M. tuberculosis* [122].

Aminoglycosides are distributed over the extracellular space. Therefore, in patients with ascites, congestive heart failure or dehydration, a dosage modification may be required. Fever [123] and anemia [124] are associated with shortened aminoglycoside half lives, related to higher glomerular blood flow. Aminoglycosides achieve good levels in bone, pleural, ascitic, synovial and peritoneal fluid. Urinary levels exceed serum levels by 100 times. High concentrations are also found in the fluids of the inner ear. The drugs distribute less well into the lung, bile, amniotic and prostatic fluids and poorly into the CSF [125].

These drugs are excreted primarily by glomerular filtration. Of a parenteral dose of streptomycin, 50–60% is renally excreted within 24 hours. Streptomycin has a half life in serum of 2–3 hours and kanamycin of 2–4 hours [125]. Aminoglycosides are removed by hemodialysis and, to a lesser extent, by peritoneal dialysis. All accumulate in renal failure, requiring decrease in dosage [122].

### 11.6.3 Adverse effects

These drugs can cause nephrotoxicity, auditory and vestibular ototoxicity and neuromuscular blockade. Streptomycin can cause as many as 20% of patients to develop vestibular damage [126]. Risk factors for developing ototoxicity include advanced age, concurrent use of other ototoxic drugs and renal impairment. Peak serum concentrations greater than 50 µg/ml of streptomycin are associated with an increased risk of ototoxicity [127]. Kanamycin ototoxicity usually manifests as hearing loss [118]. In 40% of cases, warning signs of tinnitus or fullness in the ears were detected prior to kanamycin associated auditory toxicity [128].

Kanamycin nephrotoxicity, unlike ototoxicity, is usually reversible and is associated with serum trough levels of more than 10 µg/ml and prolonged drug exposure. Risk factors for nephrotoxicity include concomitant use of other nephrotoxic agents, advanced age, shock and possibly concomitant liver disease [129–131]. Streptomycin has the lowest risk for nephrotoxicity of the aminoglycosides [127]. Although not tested in TB, a once daily dosage of aminoglycosides may reduce renal toxicity [132].

Streptomycin and kanamycin should be used in pregnancy only if the benefits outweigh the risks. Fetal abnormalities, including eighth cranial nerve damage with irreversible hearing loss, have been found when streptomycin was administered in pregnancy [133].

Neuromuscular blockade is rare [134], but has occurred as a result of intraperitoneal lavage, rapid intravenous administration, intramuscular and even oral use with bowel wall embarrassment [135]. Aminoglycosides should be avoided in patients with myasthenia gravis [125,134] and possibly in those with Parkinson's disease [136] because of this neuromuscular effect. Other CNS effects from aminoglycosides have been reported in patients with impaired renal function [137]. Intravenous streptomycin should be infused over at least 1 hour to minimize facial flushing and headache [138]. Rarely, cutaneous, hepatic and a variety of hematologic reactions may occur [121,137].

### 11.6.4 Monitoring parameters

Renal function and eighth nerve testing should be done at baseline and periodically. Peak streptomycin levels should be 20–30 µg/ml and trough levels less than 5 µg/ml. Kanamycin peak levels of 15–30 µg/ml and a trough of less than 10 µg/ml are acceptable.

### 11.6.5 Dosage

The usual dose of streptomycin is 15 mg/kg/day IM for TB treatment. This dose should be given as one dose not to exceed 1 g [50]. Although not FDA approved, the dose can be infused intravenously over 1 hour in patients who do not tolerate the IM route [138]. Elderly patients should receive 10 mg/kg/day (not to exceed 750 mg/day) [50]. Patients with creatinine clearances greater than 50 ml/min may receive the normal dose of streptomycin. Patients with clearance of 10–50 ml/min should receive the same dose but at 48–72 hour intervals and patients with a clearance of less than 10 ml/min should receive the dose at 72–96 hour intervals.

Streptomycin has also been administered on a twice weekly basis in combination with other agents. The twice weekly dose for infants, children and adolescents is 20–40 mg/kg as a single IM injection (maximum dose 1 g). The twice weekly dose for adults is 25–30 mg/kg (not to exceed 1 g) [50,73,139].

Kanamycin dosage for adults is 15 mg/kg IM with a maximal dose of 1 g. For children, the dosage is 15–30 mg/kg/day. The dose must be appropriately lowered for renal impairment [125].

## 11.7 CYCLOSERINE

Several investigative groups, working independently, discovered cyclo-serine (Figure 11.7). It now can be prepared synthetically from serine. Because of significant toxicity, use is very limited.

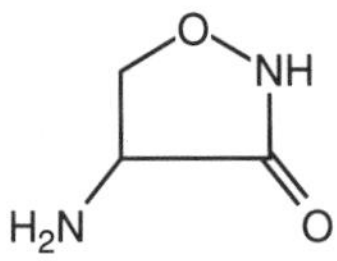

**Figure 11.7** Cycloserine.

### 11.7.1 Mechanism of action and activity

As a structural analog of D-alanine, it inhibits L-alanine racemase and D-alanyl-D-alanine synthetase. These enzymes are necessary to produce D-alanine from L-alanine and incorporate D-alanine into the peptidoglycan [140–142]. The antibacterial effects of cycloserine are antagonized by the presence of D-alanine. *In vitro* testing of sensitivity to cycloserine must be done in alanine-free medium [143]. This antagonism is found *in vivo* in tuberculous guinea pigs treated with cycloserine, as guinea pigs have significant blood levels of alanine [144].

The drug is active against TB as well as some strains of *M. bovis*, *M. marinum*, *M. ulcerans* and *M. avium-intracellulare*. The MIC for the tubercle bacillus is 5–20 µg/ml and slightly higher for non-TB mycobacteria [145]. It has activity against some bacteria, including *Staphylococcus aureus*, *Nocardia* sp., *Enterobacter* sp. and enterococci. Cycloserine resistance in TB is due to mutations in the gene for D-alanyl-D-alanine synthetase [146,147]. In *B. subtilis*, cycloserine resistance was found to be due to decreased drug uptake into the cell [148].

### 11.7.2 Pharmacokinetics

After an oral dose, 70–90% of the drug is rapidly absorbed. A serum level of 10–20 µg/ml is produced by a dose of 250 mg twice daily [144]. Cycloserine is widely distributed into most tissues and body fluids. The rate of excretion is relatively slow and higher blood levels occur with repeat dosing. CSF levels are 50–80% of those in the blood with uninflamed meninges and 80–100% in meningitis. The urine level is higher than that in serum. The drug crosses the placenta and is excreted at levels close to the serum level in breast milk [149].

Cycloserine is eliminated by glomerular filtration with a serum half life of about 10 hours with normal renal function. About 35% of the drug is not accounted for and probably reflects metabolism [150]. It is retained in patients with impaired renal function and removed by hemodialysis.

### 11.7.3 Adverse reactions

A patient taking cycloserine should avoid alcohol use, which may lower the seizure threshold. Concurrent use of cycloserine with ethionamide, INH and phenytoin increases the incidence of adverse CNS effects (seizures, dizziness, drowsiness) [151,152]. Cycloserine can increase pyridoxine requirements and it is reasonable to administer supplemental pyridoxine (100–300 mg/day) to reduce the incidence of anemia or neuritis [21].

Because of cycloserine's link with neuropsychiatric symptoms, it is best to avoid it in patients with seizures, anxiety, depression and/or psychosis. Such effects are somewhat dose-related and occur within the first 2 weeks in about 30% of patients receiving 500 mg daily. The psychiatric effects can include nightmares and potentially serious episodes of depressive psychosis with suicidal tendencies.

Since the toxic/therapeutic ratio is quite narrow and the drug is retained in renal insufficiency, extreme caution must be utilized in such patients and the drug should be avoided if at all possible in those with significant renal disease. Few data are available regarding its safety in pregnancy but the drug is best avoided.

### 11.7.4 Monitoring parameters

Close observation by family members is needed in patients taking cycloserine to recognize neurotoxic complications early. Serum levels should be kept below 30 µg/ml.

### 11.7.5 Dosage

Therapy is started at 250 mg orally every 12 hours and, after 2 weeks, dosage can be cautiously increased to 750–1000 mg/day. Doses over 500 mg/day should be monitored with serum levels.

## 11.8 CAPREOMYCIN

Capreomycin consists of four active compounds, capreomycin IA, IB, IIA and IIB [153,154] (Figure 11.8) as a group of complex cyclic polypeptides. Capreomycin is used only to treat TB that is resistant to primary drug therapy.

### 11.8.1 Mechanism of action and activity

The action of capreomycin is not totally clear but it appears to inhibit protein synthesis. It is bacteriostatic, however, and may be bacteriocidal in neutral or slightly alkaline pH. Capreomycin is only active against mycobacteria including *M. tuberculosis*, *M. bovis*, *M. kansasii* and *M. avium-intracellulare* [155]. Resistance is rare.

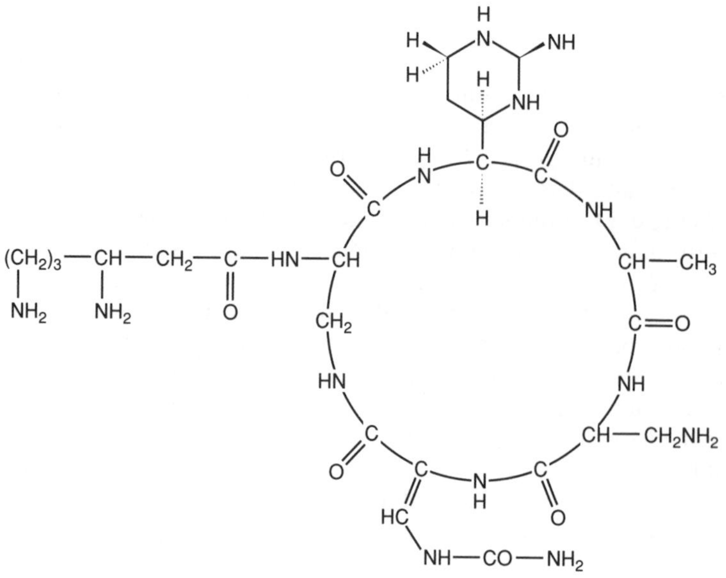

**Figure 11.8** Capreomycin IB.

### 11.8.2 Pharmacokinetics

Capreomycin has pharmacokinetics similar to the aminoglycosides. It is poorly absorbed given orally but well absorbed after IM dosing. Peak serum levels of 30–35 µg/ml are seen at 1–2 hours, 10 µg/ml at 6 hours and less than 1 µg/ml at 24 hours. Over half (50–60%) of the drug is eliminated by glomerular filtration as the unchanged drug within 24 hours [16,154].

The penetration of capreomycin into body tissues and fluids has not been studied. The drug probably does not cross meninges well and it is not known whether it crosses the placenta or is found in breast milk [154].

### 11.8.3 Adverse effects

Nephrotoxicity and ototoxicity are the most serious side effects of the drug. Concurrent use of other nephrotoxic or ototoxic agents, such as aminoglycosides or vancomycin, may have additive toxic effects [16,154].

Capreomycin therapy may be continued with caution if protein, white or red cells, or casts appear in the urine, unless there is a rise in BUN and serum creatinine. Renal tubular dysfunction has also been reported with alkalosis and electrolyte disturbances including hypokalemia, hypocalcemia and hypomagnesemia. The drug may also cause ototoxicity, including vertigo, tinnitus and deafness. Patients with compromised renal function, pre-existing hearing problems and the elderly are more at risk.

### 11.8.4 Monitoring parameters

Electrolytes (including potassium, calcium, magnesium and sodium), serum creatinine and BUN should be measured prior to initiation of therapy and repeated periodically.

### 11.8.5 Dosage

The usual dose of capreomycin is 20 mg/kg (up to 1 g) IM daily for 60–120 days followed by 1 g 2–3 times weekly. Patients with creatinine clearances of 50–80 ml/min should receive half the usual dose (500 mg) every 24 hours. Patients with clearances of 10–50 ml/min should receive 500 mg every 48–72 hours and patients with clearances less than 10 ml/min every 72–96 hours. Patients undergoing hemodialysis should receive 50–75% of the initial dose after each treatment [154].

## 11.9 PARA-AMINOSALICYLIC ACID

Para-aminosalicylic acid (PAS) is a structural analog of para-aminobenzoic acid (Figure 11.9). As with other salicylates, the drug deteriorates rapidly when exposed to moisture, heat or light. Owing to the high incidence of adverse effects, its use is reserved for patients with TB resistant to multiple drugs.

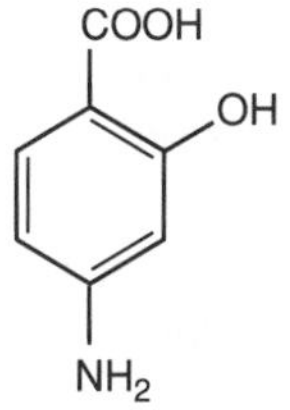

**Figure 11.9** Para-aminosalicylic acid.

### 11.9.1 Mechanism of action and activity

PAS inhibits the synthesis of folic acid by preventing the conversion of aminobenzoic acid to dihydrofolic acid and is active only against *M. tuberculosis*. Susceptible strains are inhibited by 0.5–2.0 µg/ml [156]. This limited activity is unlike sulfonamides or other structural analogs of para-aminobenzoic acid, which are broad spectrum antibacterials. As with other anti-TB agents, resistance develops rapidly when the drug is used alone, but when used in combination with other agents, resistance is delayed or prevented. There is no evidence of cross resistance with other agents [157,158].

### 11.9.2 Pharmacokinetics

PAS, available as a sodium salt, is readily absorbed orally. Peak serum levels attained after a 4 g dose are 40–75 µg/ml [159]. It diffuses into peritoneal, pleural and synovial fluids at a level approaching the serum concentration. CSF levels are 10–50% of serum levels in the presence of inflamed meninges, but PAS does not cross into the CSF when the meninges are not inflamed [160]. The ability of the drug to cross the placenta is unknown but small amounts of the drug have been found in milk [161].

The half life of PAS is about 1 hour, undergoing acetylation to inactive metabolites in the intestine and liver. These metabolites are then renally excreted by filtration and tubular secretion [159]. The elimination of PAS and its metabolites is blocked by probenecid, leading to high serum levels. The drug should be given with caution in patients with renal or hepatic insufficiency and the dose should be reduced. Although the half life of active drug is not prolonged in renal or hepatic insufficiency, the half life of the inactive metabolites is prolonged in patients with renal impairment and contributes to salicylate toxicity.

### 11.9.3 Adverse effects

PAS may decrease digoxin absorption by as much as 20%. In addition, the hypoprothrombinemic effect of warfarin may be enhanced by the drug. Diphenhydramine has been reported to decrease the absorption of PAS, therefore, these drugs should not be given together. PAS may increase INH toxicity by inhibiting acetylation and may decrease rifampin levels by decreasing absorption.

The most common side effect is gastrointestinal intolerance, occurring in 10–30% of patients, including nausea, vomiting, abdominal pain and diarrhea. Ulceration and gastric hemorrhage have also been reported. These effects may be decreased by administering PAS with food or antacids. Hypersensitivity reactions including fever, rash, pruritus, vasculitis, joint pain and eosinophilia may occur in 5–10%. Leukopenia, agranulocytosis, thrombocytopenia and hepatitis have also been reported [47,162]. A mononucleosis-like syndrome with atypical lymphocytes can occur. This sodium salt should not be given to patients on restricted salt intake.

Patients with hepatic or renal insufficiency should be given the drug with caution. Patients with a history of peptic ulcer disease may be predisposed to recurrence while on PAS. The use of PAS in patients with a history of severe allergies to Aspirin or related compounds is contraindicated [47,156]. A new non-sodium containing PAS formulation is soon to be commercially available in the USA. It is enterically coated so that the toxic metabolite, m-aminophenol, is not released in the stomach to cause gastrointestinal effects.

### 11.9.4 Monitoring parameters

Patients receiving PAS should be monitored for symptoms of peptic ulcer. CBC should be measured periodically [47,156,162].

### 11.9.5 Dosage

The usual dose of PAS is 150 mg/kg/day given in 2–4 equally divided doses.

## 11.10 FLUOROQUINOLONES

Ciprofloxacin and ofloxacin are the quinolones with the most activity against *M. tuberculosis* (Figure 11.10). Sparfloxacin, a difluorinated quinolone not yet marketed, has shown promising *in vitro* activity. Although not indicated as first line therapy for the treatment of TB, the

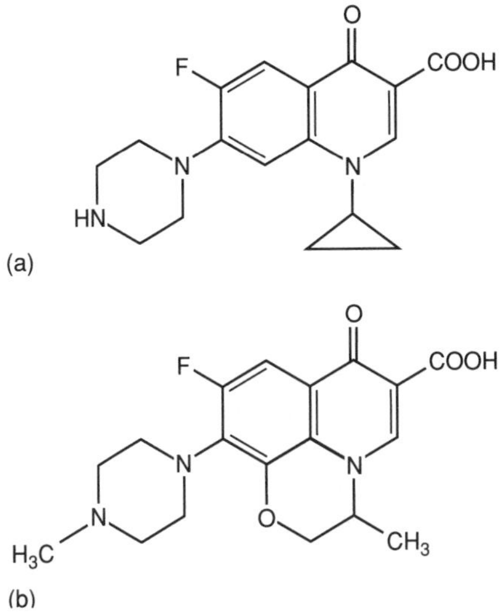

**Figure 11.10** Ciprofloxacin (a) and ofloxacin (b).

fluoroquinolones have an important role in the treatment of resistant organisms. Studies using ciprofloxacin [162a] found the drug particularly useful as an early bacteriocidal agent with a similar rate of killing as INH.

### 11.10.1 Mechanism of action and activity

The fluoroquinolones work by inhibiting the function of DNA gyrase (topoisomerase II) [163–165]. This enzyme catalyzes the introduction of negative superhelical twists into the circular bacterial DNA. The absence of such circular DNA in mammalian genomes explains the lack of an effect in human cells. These drugs have broad spectrum activity for most Gram-negative aerobic and facultative bacilli but variable streptococcal and staphylococcal and no anaerobic activity [166].

Quinolones are tuberculocidal. Ciprofloxacin and ofloxacin are about equally active *in vitro* against *M. tuberculosis* with reported $MIC_{50}$ (concentrations to inhibit 50% of strains) of 0.5 µg/ml and $MIC_{90}$ of 1.0 µg/ml [167]. Sparfloxacin has been shown to have slightly lower MICs for *M. tuberculosis* by a factor of two [168].

The quinolones have variable activity against non-TB mycobacteria [167]. *Mycobacterium bovis* is inhibited by 1 µg/ml of either ciprofloxacin or ofloxacin and the MICs of ciprofloxacin and ofloxacin for *M. avium-intracellulare* are 8–16 µg/ml. Although less active for *M. avium-intracellulare* than for TB, they retain a treatment role because of the lack of many other active drugs. *Mycobacterium scrofulaceum* is generally resistant. It appears that many of the rapid growing mycobacteria are more susceptible than the slower growers [169].

Laboratory and clinical resistance to the quinolones are well documented [166,170]. In a report of ofloxacin use in 19 patients with multiple-drug-resistant cavitary pulmonary TB, resistance emerged in those patients who did not become culture negative [171].

### 11.10.2 Pharmacokinetics

These drugs are well absorbed after oral administration. Ofloxacin has a bioavailability near 100% [170] while ciprofloxacin is somewhat lower [172]. Administration with food delays the absorption of both drugs but may not be clinically significant. It is recommended not to give ofloxacin with food [170]. Ciprofloxacin may be given without regard to meals [172].

Fluoroquinolones are distributed to most body tissues including the lung, with concentrations 1.5–4 times serum level [173]. Ofloxacin penetrates bronchial secretions and sputum better than ciprofloxacin but ciprofloxacin penetrates lung tissue at least as well as, and in some cases better than, ofloxacin [174,175]. Since *M. tuberculosis* is an intracellular pathogen, the concentration of ciprofloxacin and other quinolones in alveolar macrophages 14–18-fold greater than serum is relevant [163].

Approximately 35% of ciprofloxacin but less than 5% of ofloxacin is metabolized by the liver [170,172]. Ciprofloxacin and ofloxacin have half lives of 4 hours and 6 hours, respectively [170–172]. The dose of both ciprofloxacin and ofloxacin should be decreased in patients with creatinine clearances less than 50 ml/min.

### 11.10.3 Adverse effects and drug reactions

Ciprofloxacin has been shown to inhibit the hepatic cytochrome P450 enzyme system, resulting in a 26–35% increase in theophylline half life

[176,177]. Ofloxacin has been reported to increase plasma concentrations of theophylline by 10%, which may not be clinically significant [170]. Ciprofloxacin and, to a lesser degree, ofloxacin, may similarly increase caffeine concentrations. Patients should be advised of the potential tachycardia, tremors and hypertension from caffeine. Co-administration of ciprofloxacin with cyclosporin may result in renal toxicity. Ciprofloxacin may also inhibit the metabolism of warfarin [178].

Ciprofloxacin and ofloxacin should not be given at the same time as sucralfate [179,180] to avoid decreased absorption of the quinolones. This may be due to the aluminum cation in the compound. Other cations such as iron, magnesium, zinc and calcium found in multivitamins or antacids should also be separated from quinolones by at least 2–4 hours [170,181]. Cations in didanosine may also cause decreased absorption [182].

Gastrointestinal side effects including nausea, vomiting and/or diarrhea have been reported in 8.5% of patients [170]. CNS effects including restlessness, tremors and dizziness occur with an incidence of 4.6% [170]. Skin reactions are usually mild and transient, with pruritus being the most common. Reversible renal failure has been associated with both ciprofloxacin and ofloxacin [183]. Other side effects reported with the fluoroquinolones include rash, fever, eosinophilia, arthralgias and hepatitis [184–186].

No well-controlled trials in pregnant women have been conducted with the fluoroquinolone antibiotics, but studies conducted in dogs have demonstrated cartilage damage in the developing animal. Because of this potential, this class of medications is not approved for use in individuals under 18 years. To date, there is little clinical evidence to assess the extent of this problem in humans. A study of 634 cases (adolescents and children) found reversible arthropathy in 1.3% [187].

### 11.10.4 Monitoring parameters

All patients receiving fluoroquinolones should have baseline CBC and renal and hepatic function tests. These should be monitored periodically during treatment.

### 11.10.5 Dosage

The dose of ciprofloxacin for TB is not clearly established; 1000–1500 mg/day is sometimes recommended but 500–750 mg/day has been successfully used in combination therapy [188].

Dosage adjustments are recommended in patients with reduced creatinine clearance rates. Patients with a clearance rate of 50–100 ml/min should receive 1000–1500 mg/day in two divided doses. Patients with a clearance rate of 30–50 ml/min should receive 50% of the usual dose. In those with clearance rates less than 30 ml/min, no more than 500 mg every 18 hours is needed [189]. Ciprofloxacin is removed by peritoneal and hemodialysis. The recommended dose is 250–500 mg/day, administered after dialysis.

Doses of at least 600 mg/day of ofloxacin should be used in TB treatment. Patients with clearance rates of 50–100 ml/min should receive 300–400 mg twice daily, those with clearance rates of 10–50 ml/min should receive 300–400 mg/day and those with clearance rates of less than 10 ml/min should receive 200 mg/day [171,174].

## 11.11 MISCELLANEOUS ANTIMYCOBACTERIAL DRUGS

### 11.11.1 Rifabutin

Rifabutin (ansamycin) is a rifamycin derivative which has been shown to be useful in preventing or delaying *M. avium-intracellulare* complex bacteremia in AIDS patients [190]. It may be used in combination with other agents for *M. avium-intracellulare* infection in HIV-infected and noninfected individuals. The drug is active against some rifampin-resistant TB [191].

Although the drug induces the cytochrome P450 hepatic enzymes, it does not appear to be as significant as rifampin. Physicians with patients taking rifabutin, however, should be alert to such potential interactions. Discoloration of the skin, urine and other body fluids occurs in about two-thirds of patients on the daily dose of 300 mg/day. In patients with abdominal distress, the dose can be given in two divided doses with food.

### 11.11.2 Clofazimine

Clofazimine is a hydrophobic phenazine quinoneimine that is red in color. It is an electron acceptor and may be active by inhibiting certain mycobacterial energy yielding reactions [192]. The drug binds to nucleic acids but it is not clear if this binding is related to its activity. The drug is used at doses of 100 mg/day for *M. avium-intracellulare* and *M. leprae*. It has anti-inflammatory properties and has been used for noninfectious conditions such as pyoderma gangranosum.

Because of its hydrophobic properties, clofazimine must be given as a microcrystalline suspension in an oil–detergent base [16]. High concentrations of drug accumulate in adipose tissue, liver, lung, kidney, spleen and skin. Accumulation may result in drug crystal deposits in these tissues and red–brown discoloration of skin and conjunctiva as well as of urine, feces, sputum and sweat [193]. Dryness of the skin of the extremities may also occur.

### 11.11.3 Amikacin

Amikacin, an aminoglycoside derivative of kanamycin, is used in the treatment of *M. avium-intracellulare* and drug-resistant TB. The pharmacologic properties of amikacin and kanamycin are virtually identical, but amikacin is generally more active *in vitro* and *in vivo* [194,195]. The inhibitory concentrations of amikacin are around 16 µg/ml [196] but lower values have been reported [195]. Cidal levels are four to eight times inhibitory levels [197]. After a 0.5–1 g parenteral dose of amikacin, peak levels are 10–30 µg/ml [121], with a post-antibiotic residual effect. Intracellular killing can be significantly improved by administering entrapped amikacin in liposomes [198]. Such preparations are currently undergoing trials in humans. The use of amikacin once a day for mycobacteria has been shown to be as effective as when given more often [199].

Amikacin shares the same toxicities as the other aminoglycosides, including nephrotoxicity and ototoxicity, the latter manifesting as hearing loss. Between 3.4% and 24% of patients develop some degree of hearing loss by audiogram [200]. Although once a day dosing of aminoglycosides is thought to decrease nephrotoxicity [201], a small study indicated that ototoxicity may be increased [200].

### 11.11.4 Thiacetazone

This drug is a thiosemicarbazone found to be bacteriostatic against TB by Domagk in 1946 [202]. Because of toxicity and low potency, it is rarely used in industrialized countries and is not marketed in the USA. It has, however, been used in developing countries as a fixed combination with 150 mg of thiacetazone and 300 mg of INH.

Thiacetazone commonly causes hypersensitivity reactions including fever and skin rash. The drug may enhance streptomycin ototoxicity. Potentially serious side effects are erythema multiforme, hepatitis, hemolytic anemia and granulocytopenia [16]. Serious thiacetazone cutaneous hypersensitivity including Stevens-Johnson syndrome appears to be particularly common in individuals with TB and HIV co-infection [203].

### 11.11.5 Beta-lactam antibiotics

Although cefoxitin may be used in the treatment of *M. fortuitum* and *M. chelonae* infections at a dose of 12 g/day, the role of ß-lactam antibiotics in the treatment of TB has been small. A major reason for this is the production of ß-lactamase by mycobacteria. Lorian and Sabath [204] found that cloxacillin could inhibit the TB bacillus at attainable blood levels. In 1991, Nadler *et al.* [205] reported the utility of amoxicillin/clavulanic acid, which is resistant to the TB ß-lactamase, at doses of 2–4 g/day in combination with other agents for multi-drug-resistant TB. It has been found that the ß-lactamase production is constitutive and not inducible and BRL 42715 is active against the ß-lactamase at levels of 0.0001 µg/ml [206]. This activity is 200–500 times greater than clavulanic acid (0.05 µg/ml) which is 20 times more active than sulbactam, tazobactam and cloxacillin. Penicillins and cephalosporins, when combined with clavulanic acid or BRL 42715, merit more interest in the treatment of mycobacterial infections.

### 11.11.6 Trimethoprim/sulfamethoxazole

This fixed combination works by inhibiting sequential steps in folic acid synthesis. It can be used to treat certain infections caused by non-TB mycobacteria. *In vitro* studies reveal activity of the sulfa component for *M. fortuitum* and *M. marinum* [207], and the combination has been an acceptable treatment for superficial cutaneous *M. marinum* disease [208]. Prolonged treatment with trimethoprim/sulfamethoxazole has been shown to be effective for pulmonary disease due to susceptible strains of *M. fortuitum* [209]. Dosages of the combination used for mycobacterial infections are 10 mg/kg of trimethoprim and 50 mg/kg of sulfamethoxazole per day in two divided doses. Toxicity is related to allergy, bone marrow suppression and gastrointestinal symptoms.

### 11.11.7 Tetracyclines

Tetracyclines inhibit protein synthesis by binding to the 30S ribosomal subunit. Some tetracyclines have antibacterial effects separate from protein synthesis inhibition [209a]. The members of this group used to treat non-TB mycobacteria are tetracycline, minocycline and doxycycline. Each has been shown to be effective for cutaneous disease due to *M. marinum* [210,211]. Doxycycline has also been shown to inhibit some strains of *M. fortuitum* and *M. chelonae in vitro* [212].

Tetracycline's shorter half life mandates dosing at 6 hour intervals (usual dose 2000 mg/day) while doxycycline and minocycline can be given twice daily (usual dose 200 mg/day). Toxicity includes cutaneous hypersensitivity, photosensitization and gastrointestinal irritation. Worsening of renal failure by increasing catabolism occurs with tetracycline. Discoloration of the teeth, which is permanent, may occur when these agents are given to children. Vertigo may occur with minocycline [213]. The absorption of some tetracyclines is impaired if given with milk or with calcium, magnesium or aluminum-containing antacids. The same effect may occur with iron and iron-containing tonics.

### 11.11.8 Macrolide group

The macrolide agents inhibit protein synthesis via binding to the 50S ribosomal subunit. Members of this group which have been used to treat non-TB mycobacterial infections are erythromycin, clarithromycin and azithromycin.

Erythromycin inhibits *M. kansasii, M. scrofulaceum* and some strains of *M. avium-intracellulare in vitro* at readily achievable concentrations [214]. The newer macrolides, clarithromycin and azithromycin, have been reviewed [215]. Since these agents are concentrated intracellularly, their activity is greater *in vivo* than that predicted by *in vitro* testing and usual serum levels. Clarithromycin is more active than azithromycin for mycobacteria. *In vitro* testing shows clarithromycin to be active against *M. gordonae, M. scrofulaceum, M. szulgai, M. kansasii, M. marinum* and *M. avium-intracellulare* and inactive against *M. simiae* [216].

Clarithromycin appears to be quite effective in disseminated *M. avium-intracellulare* infection in AIDS patients. It is often combined with clofaz-imine and/or ethambutol to minimize the development of resistance during therapy [217]. The dose of clarithromycin used is 500–1000 mg twice daily. The new macrolides have also been shown to have good *in vitro* activity for *M. fortuitum* and *M. chelonae*, with clarithromycin being the most effective [218].

## 11.12 SUMMARY

This chapter provides basic and clinical information so that the clinician can more appropriately utilize anti-TB chemotherapy. For the reader's convenience, a number of tables are provided to classify toxicities and interactions. Table 11.2 lists the dosage modifications required in hepatic

**Table 11.2** Antituberculous agents requiring dose modification in renal or hepatic insufficiency

| | Condition[a] | |
|---|---|---|
| Drug | Kidney failure | Liver failure |
| Amikacin | + | − |
| Capreomycin | + | − |
| Ciprofloxacin | + | − |
| Cycloserine | + | − |
| Ethambutol | + | − |
| Ethionamide | − | + |
| Isoniazid | + | + |
| Kanamycin | + | − |
| Ofloxacin | + | − |
| Para-aminosalicylic acid | + | + |
| Pyrazinamide | + | + |
| Rifampin | − | + |
| Streptomycin | + | − |

[a] +, requires dose adjustment; −, does not require dose adjustment.

or renal failure. Table 11.3 classifies the agents by significant hepato-toxicity. Table 11.4 organizes the medications regarding other toxicities. Table 11.5 summaries the use of anti-TB agents in pregnancy. Finally, Table 11.6 lists recognized drug–drug interactions between these agents.

**Table 11.3** Hepatotoxic antituberculous agents

| *Hepatotoxic* | *Non-hepatotoxic[a]* |
|---|---|
| Isoniazid | Ethambutol |
| Rifampin | Streptomycin |
| Pyrazinamide | Kanamycin |
| Ethionamide | Amikacin |
| Para-aminosalicylic acid | Cycloserine |
| | Capreomycin |
| | Fluoroquinolones |

[a]   Rare hepatotoxic reactions may occur.

**Table 11.4** Characteristic toxicities related to antituberculous agents

**CNS effects**
- Isoniazid
- Ethionamide
- Cycloserine

**Peripheral neuropathy**
- Isoniazid
- Ethionamide
- Cycloserine
- Aminoglycosides[a]

**Hyperuricemia**
- Pyrazinamide
- Ethambutol

**Body fluid/tissue color**
- Rifampin
- Rifabutin
- Clofazimine

**Optic neuritis**
- Ethambutol
- Isoniazid
- Aminoglycosides
- Ethionamide

**Pellagra**
- Isoniazid
- Ethionamide

**Pyridoxine deficiency**
- Isoniazid
- Ethionamide
- Cycloserine

**Nephrotoxicity/ototoxicity**
- Aminoglycosides
- Capreomycin

[a]   Neuromuscular block.

**Table 11.5** Antituberculous agents in pregnancy

**Appropriate for use**
- Isoniazid
- Rifampin

**Use if needed**[a]
- Pyrazinamide
- Ethambutol

**Not for use**[b]
- Ethionamide
- Aminoglycosides
- Cycloserine
- Capreomycin
- Fluoroquinolones

[a] These agents can be used if benefit is likely to outweigh risks.
[b] These agents may be used only if no alternatives exist.

**Table 11.6** Antituberculous agent drug–drug interactions

| | |
|---|---|
| Isoniazid – rifampin | ↑ hepatotoxicity |
| Isoniazid – PAS | ↑ INH level by ↓ acetylation |
| Rifampin – PAS | ↓ absorption of rifampin |
| Rifampin – clofazimine | ↓ absorption of rifampin |
| Ethionamide – isoniazid | ↑ CNS toxicity |
| Ethionamide – cycloserine | ↑ CNS toxicity |
| Ethambutol – ethionamide | ↑ optic neuritis |
| Aminoglycoside – ethionamide | ↑ optic neuritis |
| Cycloserine – isoniazid | ↑ CNS toxicity |

## REFERENCES

1. Fox, H.H. (1953) The chemical attack on tuberculosis. *Trans NY Acad Sci*, **15**, 234–42.
2. Davidson, L.A. and Takayama, K. (1979) Isoniazid inhibition of the synthesis of monounsaturated long-chain fatty acids in Mycobacterium tuberculosis H37Ra. *Antimicrob Agents Chemother*, **16**, 104–5.
3. Takayama, K., Schnoes, J.K., Armstrong, E.L. and Boyle, R.W. (1975) Site of inhibitory activity of isoniazid in the synthesis of mycolic acids in *Mycobacterium tuberculosis*. *J Lipid Res*, **16**, 308–72.
4. Zhang, Y., Heym, B., Allen, B. *et al.* (1992) The catalase–peroxidase gene and isoniazid resistance of *Mycobacterium tuberculosis*. *Nature*, **358**, 591–3.
5. Krivis, A.F. and Rabb, J.M. (1969) Cuprous complexes formed with isonicotinic hydrazide. *Science*, **164**, 1064–5.

6. Herman, R.P. and Weber, M.M. (1980) Site of action of isoniazid on the electron transport chain and its relationship to nicotinamide adenine dinucleotide regulation in *Mycobacterium phlei*. *Antimicrob Agents Chemother*, **17**, 450–4.

6a. Jindani, A., Aber, V.R., Edwards, E.A. and Mitchison, D.A. (1980) The early bactericidal activity of drugs in patients with pulmonary tuberculosis. *Am Rev Respir Dis*, **121**, 939–49.

7. Dutt, A.K. and Stead, W.W. (1982) Medical perspective: present chemotherapy for tuberculosis. *J Infect Dis*, **146**, 698–704.

8. Costello, H.D., Caras, G.J. and Snider, D.E. (1980) Drug resistance among previously treated tuberculosis patients: a brief report. *Am Rev Respir Dis*, **121**, 313–6.

9. Carpenter, J.L., Covelli, H.D., Avant, M.E. *et al.* (1982) Drug resistant *Mycobacterium tuberculosis* in Korean isolates. *Am Rev Respir Dis*, **126**, 1092–5.

9a. Altamirano, M., Marostenmaki, J., Wong, A. *et al.* (1994) Mutations in the catalase-peroxidase gene from isoniazid-resistant *Mycobacterium tuberculosis* isolates. *J Infect Dis*, **165**, 1162–5.

9b. Banerjee, A., Dubnau, E., Quemard, A. *et al.* (1994) *inhA*, a gene encoding a target for isoniazid and ethionamide in *Mycobacterium tuberculosis*. *Science*, **263**, 227–30.

10. Holdiness, M.R. (1984) Clinical pharmacokinetics of antitubercular drugs. *Clin Pharmacokinet*, **9**, 511–44.

11. Olson, W.A., Pruitt, A.W. and Dayton, P.G. (1987) Plasma concentrations of isoniazid in children with tuberculous infections. *Pediatrics*, **67**, 876–8.

12. Hurwitz, A. and Schlozman, D.L. (1974) Effects of antacids on gastrointestinal absorption of isoniazid in rat and man. *Am Rev Respir Dis*, **109**, 41–7.

13. Robson, J.M. and Sullivan, F.M. (1963) Antituberculosis drugs. *Pharmacol Rev*, **15**, 169–223.

14. Weber, W.W. and Hein, D.H. (1985) Acetylation pharmacogenetics. *Pharmacol Rev*, **37**, 25–79.

15. La Du, B.N. (1972) Isoniazid and pseudocholinesterase polymorphism. *Fed Proc*, **31**, 1276–85.

16. Pratt, W.E. and Fekety, R. (1986) Drugs that act on mycobacteria, in *The Antimicrobial Drugs*, Oxford University Press, New York, pp. 277–314.

17. Ellard, G.A. (1976) Variations between individuals and populations in the acetylation of isoniazid and its significance for the treatment of pulmonary tuberculosis. *Clin Pharm Ther*, **19**, 610–25.

18. Sarma, G.R., Kailasam, S., Nair, N.G.K. *et al.* (1980) Effect of prednisolone and rifampin on isoniazid metabolism in slow and rapid inactivators of isoniazid. *Antimicrobial Agents Chemother*, **18**, 661–6.

19. Acocella, G., Bonollo, L., Gaimoldi, M. *et al.* (1972) Kinetics of rifampicin and isoniazid administered alone and in combination to normal subjects and patients with liver disease. *Gut*, **13**, 47–53.

20. Muakkassah, S.F., Bidlack, W.R. and Yarg, W.C.T. (1981) Mechanism of the inhibitory action of isoniazid on microsomal drug metabolism. *Biochem Pharmacol*, **30**, 1651–8.

21. Kutt, H., Winters, W. and McDowell, F.H. (1966) Depression of parahydroxylation of diphenylhydantoin by antituberculous chemotherapy. *Neurology*, **16**, 594–602.

22. Garibaldi, R.A., Drusin, R.E., Ferebee, S.H. and Gregg, M.B. (1972) Isoniazid-associated hepatitis. Report of an outbreak. *Am Rev Respir Dis*, **106**, 357–65.
23. Kopanoff, D.E., Snider, D.E. and Caras, G.J. (1978) Isoniazid-related hepatitis. A U.S. Public Health Service Cooperative surveillance study. *Am Rev Respir Dis*, **117**, 991–1001.
24. Bailey, W.C., Weil, H., DeRouen, T.A. *et al.* (1974) The effect of isoniazid on transaminase levels. *Ann Intern Med*, **81**, 200–2.
25. Mitchell, J.R., Long, M.W., Thorgeirsson, U.P. and Hollow, D.J. (1975) Acetylation rates and monthly liver function tests during one year of isoniazid preventive therapy. *Chest*, **68**, 181–90.
26. Byrd, R.B., Horn, B.R., Griggs, G.A. and Solomon, D.A. (1977) Isoniazid chemoprophylaxis. Association with detection and incidence of liver toxicity. *Arch Intern Med*, **137**, 1130–3.
27. Black, M., Mitchell, J.R., Zimmerman, H.J. *et al.* (1975) Isoniazid-associated hepatitis in 114 patients. *Gastroenterology*, **69**, 289–302.
28. Stein, M.T. and Liang, D. (1979) Clinical hepatotoxicity of isoniazid in children. *Pediatrics*, **64**, 499–505.
29. Vanderhoof, J.A. and Ament, M.E. (1976) Fatal hepatic necrosis due to isoniazid chemoprophylaxis in a 15-year-old girl. *J Pediatr*, **88**, 867–8.
30. McGlynn, K.A., Lustabader, E.D., Sharrar, R.G. *et al.* (1986) Isoniazid prophylaxis in hepatitis B carriers. *Am Rev Respir Dis*, **134**, 666–8.
31. Maddrey, W.C. and Baitnott, J.K. (1973) Isoniazid hepatitis. *Ann Intern Med*, **79**, 1–12.
32. Mitchell, J.R., Thorgeirsson, U.P., Black, M. *et al.* (1975) Increased incidence of isoniazid hepatitis in rapid acetylators: possible relation to hydrazine metabolites. *Clin Pharm Ther*, **18**, 70–9.
33. Singapore Tuberculosis Service/British Medical Research Council (1977) Controlled trial of intermittent regimens of rifampin plus isoniazid for pulmonary tuberculosis in Singapore. The results of up to 30 months. *Am Rev Respir Dis*, **116**, 807–20.
34. Ellard, G.A., Girling, D.J. and Nunn, A.J. (1981) The hepatotoxicity of isoniazid among the three acetylator phenotypes. *Am Rev Respir Dis*, **123**, 568.
35. Dickinson, D.S., Bailey, W.C., Hirschowitz, G.I. *et al.* (1981) Risk factors for isoniazid (INH)-induced liver dysfunction. *J Clin Gastroenterol*, **3**, 271–9.
36. Ellard, G.A. and Gammon, P.T. (1976) Pharmacokinetics of isoniazid metabolism in man. *J Pharmacokinet Biopharm*, **4**, 83–113.
37. Pessayre, D., Bentata, M., Degott, C. *et al.* (1977) Isoniazid-rifampin fulminant hepatitis. A possible consequence of the enhancement of isoniazid hepatotoxicity by enzyme induction. *Gastroenterology*, **72**, 284–9.
38. Gangadharam, P.R.J. (1986) Isoniazid, rifampin, and hepatotoxicity. *Am Rev Respir Dis*, **133**, 963–5.
39. Krishna Murti, C.R. (1975) Isonicotinic acid hydrazide, in *Antibiotics III* (eds J.W. Corcoran and F.E. Hahn), Springer-Verlag, New York, pp. 623–52.
40. Wason, S., Lacouture, P.G. and Lovejoy, F.H. (1981) Single high-dose pyridoxine treatment for isoniazid overdose. *JAMA*, **246**, 1102–4.
41. Goldman, A.L. and Braman, S.S. (1972) Isoniazid: a review with emphasis on adverse effects. *Chest*, **62**, 71–7.
42. Alarcón-Segovia, D. (1969) Drug-induced lupus syndromes. *Mayo Clin Proc*, **44**, 664–81.

43. Rothfield, N.F., Blerer, W.F. and Garfield, J.W. (1978) Isoniazid induction of antinuclear antibodies. *Ann Intern Med*, **88**, 650–2.

44. Jacobs, N.F. and Thompson, S.E. (1977) Spiking fever from isoniazid simulating a septic process. *JAMA*, **238**, 1759–60.

45. Brodie, M.J., Boobis, A.R., Hillyard, C.J. *et al.* (1981) Effect of isoniazid on vitamin D metabolism and hepatic monooxygenase activity. *Clin Pharmacol Ther*, **30**, 363–7.

46. Smith, C.K. and Durack, D.T. (1978) Isoniazid and reaction to cheese. *Ann Intern Med*, **88**, 520–1.

47. Girling, D.J. (1982) Adverse effects of antituberculous drugs. *Drugs*, **23**, 56–74.

48. Byrd, R.B., Horn, B.R., Solomon, D.A. and Griggs, G.A. (1979) Toxic effects of isoniazid in tuberculous chemoprophylaxis. *JAMA*, **241**, 1239–41.

49. Bowersox, D.W., Winterbauer, R.H., Steward, G.L. *et al.* (1973) Isoniazid doses in patients with renal failure. *N Engl J Med*, **289**, 84–7.

50. Mandell, G.L and Sande, M.A. (1990) Antimicrobial agents: Drugs used in the chemotherapy of tuberculosis and leprosy, in *Goodman and Gilman's The Pharmacologic Basis of Therapeutics* (eds A.G. Gilman, T.W. Ral, A.S. Nies and P. Taylor), Pergamon Press, New York, pp. 1149–52.

51. Wehrli, W. (1983) Rifampin: mechanisms of action and resistance. *Rev Infect Dis*, **5** (suppl 3), S407–11.

52. Thornsberry, C.M., Hill, B.C., Swenson, J.M. and McDougal, L.K. (1983) Rifampin: spectrum of antibacterial activity. *Rev Infect Dis*, **5** (suppl 3), S412–7.

53. Dickinson, J.M. and Mitchison, D.A. (1981) Experimental models to explain the high sterilizing activity of rifampin in the chemotherapy of tuberculosis. *Am Rev Respir Dis*, **123**, 367–71.

54. McCracken, G.H., Ginsburg, C.M., Zweighaft, T.C. and Clahsen, J. (1980) Pharmacokinetics of rifampin in infants and children: relevance to prophylaxis against *Haemophilus influenzae* type b disease. *Pediatrics*, **66**, 17–21.

55. Radner, D.B. (1973) Toxicologic and pharmacologic aspects of rifampin. *Chest*, **64**, 213–6.

56. Acocella, G. (1978) Clinical pharmacokinetics of rifampicin. *Clin Pharmacokinet*, **3**, 108–27.

57. Sippel, J.E., Mikhail, I.A., Girgis, N.I. and Youssef, J.J. (1974) Rifampin concentrations in cerebrospinal fluid of patients with tuberculous meningitis. *Am Rev Respir Dis*, **109**, 579–80.

58. Allen, B.W., Ellard, G.A., Cammon, P.T. *et al.* (1975) The penetration of dapsone, rifampicin, isoniazid and pyrazinamide into peripheral nerves. *Br J Pharmacol*, **55**, 151–5.

59. Kenwright, S. and Levi, A.J. (1974) Sites of competition in the selective hepatic uptake of rifamycin-SV, flavaspidic acid, bilirubin and bromsulphthalein. *Gut*, **15**, 220–6.

60. Baciewicz, A.M., Self, T.H. and Bekemeyer, W.B. (1987) Update on rifampin drug interactions. *Arch Intern Med*, **147**, 565–8.

61. Baron, D.N. and Bell, J.L. (1974) Serum enzyme changes in patients receiving antituberculosis therapy with rifampicin or p-aminosalicyclic acid, plus isoniazid and streptomycin. *Tubercle*, **55**, 115–20.

62. Gronhagen-Riska, C., Hellstrom, P.E. and Froseth, B. (1979) Predisposing factors in hepatitis induced by isoniazid-rifampin treatment of tuberculosis.

*Am Rev Respir Dis*, **118**, 461–6.

63. Newman, R., Doster, B.E., Muray, F.J. and Woolpert, S.F. (1974) Rifampin in initial treatment of pulmonary tuberculosis. A U.S. Public Health Service tuberculosis trial. *Am Rev Resp Dis*, **109**, 216–32.

64. Girling, D.J. and Hitze, K.L. (1979) Adverse reactions to rifampicin. *Bull WHO*, **57**, 45–9.

65. Grosset, J. and Leventis, S. (1983) Adverse effects of rifampin. *Rev Infect Dis*, **5** (suppl 3), S440–6

65a. Matz, J., Borish, L.C., Routes, J.M. and Rosenwasser, L.J. (1994) Oral desensitization to rifampin and ethambutol in mycobacterial disease. *Am J Respir Crit Care Med*, **149**, 815–7.

66. Stern, J.S.M. and Stainton-Ellis, D.M. (1977) Rifampicin in pregnancy. *Lancet*, **2**, 604–5.

67. Eggermont, E., Logghe, N., Van De Cassey, W. *et al.* (1976) Haemorrhagic disease of the newborn in the offspring of rifampicin and isoniazid treated mothers. *Acta Paediatr Belg*, **29**, 87–90.

68. Medchill, M.T. and Gillum, M. (1989) Diagnosis and management of tuberculosis during pregnancy. *Obstet Gynecol Surv*, **44**, 81–4.

69. Snider, D.E., Layde, P.M., Johnson, M.W. and Lyle, M.A. (1980) Treatment of tuberculosis during pregnancy. *Am Rev Respir Dis*, **122**, 65–79.

70. American Thoracic Society (1986) Treatment of tuberculosis and tuberculosis infection in adults and children. *Am Rev Respir Dis*, **134**, 355–63.

71. Committee on Drugs, American Academy of Pediatrics (1989) Transfer of drugs and other chemicals into human milk. *Pediatrics*, **84**, 924–36.

72. Ji, B., Truffot-Pernot, C., Lacroix, C. *et al.* (1993) Effectiveness of rifampin, rifabutin, and rifapentine for preventive therapy of tuberculosis in mice. *Am Rev Respir Dis*, **148**, 1541–6.

73. Goldberger, M.J.(1988) Antituberculosis agents. *Med Clin North Am*, **72**, 661–8.

74. Rieder, H.L., Cauthen, G.M., Kelley, G.D. *et al.* (1989) Tuberculosis in the United States. *JAMA*, **262**, 385–9.

75. Davidson, P.T. and Quoc, L.H. (1992) Drug treatment of tuberculosis. *Drugs*, **43**, 651–73.

76. Ellard, G.A. (1969) Absorption, metabolism and excretion of pyrazinamide in man. *Tubercle*, **50**, 144–58.

77. McDermott, W., Ormond, L., Muschenheim, C. *et al.* (1954) Pyrazinamide-isoniazid in tuberculosis. *Am Rev Tuberc*, **69**, 319–33.

78. Mitchison, D.A. (1979) Basic mechanisms of chemotherapy. *Chest*, **76**(suppl), 771–81.

79. Stottmeier, K.D., Beam, R.E. and Kubica, G.P. (1968) The absorption and excretion of pyrazinamide. *Am Rev Respir Dis*, **98**, 70–4.

80. Forgan-Smith, R., Ellard, G.A., Newton, D. and Mitchison, D.A. (1973) Pyrazinamide and other drugs in tuberculous meningitis. *Lancet*, **2**, 374.

81. Girling, D.J. (1978) The hepatic toxicity of antituberculous regimens containing isoniazid, rifampicin and pyrazinamide. *Tubercle*, **59**, 13–32.

82. Zierski, M. and Bek, E. (1980) Side effects of drug regimens used in short course chemotherapy for pulmonary tuberculosis. A controlled study. *Tubercle*, **61**, 41–9.

83. Pilheu, J.A., DeSalvo, M.C. and Koch, O. (1981) Liver alternations in anti-tuberculosis regimens containing pyrazinamide. *Chest*, **80**, 720–4.

84. Yu, T.F., Perel, J., Berger, L. *et al.* (1977) The effect of the interaction of pyrazinamide and probenicid on urinary uric acid excretion in man. *Am J Med*, **63**, 723–8.

85. Hong Kong Tuberculosis Treatment Services/British Medical Research Council (1976) Adverse reactions to short course regimens containing streptomycin, isoniazid, pyrazinamide and rifampicin in Hong Kong. *Tubercle*, **57**, 81–95.

86. Centers for Disease Control (1993) Tuberculosis among pregnant women – New York City, 1985–1992. *MMWR*, **42**, 605, 611–12.

87. Committee on Infectious Diseases (1992) Chemotherapy for tuberculosis in infants and children. *Pediatrics*, **89**, 161–5.

88. Crowle, A.J., Sbarbaro, J.A., Judson, F.N. *et al.* (1985) The effect of ethambutol on tubercle bacilli within cultured human macrophages. *Am Rev Respir Dis*, **132**, 742–5.

89. Takayama, K., Armstrong, E.L., Kunugi, K.A. and Kilburn, J.O. (1979) Inhibition by ethambutol of mycolic acid transfer into the cell wall of *Mycobacterium smegmatis*. *Antimicrob Agents Chemother*, **16**, 240–2.

90. Karlson, A. (1961) The *in vitro* activity of ethambutol (dextro-2,2'-(ethylethylenedimino)-di-1-butanol) against tubercle bacilli and other microorganisms. *Am Rev Respir Dis*, **84**, 905–6.

91. Kuze, F., Kurasawa, T., Bando, K. *et al.* (1981) *In vitro* and *in vivo* susceptibility of atypical mycobacteria to various drugs. *Rev Infect Dis*, **3**, 885–97.

92. Peets, E.A., Sweeney, W.M., Place, V.A. and Buyske, D.A. (1965) The absorption, excetion and metabolic fate of ethambutol in man. *Am Rev Respir Dis*, **91**, 51–8.

93. DeSol, C.A. and Umans, J.G. (1992) Principles of drug therapy in renal failure. *Hosp Formul*, **27**, 164–80.

94. Campbell, I.A. and Ormerod, L.P. (1988) Ethambutol and the eye. *Lancet*, **2**, 113–14.

95. Citron, K.M. and Thomas, G.O. (1986) Ocular toxicity from ethambutol. *Thorax*, **41**, 737–9.

96. Centers for Disease Control (1980) Guidelines for short course tuberculosis chemotherapy. *MMWR*, **29**, 97–105.

97. Centers for Disease Control (1980) Follow-up on guidelines for short course tuberculosis chemotherapy. *MMWR*, **29**, 183–9.

98. Warkany, J. (1979) Antituberculosis drugs: teratogen update. *Teratology*, **20**, 133–7.

99. Jacobs, R.F. and Abernathy, R.S. (1988) Management of tuberculosis in pregnancy and the newborn. *Clin Perinatal*, **15**, 305–19.

100. Postletwaite, A.E., Bartel, A.G. and Kelley, W.N. (1972) Hyperuricemia due to ethambutol. *N Engl J Med*, **286**, 761–2.

101. Bennett, W.M. (1980) Drug therapy in renal failure: dosing guidelines for adults. *Ann Intern Med*, **93**, 62–89.

102. Mandell, G.L. and Sande, M.A. (1990) Drugs used in the chemotherapy of tuberculosis and leprosy, in *Goodman and Gilman's The Pharmacologic Basis of Therapeutics* (eds A.G. Gilman, T.W. Ral, A.S. Nies, and P. Taylor), Pergamon Press, New York, pp. 1154–5.

103. Schwartz, W.S. (1966) Comparison of ethionamide with isoniazid in original treatment cases of pulmonary tuberculosis, XIV. A report of the Veterans

Administration – Armed Forces Cooperative Study. *Am Rev Respir Dis*, **93**, 685–92.

104. McEvoy, G.K. (ed.) (1993) *AHFS Drug Information '93*, American Society of Hospital Pharmacists, Bethesda, MD, p. 353.

105. United States Pharmacopeial Convention (1993) *Drug Information for the Health Care Professional: USP–DI*, United States Pharmacopeial Convention, Rockville, MD, p. 1360.

106. Rist, N., Grumbach, R. and Libermann, D. (1959) Experiments on the antituberculous activity of alpha-ethyl-thioisonicotinamide. *Am Rev Tuberc*, **79**, 1–5.

107. Lees, A.W. (1967) Ethionamide, 500 mg daily, plus isoniazid, 500 mg or 300 mg daily in previously untreated patients with pulmonary tuberculosis. *Am Rev Respir Dis*, **95**, 109–11.

108. Kucus, A. and Bennett, N.McK. (1987) *The Use of Antibiotics: A Comprehensive Review with Clinical Emphasis*, J.B. Lippincott, Philadelphia, PA, p. 1426.

109. Swash, M., Roberts, A.H. and Murnaghan, D.J. (1972) Reversible pellagralike encephalopathy with ethionamide and cycloserine. *Tubercle*, **53**, 132–6.

110. Simon, E., Veres, E. and Bánki, G. (1969) Changes in SGOT activity during treatment with ethionamide. *Scand J Resp Dis*, **50**, 314–18.

111. Phillips, S. and Tashman, H. (1963) Ethionamide jaundice. *Am Rev Respir Dis*, **87**, 896–8.

112. Weinstein, H.J., Hallet, W.Y. and Sarauw, A.S. (1962) The absorption and toxicity of ethionamide. *Am Rev Respir Dis*, **86**, 576–8.

113. Fox, W., Robinson, D.K., Tall, R. *et al.* (1969) A study of acute intolerance to ethionamide, including a comparison with prothionamide, and of the influence of vitamin B-complex additive in prophylaxis. *Tubercle*, **50**, 125–43.

114. Moulding, T. and Fraser, R. (1970) Hypothyroidism relating to ethionamide. *Am Rev Respir Dis*, **101**, 90–4.

115. Drucker, D., Eggo, M.C., Salit, I.E. and Burrow, G.N. (1984) Ethionamide-induced goitrous hypothyroidism. *Ann Intern Med*, **100**, 837–9.

116. Rinehart, K.L. (1969) Comparative chemistry of the aminoglycosides and aminocyclitol antibiotics. *J Infect Dis*, **119**, 345–50.

117. Comroe, J.H. (1978) Pay dirt: The story of streptomycin Part I. From Waksman to Waksman. *Am Rev Respir Dis*, **117**, 773–81.

118. Finegold, S.M. (1959) Kanamycin. *Arch Intern Med*, **104**, 15–28.

119. Moellering, R.C. (1983) In vitro antibacterial activity of the aminoglycoside antibiotics. *Rev Infect Dis*, **5(Suppl 2)**, S212–30.

120. Limon, L. (1988) Current concepts in tuberculosis. Part II. *Am Pharmacy News*, **28**, 37–42.

121. Phillips, I. (1982) Aminoglycosides. *Lancet*, **2**, 311–14.

122. Suter, E. (1952) Multiplication of tubercle bacilli within phagocytes cultivated in vitro, and effect of streptomycin and isonicotinic acid hydrazine. *Am Rev Tuberc*, **65**, 775–6.

123. Siber, G.R., Echeverria, P., Smith, A.L. *et al.* (1975) Pharmacokinetics of gentamicin in children and adults. *J Infect Dis*, **132**, 637–51.

124. Barza, M., Brown, R.B., Shen, D. *et al.* (1975) Predictability of blood levels of gentamicin in man. *J Infect Dis*, **132**, 165–74.

125. Edson, R.S. and Terrell, C.L. (1991) The aminoglycosides. *Mayo Clin Proc*, **66**, 1158–64.

126. Wilson, W.R., Wilkowske, C.J., Wright, A.J. *et al.* (1984) Treatment of streptomycin-susceptible and streptomycin-resistant enterococcal endocarditis. *Ann Intern Med*, **100**, 816–23.

127. McCracken, G.H. (1986) Aminoglycoside toxicity in infants and children. *Am J Med*, **80(Suppl 6B)**, 172–8.

128. Johnson, A.H. and Hamilton, C.H. (1970) Kanamycin ototoxicity – possible potentiation by other drugs. *South Med J*, **63**, 511–13.

129. Moore, R.D., Smith, C.R., Lipsky, J.J. *et al.* (1984) Risk factors for nephrotoxicity in patients treated with aminoglycosides. *Ann Intern Med*, **100**, 352–7.

130. Lietman, P.S. (1988) Liver disease, aminoglycoside antibiotics and renal dysfunction. *Hepatology*, **8**, 966–8.

131. Moore, R.D., Smith, C.R. and Lietman, P.S. (1986) Increased risk of renal dysfunction due to interaction of liver disease and aminoglycosides. *Am J Med*, **80**, 1093–7.

132. Gilbert, D.N. (1991) Once daily aminoglycoside therapy. *Antimicrob Agents Chemother*, **35**, 399–405.

133. Robinson, G.C. and Cambon, K.G. (1964) Hearing loss in infants of tuberculous mothers treated with streptomycin during pregnancy. *Med Intell*, **271**, 949–51.

134. McQuillen, M.P., Cantor, H.E. and O'Rourke, J.R. (1968) Myasthenic syndrome associated with antibiotics. *Arch Neurol*, **18**, 402–15.

135. Cooper, E.A. and Hanson, R.G. (1963) Oral neomycin and anaesthesia. *Brit Med J*, **2**, 1527–8.

136. Holtzman, J.L. (1976) Gentamicin and neuromuscular blockage. *Ann Intern Med*, **84**, 55.

137. Anonymous (1988) Streptomycin package insert, Eli Lilly, Indianapolis, IN.

138. Driver, A.G. and Worder, J.P. (1990) Intravenous streptomycin. *Ann Pharmacother*, **24**, 826–8.

139. Committee on Infectious Diseases (1992) Chemotherapy for tuberculosis in infants and children. *Pediatrics*, **89**, 161–5.

140. Strominger, J.L. and Tipper, D.J. (1965) Bacterial cell wall synthesis and structure in relation to the mechanism of action of penicillin and other antibacterial agents. *Am J Med*, **39**, 708–21.

141. Strominger, J.L. (1960) Competitive inhibition of enzymatic reactions by oxamycin. *J Am Chem Soc*, **82**, 998–9.

142. Strominger, J.L. (1959) Oxamycin, a competitive antagonist of the incorporation of D-alanine into a uridine nucleotide in *Staphylococcus aureus*. *J Am Chem Soc*, **81**, 3803–4.

143. United States Pharmacopeial Convention. (1993) *Drug Information for the Health Care Professional: USP–DI*, United States Pharmacopeial Convention Inc., Rockville, MD, p. 1099.

144. Hoeprich, P.D. (1964) Alanine: cycloserine antagonism. I. Significant of phenomenon in testing susceptibility to cycloserine. *Am J Clin Path*, **41**, 140–9.

145. Epstein, I.G., Nair, K.G.S. and Boyd, L.J. (1956) The treatment of human pulmonary tuberculosis with cycloserine: a year's progress. *Dis Chest*, **29**, 241–57.

146. Weiss, C. (1956) Some new antibiotics: penicillin V, cycloserine and candicidin. *J Albert Einstein Med Cent*, **4**, 66–70.

147. David, H.L. (1977) Resistance to d-cycloserine in the tubercle bacillus: muta-

tion rate and transport of alanine in parenteral cells and drug-resistant mutants. *Appl Microbiol*, **21**, 888–92.

148. Clark, V.L. and Young, F.E. (1977) Inducible resistance to d-cycloserine in *Bacillus subtilis* 168. *Antimicrob Agents Chemother*, **11**, 871–6.

149. Welch, H., Putnam, L.E. and Randall, W.A. (1955) Antibacterial activity and blood and urine concentrations of cycloserine, a new antibiotic, following oral administration. *Antibiot Med*, **1**, 72–9.

150. Conzelman, G.M. (1956) The physiologic disposition of cycloserine in the human subject. *Am Rev Tuberc*, **74**, 739–46.

151. Snider, D.E. and Powell, K.E. (1984) Should women taking antituberculosis drugs breast-feed? *Arch Intern Med*, **144**, 589–90.

152. Mattila, M.J., Nieminen, E., and Tiitinen, H. (1969) Serum levels, urinary excretion, and side-effects of cycloserine in the presence of isoniazid and p-aminosalicylic acid. *Scand J Resp Dis*, **50**, 291–300.

153. Bycroft, B.W., Cameron, D., Croft, L.R. *et al.* (1971) Total structure of capreomycin IB, a tuberculostatic peptide antibiotic. *Nature*, **231**, 301–2.

154. McEvoy G.K. (ed.) (1993) *AHFS Drug Information '93*, American Society of Hospital Pharmacists, Inc., Bethesda, MD, p. 1153.

155. Wilson, T.M. (1967) Current therapeutics: Capreomycin and ethambutol. *Practitioner*, **199**, 817–24.

156. Lehmann, J. (1946) Para-aminosalicylic acid in the treatment of tuberculosis. *Lancet*, **1**, 15–16.

157. Hobby, G., Johnson, P.M. and Boytar-Papirnyik, V. (1971) Primary drug resistance: a continuing study of drug resistance in tuberculosis in a veteran population within the United States IX. September 1969-September 1970. *Am Rev Respir Dis*, **103**, 842–4.

158. Hobby, G., Johnson, P.M., and Boytar-Papirnyik, V. (1974) Primary drug resistance: a continuing study of drug resistance in tuberculosis in a veteran population within the United States X. September 1970–September 1973. *Am Rev Respir Dis*, **110**, 95–8.

159. Way, E.L., Smith, P.K., Howie, D.L. *et al.* (1948) The absorption, distribution, excretion and fate of para-aminosalicylic acid. *J Pharmacol Exp Ther*, **93**, 368–82.

160. Spector, R. and Lorenzo, W.V. (1973) The active transport of para-aminosalicylic acid from the cerebrospinal fluid. *J Pharmacol Exp Ther*, **185**, 642–8.

161. Schneinhorn, D.J. and Angelillo, V.A. (1977) Antituberculosis therapy in pregnancy. Risk to the fetus. *West J Med*, **127**, 195–8.

162. Simpson, D.G. and Walker, J.H. (1960) Hypersensitivity to para-aminosalicylic acid. *Am J Med*, **29**, 297–306.

162a.Kennedy, N., Fox, R., Kisyombe, G.M. *et al.* (1993) Effectiveness bactericidal and sterilizing activities of ciprofloxacin in pulmonary tuberculosis. *Am Rev Respir Dis*, **148**, 1547–51.

163. Walker, R.C. and Wright, A.J. (1991) The fluoroquinolones. *Mayo Clin Proc*, **66**, 1249–59.

164. Smith, J.T. and Lewis, C.S. (1988) Chemistry and mechanism of action of the quinolone antimicrobials, in *The Quinolones*, Academic Press, New York, pp. 23–82.

165. Shen, L.L., Kohlbrenner, W.E., Weigl, D. and Baranowski, J. (1989) Mechanism of quinolone inhibition of DNA gyrase. *J Biol Chem*, **264**, 2973–8.

166. Schwartz, M.N. (1987) Mechanisms of action of and resistance to ciprofloxacin. *Am J Med*, **82** (Suppl 4A), 12–20.

167. Neu, H.C. (1987) Ciprofloxacin: an overview and prospective appraisal. *Am J Med*, **82** (Suppl 4A), 395–404.

168. Rastogi, N. and Goh, K.S. (1991) In vitro activity of the new difluorinated quinolone sparfloxacin (AT-4140) against *Mycobacterium tuberculosis* compared with activities of ofloxacin and ciprofloxacin. *Antimicrob Agents Chemother*, **35**, 1933–6.

169. Leysen, D.C., Haemers, A. and Pattyn, S. (1989) Mycobacteria and the new quinolones. *Antimicrob Agents Chemother*, **33**, 1–5.

170. Todd, P.A. and Faulds, D. (1991) Ofloxacin: A reappraisal of its antimicrobial activity, pharmacology and therapeutic use. *Drugs*, **42**, 825–76.

171. Tsukamura, M., Nakamura, E., Yoshii, S. and Amano, H. (1985) Therapeutic effect of a new antibacterial substance ofloxacin (DL8280) on pulmonary tuberculosis. *Am Rev Respir Dis*, **131**, 352–6.

172. Hoffken, G., Lode, H., Prinzing, C. *et al.* (1985) Pharmacokinetics of ciprofloxacin after oral and parenteral administration. *Antimicrob Agents Chemother*, **27**, 375–9

173. Ritrovato, C.A. and Deeter, R.G. (1991) Respiratory tract penetration of quinolone antimicrobials: A case in study. *Pharmacotherapy*, **11**, 38–49.

174. Wolfson, J.S. and Hooper, D.C. (1989) Comparative pharmacokinetics of ofloxacin and ciprofloxacin. *Am J Med*, **87** (suppl 6C), 31S–36S.

175. Wise, R., Baldwin, D.R., Andrews, J.M. and Honeybourne, D. (1991) Comparative pharmacokinetic disposition of fluoroquinolones in the lung. *J Antimicrob Chemother*, **28** (Suppl C), 65–71.

176. Davis, R.L., Quenzer, R.W., Kelly, H.W. and Powell, J.R. (1992) Effect of the addition of ciprofloxacin on theophylline pharmacokinetics in subjects inhibited by cimetidine. *Ann Pharmacother*, **26**, 11–13.

177. Spivey, J.M., Laughlin, P.H., Gross, T.F. and Nix, D.E. (1991) Theophylline toxicity secondary to ciprofloxacin administration. *Ann Emerg Med*, **20**, 1131–4.

178. Renzi, R. and Finkbeiner, S. (1991) Ciprofloxacin interaction with sodium warfarin. *Am J Emerg Med*, **9**, 551–2.

179. Garrelts, J.C., Godley, P.J., Peterie, J.D. *et al.* (1990) Sucralfate significantly reduces ciprofloxacin concentrations in serum. *Antimicrob Agents Chemother*, **34**, 931–3.

180. Van Slouten, A.D., Nix, D.E., Wilton, J.H. *et al.* (1991) Combined use of ciprofloxacin and sucralfate. *Ann Pharmacother*, **25**, 578–82.

181. Polk, R.E., Healy, D.P., Sahai, J. *et al.* (1989) Effect of ferrous sulfate and multivitamins with zinc on absorption of ciprofloxacin in normal volunteers. *Antimicrob Agents Chemother*, **33**, 1841–4.

182. Sahai, J., Gallicano, K., Oliveras, L. *et al.* (1993) Cations in the didanosine tablet reduce ciprofloxacin availability. *Clin Pharmacol Ther*, **53**, 292–7.

183. Lo, W.K., Rolston, K.V.I., Rubenstein, E.B. and Bodey, G.P. (1993) Ciprofloxacin induced nephrotoxicity in patients with cancer. *Arch Intern Med*, **153**, 1258–62.

184. Hooper, D.C. and Wolfson, J.S. (1991) Fluoroquinolone antimicrobial agents. *N Engl J Med*, **324**, 384–94.

185. Aoun, M., Jacquy, C., Debusscher, L. *et al.* (1992) Peripheral neuropathy associated with fluoroquinolones. *Lancet*, **340**, 127.

186. Fennig, S. and Mauas, L. (1992) Ofloxacin induced delirium. *J Clin Psychiatry*, **53**, 137–8.

187. Chysky, V., Kapila, K., Hullman, R. *et al.* (1991) Safety of ciprofloxacin in children: worldwide clinical experience based on compassionate use. Emphasis on joint evaluation. *Infection*, **19**, 289–96.

188. Kahana, L.M. and Spino, M. (1991) Ciprofloxacin in patients with mycobacterial infections: experience in 15 patients. *Ann Pharmacother*, **25**, 919–24.

189. Gasser, T.C., Ebert, S.C., Graversen, P.H. and Madsen, P.O. (1987) Pharmacokinetic study of ciprofloxacin in patients with impaired renal function. *Am J Med*, **82** (suppl 4A), 139–41.

190. Nightingale, S.D., Cameron, D.W., Gordin, F.M. *et al.* (1993) Two placebo controlled trials of rifabutin prophylaxis against *Mycobacterium avium* complex infection in AIDS patients. *N Engl J Med*, **329**, 828–33.

191. Yoder, L.J., Jacobson, R.R. and Hastings, R.C. (1991) The activity of rifabutin against *Mycobacterium leprae*. *Lepr Rev*, **62**, 280–7.

192. Rhodes, P.M. and Wilkie, G.M. (1973) Antimitochondrial activity of Lampren in *Saccharomyces cerevisiae*. *Biochem Pharmacol*, **22**, 1047–56.

193. Levy, L. and Randall, H.P. (1970) A study of skin pigmentation by clofazimine. *Int J Lepr*, **38**, 404–16.

194. Kirby, W.M.M., Clarke, J.T., Libke, R.D. and Regamey, C. (1976) Clinical pharmacology of amikacin and kanamycin. *J Infect Dis*, **134**, 312–22.

195. Sanders, W.E., Hartwig, C., Schneider, N. *et al.* (1982) Activity of amikacin against mycobacteria *in vitro* and in murine tuberculosis. *Tubercle*, **63**, 201–8.

196. DeLalla, F., Maserati, R., Scarpellini, P. *et al.* (1992) Clarithromycin-ciprofloxacin-amikacin for therapy of *Mycobacterium avium–Mycobacterium intracellulare* bacteremia in patients with AIDS. *Antimicrob Agents Chemother*, **36**, 1567–9.

197. Yajko, D.M., Nassos, P.S. and Hadley, W.K. (1987) Therapeutic implications of inhibition vs. killing of *Mycobacterium avium* complex by antimicrobial agents. *Antimicrob Agents Chemother*, **31**, 117–20.

198. Bermudez, L.E.M., Wu, M. and Lowell, S.Y. (1987) Intracellular killing of *Mycobacterium avium* complex by rifapentine and liposome encapsulated amikacin. *J Infect Dis*, **156**, 510–3.

199. Bermudez, L.E., Wu, M., Young, L.S. and Inderlied, C.B. (1992) Post-antibiotic effect of amikacin and rifapentine against *Mycobacterium avium* complex. *J Infect Dis*, **166**, 923–6.

200. Kibbler, C.C., McWhinney, P.H.M., Warner, P. and Prentice, H.G. (1992) Ototoxicity associated with a once daily dose amikacin regimen in febrile neutropenic patients. *J Antimicrob Chemother*, **29**, 463–4.

201. DeBroe, M.E., Verbist, L. and Verpooten, G.A. (1991) Influence of dosage schedule in renal cortical accumulation of amikacin and tobramycin in man. *J Antimicrob Chemother*, **27**, 41–7.

202. Domagk, G., Behnish, R., Mietasch, F. and Schmidt, H. (1946) Über eine neue gegen tuberkelbazillon in vitro wirksame berbindungs klasse. *Naturwiss*, **33**, 315.

203. Chintu, C., Luo, C., Bhat, G. *et al.* (1993) Cutaneous hypersensitivity reactions due to thiacetazone in the treatment of tuberculosis in Zambian children infected with HIV-I. *Arch Dis Child*, **68**, 665–8.

204. Lorian, V. and Sabath, L.D. (1972) The effect of some penicillins on *Mycobacterium tuberculosis*. *Am Rev Respir Dis*, **105**, 632–7.

205. Nadler, J.P., Berger, J., Nord, C.A. *et al.* (1991) Amoxicillin-clavulanic acid for treating drug-resistant *Mycobacterium tuberculosis*. *Chest*, **99**, 1025–6.

206. Zhang, Y., Steingrube, V.A. and Wallace, R.J. (1992) Beta-lactam inhibitors and the inducibility of the beta-lactamase of *Mycobacterium tuberculosis*. *Am Rev Respir Dis*, **145**, 657–60.

207. Wallace, R.J., Wiss, K., Bushby, M.B. and Hollowell, D.C. (1982) *In vitro* activity of trimethoprim and sulfamethoxazole against the nontuberculous mycobacteria. *Rev Infect Dis*, **4**, 326–30.

208. Wallace, R.J., O'Brien, R., Glassroth, J. *et al.* (1987) Diagnosis and treatment of disease caused by nontuberculous mycobacteria. *Am Rev Respir Dis*, **142**, 940–53.

209. Pacht, E.R. (1990) *Mycobacterium fortuitum* lung abscess: resolution with prolonged trimethoprim/sulfamethoxazole therapy. *Am Rev Respir Dis*, **141**, 1599–1601.

209a. Chopra, I. (1994) Tetracycline analogs whose primary target is not the bacterial ribosome. *Antimicrob Agents Chemother*, **38,** 637–40.

210. Loria, P.R. (1976) Minocycline hydrochloride for atypical acid-fast infection. *Arch Dermatol*, **112**, 517–9.

211. Izumi, A.K., Hanke, W. and Higaki, M. (1977) *Mycobacterium marinum* infections treated with tetracycline. *Arch Dermatol*, **113**, 1067–8.

212. Dalovisio, J.R. and Pankey, G.A. (1978) *In vitro* susceptibility of *Mycobacterium fortuitum* and *Mycobacterium chelonei* to amikacin. *J Infect Dis*, **137**, 318–21.

213. Fanning, W.L., Gump, D.W. and Sufferman, P.A. (1977) Side effects of minocycline: a double blind study. *Antimicrob Agents Chemother*, **11**, 712–17.

214. Malavi, A. and Weinstein, L. (1971) *In vitro* activity of erythromycin against atypical mycobacteria. *J Infect Dis*, **123**, 216–9.

215. Whitman, M.S. and Tunkel, A.R. (1992) Azithromycin and clarithromycin. Overview and comparison with erythromycin. *Infect Control Hosp Epidemiol*, **13**, 357–68.

216. Brown, B.A., Wallace, R.J. and Onyi, G.O. (1992) Activities of clarithromycin against eight slowly growing species of nontuberculous mycobacteria determined by using a broth microdilution MIC system. *Antimicrob Agents Chemother*, **36**, 1987–90.

217. Dautzenberg, B., Saint Marc, T., Meyohas, M.L. *et al.* (1993) Clarithromycin and other antimicrobial agents in the treatment of disseminated *Mycobacterium avium* infection in patients with Acquired Immunodeficiency Syndrome. *Arch Intern Med*, **153**, 368–72.

218. Brown, B.A., Wallace, R.J., Onyi, G.O. *et al.* (1992) Activities of four macrolides including clarithromycin against *Mycobacterium fortuitum, Mycobacterium chelonei* and *M. chelonei*-like organisms. *Antimicrob Agents Chemother*, **36**, 180–4.

# Antituberculous therapy

Jeremy D. Gradon

## 12.1 HISTORY OF TUBERCULOSIS THERAPY

### 12.1.1 Antibiotic era

In 1946, the introduction of streptomycin (the first effective antituberculous agent) had a dramatic effect on patients with pulmonary tuberculosis (TB) and those with the previously uniformly fatal miliary and meningeal forms [1]. Prior to the introduction of this therapy, approximately half of patients with pulmonary TB died. The mortality dropped to 7% with the introduction of specific anti-TB therapy. The combination of streptomycin and para-aminosalicylic acid (PAS) was found to be more efficacious than treatment with either agent alone as well as being able to suppress the emergence of resistance.

Isoniazid (INH) and pyrazinamide (PZA) were both introduced in 1952, and resulted in the cure of the majority of treated patients. INH remained the mainstay of therapy until 1967 when rifampin was introduced into trials for the treatment of TB. This agent was shown to be as effective as INH, and combination therapy with the two agents allowed a decrease in the duration of treatment from 18 to 9 months. With extensive clinical trial experience, the duration of therapy to achieve cure could become even shorter; currently it is 6 months.

### 12.1.2 The 1990s

In the early 1980s, the US Public Health Service considered that TB had been vanquished. As a result, the time, effort and funding expended on TB dramatically decreased [2,3]. The onset of the AIDS epidemic, combined with the decreased efforts directed against TB, have led to an increase in the incidence of new cases of the disease in the USA and other developed countries [4–8]. The World Health Organization (WHO) has declared TB to be a global public Health emergency and has implemented programs to decrease by half the mortality from TB by the year 2003 [9].

The incidence of drug-resistant TB isolates is also increasing [10,11]. This has greatly affected the choice of empiric initial therapy. Both the Infectious Disease Society of America and the Centers for Disease Control (CDC) have strongly advocated the use of 'second line' agents such as amikacin and fluoroquinolones together with ethambutol and pyrazinamide in persons in whom drug-resistant isolates are suspected or found (Chapter 13). Some referral centers have had to resort to collapse therapies in selected cases of resistant TB, even in the 1990s [12]. This difficult clinical environment is further complicated by the non-availability (at least intermittently) of some agents, such as the classical injectable drug streptomycin [13]. Many areas of the USA and the world, however, have not experienced as much of a change in case numbers or resistance patterns. This chapter will attempt to deal with the approach to treatment of non-drug-resistant TB in the immunocompetent host.

## 12.2 CLINICAL USE OF ANTITUBERCULOUS AGENTS

The basic principles of TB treatment are given in Table 12.1. The two basic tenets of the medical therapy for TB are [14]:

- combinations of agents must be used so that clinically apparent infection is never treated with a single drug
- drug ingestion must continue uninterrupted for an adequate length of time to eradicate the infection.

**Table 12.1** Basic principles of tuberculosis treatment

- Never use a single agent
- Never treat for less than 6 months
- Ensure that patient takes the medication prescribed
- Carefully review other medications that the patient is taking and anticipate drug interactions

The American Thoracic Society (ATS) feels that the goals of therapy can be described simply as being the provision of the most effective therapy in the shortest period of time with the most effective utilization of available resources [14]. An effective TB control program will focus not only on drug therapy but also on the social aspects of the treatment regimen. These, like drug therapies, will need to be individually tailored to each patient.

## 12.2.1 Approaches to chemotherapy

TB patients, active or latent, harbor organisms at varying levels of metabolic activity. Organisms in well oxygenated areas can divide rapidly, those in less well oxygenated and more acidic areas (e.g. caseous material) will divide more slowly, while within the macrophage, virtual cessation of metabolic activity can occur [1]. Slower dividing organisms, and those in harder to penetrate areas such as caseous material, are more difficult to eradicate. No initial form of drug therapy exists that can eliminate all organisms at the same time. A cure is achieved in stages as the various subpopulations of tubercle bacilli are killed. Certain agents, especially INH, are particularly active as early bacteriocidal drugs whereas other agents, especially PZA, are active as sterilizing agents for residual bacterial populations [14a].

Underlying the problem of multiple drug resistance (MDR) (Chapter 13) is an innate developmental resistance to certain drugs despite the bacilli never having been exposed to these agents [15]. This natural resistance is a statistical phenomenon based on the number of organisms present in the host. The probability of resistance differs for the various drugs as discussed in Chapters 7 and 13.

To prevent the selection and clinical expression of such naturally resistant strains, active TB is never treated with a single agent. In general, innate resistance to one agent does not directly lead to resistance to other agents [16]. It is the case, however, in patients who are noncompliant with medication that it can be easier to select for resistant strains.

## 12.2.2 Combination chemotherapy

As a result of more than 30 years of research in the treatment of TB [17–20] it has been clearly demonstrated that combination chemotherapy is important. Table 12.2 summarizes the major concepts involved in TB therapy in individuals with non-drug-resistant infection [14, 17–29]. A review of some of the major studies can put the data that these trials generated into perspective. Many thousands of persons have participated in these trials and the experience gained provides a solid basis for the current recommendations.

**Table 12.2** Current concepts in tuberculosis therapy (non MDR-TB)

- All regimens should contain isoniazid due to effectiveness, low cost and tolerance
- Treatment for less than 6 months leads to unacceptably high relapse rates
- Pyrazinamide should be used with isoniazid and rifampin for the first 2 months of treatment
- Intermittent therapy is as effective as daily therapy if adequately supervised

Snider *et al.* [20] studied 213 patients with sputum smear positive pulmonary TB treated either with INH/rifampin/PZA/streptomycin (IRPS) daily for 2 months followed by INH/rifampin twice weekly for 4 months or IRP daily for 2 months followed by the same twice weekly INH/rifampin (IR). Essentially all patients with or without streptomycin had smear and culture negative sputum at the end of treatment. The study demonstrated that both regimens were highly efficacious in the treatment of drug sensitive sputum smear positive TB. There was a higher drop out rate in the group receiving streptomycin, with 86% of those not receiving streptomycin completing therapy compared with 72% of those receiving it.

Cohn *et al.* [21] studied 160 patients with both pulmonary (81%) (both sputum smear positive and smear negative) and extrapulmonary TB (19%) and treated them with the following regimen: IRPS daily for 2 weeks, followed by IRPS twice weekly for 6 weeks finishing with 18 weeks of IR. The sputum became culture negative at a mean time of 4 weeks of therapy with 100% negative at 20 weeks. The regimen was well tolerated as well as efficacious.

The Hong Kong Chest Service [22] evaluated 1386 patients with sputum smear positive pulmonary TB. The results indicated that there might be value in adding streptomycin to the first 2 months of therapy in sputum smear positive patients when an intermittent drug regimen (IRP) is used. Four of 224 persons not receiving streptomycin failed initial therapy compared with none who were receiving the drug. The authors, however, did state that more studies are needed to evaluate this further.

The same group [25] reported the results of a 5 year follow-up of 833 sputum smear positive cases treated with various combinations of 'first-line' agents including ethambutol (E) in combinations that included IRPSE, IRPS, IRPE and IRSE. The results demonstrated that for drug susceptible TB strains, regimens containing PZA had a lower relapse rate at 5 year follow-up than did non-PZA containing regimens (3.4% versus 10.3%).

The Singapore TB Service [23] reported a similar 5 year follow-up of patients treated for sputum smear positive pulmonary TB. In patients with drug susceptible bacilli, only 3 of 297 patients relapsed by 5 years. The patients were treated with one of three initial induction regimens (IRPS for 2 months, IRPS for 1 month, IRP for 2 months) followed by IR three times a week up to 6 months. All three regimens were equally efficacious, demonstrating no need for the addition of streptomycin in the initial induction therapy regimen.

The same group from Singapore evaluated the use of a combined IRP preparation (Rifater) in 310 patients with smear positive pulmonary TB, compared with the same drugs given separately with or without streptomycin [28]. The initial cure rates were the same among all the treatment groups, as was the incidence of side effects. However, at 18 months of follow-up, there was a statistically higher relapse rate in the Rifater group

(8% bacteriologic relapse compared with 0–3% for the other regimens ($p = 0.04$)). The authors conclude that further evaluation of the combined preparation is indicated.

The US Public Health Service [29] compared 9 months of IR therapy with 2 months of IRP therapy followed by 4 months of IR for the treatment of pulmonary TB. The 1451 patient study showed that both regimens were equally efficacious (94% and 90% converted, respectively). A statistically greater proportion of those taking the 6 month therapy completed a full treatment course. It was concluded that a 6 month course of therapy is adequate for pulmonary TB.

The application of these studies in practical terms results in several general recommendations. A patient with TB that is not suspected to be drug resistant should initially be treated with at least three drugs for a minimum of 6 months. The initial drug combination should be INH, rifampin and PZA. The PZA component should only be used in the first 2 months. Subsequent therapy, which should be supervised, particularly in unreliable patients (see below), can be given on an intermittent basis. It is acceptable to add streptomycin or ethambutol to the initial IRP treatment for drug-sensitive TB infections. However, as discussed, data suggest that such an addition adds no therapeutic benefit in this setting [30].

If, for any reason, rifampin cannot be used, then an alternative regimen for drug-sensitive pulmonary TB is 18–24 months of INH and ethambutol with streptomycin given during the first 2 months. This can be used in a setting where cost containment is important or pre-existing liver disease mandates against the use of potentially hepatotoxic agents. This prolonged regimen is effective, but less attractive than the IRP combination in otherwise uncomplicated cases [31,32].

Intermittent regimens that have been demonstrated to be efficacious are all of 6 months' duration [33,34] and are shown in Table 12.3.

It should be noted that when therapy is given intermittently, the doses of all agents are increased except for rifampin [15]. These doses are shown in Table 12.4.

**Table 12.3** Acceptable six month intermittent treatment regimens

- Isoniazid, rifampin, pyrazinamide, streptomycin daily for 2 weeks, then
  isoniazid, rifampin, pyrazinamide twice weekly for 6 weeks, then
  isoniazid, rifampin twice weekly for 18 weeks
- Isoniazid, rifampin, pyrazinamide, streptomycin 3 times a week for 26 weeks
- Isoniazid, rifampin, pyrazinamide 3 times a week for 26 weeks

The current recommendation by the CDC Advisory Council for the Elimination of Tuberculosis is to begin all TB patients on a four-drug regimen until susceptibility testing results are available, unless the incidence

**Table 12.4** Dosages of antituberculous drugs (mg/kg/day)

| Drug | Daily therapy | Twice weekly | Maximum dose |
|---|---|---|---|
| **Adults** | | | |
| Isoniazid | 5 | 15 | Daily 300 mg<br>Twice weekly 900 mg |
| Rifampin | 10 | 10 | 600 mg |
| Pyrazinamide | 15–30 | 50–70 | Daily 2 g<br>Twice weekly 3.5 g |
| Streptomycin | 15 | 25–30 | Daily 1 g<br>Twice weekly 1.5 g |
| Ethambutol | 15–25 | 50 | 2.5 g |
| Ethionamide | 10–20 | – | 1 g |
| Capreomycin | 15 | – | 1 g |
| **Children**[a] | | | |
| Isoniazid | 10–15 | 20–40 | Daily 300 mg<br>Twice weekly 900 mg |
| Rifampin | 10–20 | 10–20 | 600 mg |
| Pyrazinamide | 20–30 | 40–50 | Daily 2 g<br>Twice weekly 3 g |
| Streptomycin | 20–30 (IM) | 25–30 (IM) | 1 g |
| Ethambutol | 15–25 | 30–50 | 2.5 g |
| Ethionamide | 15–20 | – | 1 g |
| Capreomycin | 15–30 (IM) | – | 1 g |

[a] Derived from Starke, J.R. (1992) Current chemotherapy for tuberculosis in children. *Infect Dis Clin NA*, **6**, 215–238 with permission of the publisher, and from recommendations of the City of New York, Department of Health. Applies to children under the age of 12 years. For children aged ≥ 12 years refer to adult doses.

of INH resistance in the locale is less than 4%. Four drugs are likely to be needed in most areas of the USA where there are substantial numbers of patients with TB. In circumstances where multi-drug-resistant infection is suspected, a five or six-drug regimen may be indicated even before susceptibility results are available (Chapter 13).

### 12.2.3 Duration of therapy

Various regimens have proved efficacious when given for varying times. In general, any regimen that is less than 6 months in length has an unacceptable relapse rate [14]. Thus, 6 months is the minimum acceptable duration of therapy. Within this framework, options include either daily or intermittent therapy. Based on cost considerations, patient reliability and extent of disease, the physician must choose the most appropriate regimen for the patient. All options discussed are acceptable and produce equally good results in comparable patients.

## 12.3 DIRECTLY OBSERVED TREATMENT STRATEGIES

Once active TB disease is found and treatment started, the physician's mission has just begun. It is paramount, both to the patient and to the community, that the prescribed course is completed. Factors mitigating against completion are the long duration, cost and the disenfranchized nature of many patients with TB. Many patients are recent immigrants (often illegal aliens with no access to medical care), they may have problems of homelessness, alcoholism, drug abuse or a combination of these factors [35]. The medical community must reach out to these groups to ensure compliance. This benefits not only those infected but also society as there will be less secondary spread.

Directly observed therapy (DOT), in which medication is taken at a facility under observation or a care provider brings the medications and observes that it is taken, is the most cost effective method for improving adherence to treatment [36–38]. CDC reported that DOT produced 97% compliance in noncompliant patients in South Carolina [39]. The cost was about $650 per patient for DOT, compared with about $10 700 per patient for commitment to a long term care facility to ensure compliance. The Denver, Colorado experience found DOT costs about $400 per patient [40].

The importance of DOT's contribution to improving TB therapy is shown by the fact that both the CDC and ATS recommend that consideration of DOT be made for all patients with active TB [41]. It has been suggested that society stands to lose much should DOT not become universally introduced [40]. The ability to quarantine a non-compliant patient to enforce adequate therapy is endorsed by the CDC [41] providing that due consideration is given to the patient's civil and legal rights [42,43]. DOT is further discussed in Chapter 9 and ethical issues related to TB are considered in Chapter 10.

## 12.4 MONITORING PATIENTS ON ANTITUBERCULOUS MEDICATIONS

### 12.4.1 Monitoring for adverse drug reactions

There is little doubt that DOT provides the most direct means of ensuring compliance with therapy. The physician is also responsible for monitoring to ensure therapy safety.

Monitoring for adverse reactions to therapy should be performed in the following manner:

- An inventory of current medications should be taken to anticipate any possible drug–drug interactions that may result from the initiation of TB treatment. Serum levels of drugs that can be affected by TB drugs should be measured.

- A history of drug allergy or intolerance should be obtained to guide in the selection of appropriate agents.
- Baseline liver function tests, renal function indexes and a complete blood count should be obtained.
- If PZA or ethambutol is to be used, serum uric acid should be measured.
- If ethambutol is to be used, baseline visual acuity testing should be performed.
- If an aminoglycoside or capreomycin is to be used, baseline testing of both vestibular and cochlear functioning of the eight cranial nerve should be performed.

This information is obtained at the onset of therapy so any change can be found while taking therapy. A significant change may necessitate a change of drug to one with alternative toxicities.

Patients should be monitored clinically for adverse reactions during therapy [1,14]. Patients should be informed of the common side effects of therapy and be told to notify their physician if any suspicious symptoms occur. Routine repeat laboratory testing to detect subclinical abnormalities is not recommended [14]. However, patients should be seen monthly while on therapy, and questioned specifically about relevant symptoms. It is the clinical practice of many physicians to follow tests of liver function on a monthly basis while patients are taking treatment. Reasons include doubt that the patient can be relied on to report suspicious symptoms promptly and the fear of the medicolegal consequences in a patient with an adverse reaction.

### 12.4.2 Monitoring the effect of therapy

*(a) Patients with smear positive sputum*

ATS recommends that patients with smear positive sputum should have sputum specimens examined monthly until they are negative [14] (Table 12.5) Following 3 months of therapy with INH and rifampin, more than 90% of such patients should be smear negative.

Should the sputum remain smear positive at 3 months, consideration should be given to whether the patient is complying with therapy. Should noncompliance be an issue, either DOT or forced quarantine with therapy will need to be considered. If the patient is known to be compliant, drug resistant TB is a concern and two new drugs should be added to the treatment while awaiting susceptibility testing. Rarely, malabsorption has resulted in treatment failure [44]. The symptoms suggestive of continuing active TB include cough, weight loss, fever and an impaired sense of well being. If these symptoms resolve, it is likely that the treatment will be successful if the regimen is completed.

**Table 12.5** Monitoring tuberculosis therapy in smear positive patients

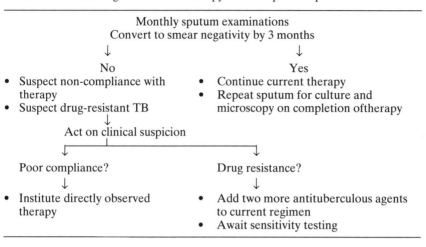

Monthly sputum examinations
Convert to smear negativity by 3 months

| No | Yes |
|---|---|
| • Suspect non-compliance with therapy<br>• Suspect drug-resistant TB | • Continue current therapy<br>• Repeat sputum for culture and microscopy on completion of therapy |

Act on clinical suspicion

| Poor compliance? | Drug resistance? |
|---|---|
| • Institute directly observed therapy | • Add two more antituberculous agents to current regimen<br>• Await sensitivity testing |

Once sputum is smear negative, a final sputum test for acid-fast bacilli (AFB) smear and culture is obtained on completion of therapy. Some physicians will obtain a chest X-ray as a baseline for comparison with any future films obtained. No specific follow-up is necessary on completion of therapy owing to the high rates of success [45]. The patient should be instructed, however, to seek attention if symptoms suggestive of recurrent TB occur. Some feel that, despite the high success rates of current therapy, patients who have successfully completed therapy should be followed up with sputum examinations and chest X-rays every 3–6 months for the initial 2 years after therapy [1].

### (b) Patients with smear negative sputum

In this group of patients, the chest X-ray appearance is of major importance in assessing therapy (Table 12.6). An improvement in the radiographic picture should have occurred by 3 months. Should no improvement occur, the disease is either not due to TB, the organism is drug-resistant, or the patient is noncompliant.

## 12.5 CORTICOSTEROIDS

In general, corticosteroids are not indicated for the treatment of pulmonary TB. However, in specific clinical settings, steroids may have a role in therapy. The topic has been reviewed by an expert committee the Infectious Disease Society of America (IDSA) [46]. The following is a distillation of the recommendations made on the basis of a review of published trials.

**Table 12.6** Monitoring tuberculosis therapy in smear negative patients

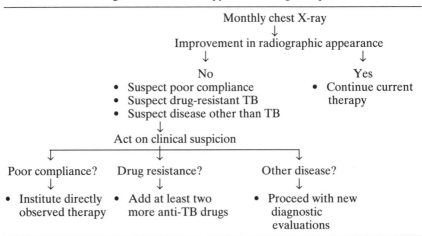

In the setting of TB pericarditis, there is strong evidence in favor of the use of corticosteroid therapy based on evidence obtained from a randomized, controlled trial [47]. In this study, the addition of 40–80 mg/day of prednisolone to the anti-TB chemotherapy (INH, rifampin, streptomycin and PZA for 14 weeks followed by INH/rifampin for 12 weeks) resulted in fewer deaths and a more rapid clinical improvement in the steroid treated group. In addition, the subsequent pericardiectomy rate was higher in the non-steroid group.

For meningitis, the committee concluded that there is moderate evidence to favor of the use of corticosteroids. Their conclusion was based on a controlled nonrandomized trial from India [48]. This study demonstrated that dexamethasone plus INH and streptomycin led to a more rapid fall in cerebrospinal fluid opening pressure than did anti-TB therapy alone. The beneficial effects of the steroids were thought to be in preventing arachnoiditis and spinal fluid block. An Egyptian study [cited in 48] demonstrated a survival advantage in the steroid treated group (5/11 survivors in the steroid treated group compared with 3/12 in the non-steroid group).

There was poor evidence, in the opinion of the expert committee, for the use of corticosteroids in the treatment of severe hypoxia, pleurisy or peritonitis caused by infection with *Mycobacterium tuberculosis*.

A second recently published review also examined the use of steroids in the treatment of TB [49]. The conclusions were similar to those of the IDSA in that there was a definite role for the use of steroids in the treatment of TB pericarditis and meningitis. In addition, pleural TB might be a situation where steroids are of benefit, especially if the patient has a very large effusion or 'high fevers'. The authors also suggested that clinically significant fever in a patient with TB might respond to a 6 week tapering course of corticosteroids, but there are no controlled trials to support this contention.

## 12.6 THERAPY IN SPECIAL SITUATIONS

### 12.6.1 Pregnancy and lactation

TB that occurs during pregnancy should be treated as soon as it is diagnosed. Treatment should not be deferred until after delivery of the baby [50]. INH, rifampin and ethambutol are thought to be safe for use in gestation [1,5]. Too few data exist to recommend the use of PZA [1]. Streptomycin should be avoided because of the possible toxic effects on the eighth cranial nerve of the fetus. Pregnant women taking INH should also take pyridoxine supplementation.

Lactating women taking anti-TB therapy may continue to breast-feed the infant [51]. The amount of each drug present in breast milk is too small to pose any threat to the child. The drug concentrations are also not sufficient to treat the child should that be deemed necessary [14].

### 12.6.2 Extrapulmonary tuberculosis

Clinical trials for the treatment of extrapulmonary TB infection of the magnitude of those carried out in patients with pulmonary TB have not been performed. However, over 4000 cases/year of extrapulmonary TB occur in the USA [52] making it a significant problem. The number will continue to increase in parallel with the increasing number of patients with HIV infection [53].

The general principles governing the treatment of extrapulmonary TB are the same as for the pulmonary form. The logic underlying this is that no form of extrapulmonary disease is associated with a higher organism load than the cavitary pulmonary form. Hence, since successful therapy is available for the latter, the former should be similarly, or even more readily treatable. When the infection is in a life threatening anatomical location (e.g. intracranial, paraspinal or pericardial), maximal aggressive therapy is applied. Other anatomical locations respond well to 'less aggressive' treatment regimens.

### (a) Tuberculous meningitis

Following rupture of a subependymal tubercle into the subarachnoid space, TB meningitis can ensue [54]. In the presence of meningeal inflammation, the concentration of INH in the cerebrospinal fluid equals that in the blood. Rifampin and PZA penetrate less well, but also achieve levels greater than those needed to kill tubercle bacilli in the fluid. Triple therapy with INH, rifampin and PZA, therefore (perhaps plus steroids) should be given. The steroid treatment can usually be tapered after 6 weeks.

A recent study of 53 children with TB meningitis demonstrated that aggressive therapy for 6 months with a regimen that included PZA was more efficacious than 9 or 12 months without PZA [55]. The study reported that four of eight patients not receiving a PZA-containing regimen died while only seven of 45 receiving a course containing that agent died. It has recently been reported that about 20% of children who survived TB meningitis developed hypopituitarism [56]. The authors concluded that early, aggressive treatment may reduce the incidence of this late sequela.

### (b) Intracranial tuberculoma

Although uncommon, intracranial tuberculomas are worthy of comment as they may cause great confusion by presenting or expanding during anti-TB chemotherapy [57–59]. In general, once recognized, they are better treated with medical rather than surgical therapy [60,61].

### (c) Tuberculous paraspinal infections

When this condition is recognized in a patient presenting with signs and symptoms consistent with spinal cord compression, urgent surgical decompression coupled with aggressive medical therapy is indicated [62]. The same drugs that are used for TB meningitis are indicated in this setting. If the tuberculoma is resected, medical therapy is given for 12 months. Should the patient be managed with conservative medical treatment, it is prudent to treat for 18–24 months. The role of steroids in this setting remains to be defined [62].

### (d) Tuberculous pericarditis

TB pericarditis usually occurs as a result of the rupture of a caseous node into the pericardium. It may occasionally complicate hematogenous disease [1]. The treatment is the same as for pulmonary TB although the addition of corticosteroids is of benefit [46,49]. Surgical intervention is warranted if either pericardial tamponade or constriction occurs.

### (e) Other forms of extrapulmonary tuberculosis

The treatment of other major forms of extrapulmonary TB is outlined in Table 12.7 [63–73].

## 12.7 'CHEMOPROPHYLAXIS'

Once it was shown that INH was a relatively safe drug to use, a move was made from treating only those persons with active TB to additionally treating those with evidence of infection with *M. tuberculosis* (i.e. with a positive skin test reaction to tuberculin) without clinical disease. It is

**Table 12.7** Therapy of extrapulmonary tuberculosis[a]

| | |
|---|---|
| • Miliary tuberculosis | Isoniazid, rifampin ± steroids (12–18 months) |
| • Pleural tuberculosis | Isoniazid, rifampin (9 months)<br>Isoniazid, ethambutol (18 months) |
| • Tuberculous spondylitis | Isoniazid, rifampin, ethambutol, pyrazinamide (24 months)<br>Surgical intervention as indicated |
| • Renal tuberculosis | Isoniazid, rifampin + one other drug for 9 months (UK opinion) or 24 months (US opinion) |
| • Tuberculous peritonitis | Isoniazid, rifampin (6 months) |
| • Tuberculous lymphadenitis | Isoniazid, rifampin<br>Surgical excision if needed |

[a] For fully sensitive organisms.

apparent that the same idea was generated independently in several countries and that no one individual can claim to have invented the concept.

It should be noted that despite general acceptance of the term prophylaxis, it is an incorrect use of the word. The people eligible for such therapy harbor tubercle bacilli in their bodies and are thus infected, albeit subclinically. The administration of INH is directed against these clinically inapparent organisms with the intention of eradicating all or most of them prior to disease development.

The risk of infection becoming a clinical problem is greatest within the first 2 years of acquisition. Clinical status and age are variables, with young children and the immunosuppressed having the greatest incidence of disease development. Overall, about 3% of people infected develop TB within a year of infection, and a total of about 10% will do so throughout their lives [74]. Intervention that is begun prior to the development of clinical disease should, at least theoretically, be capable of decreasing this lifetime risk of clinical TB. INH therapy has been shown to be both safe and cost effective when used in the appropriate prophylactic setting [75].

The early trials that were carried out worldwide were reviewed by Ferebee in an extensive monograph published in 1970 [76]. In this work, the author reviewed the controlled chemoprophylaxis trials carried out previously by the U.S. Public Health Service and the Danish Tuberculosis Index. In addition, the studies carried out by Tunisian, Kenyan, Japanese, Dutch and Philippine investigators are also reviewed. All the trials were carried out between the years 1955 and 1964. The general consensus of all the data collected was that: INH prophylactic therapy greatly reduced the incidence of clinically apparent cases of TB compared with placebo recipients; INH was well tolerated by these generally healthy persons; and therapy did not cause reversion of a positive tuberculin skin test to negative.

Current recommendations have been based on an assessment of the risk to benefit ratio of administering INH to asymptomatic persons in each specific category. The incidence of hepatotoxicity from INH increases in persons aged over 35 years and peripheral neuropathy is more likely to occur in persons who are malnourished, alcoholic or diabetic. A California report on 20 INH associated deaths over a 14-year period found that the majority of these deaths were caused by management errors in INH use (failure to stop the drug immediately when symptoms developed) and concluded that careful reconsideration be given to the use of prophylactic INH [77]. This conclusion is challenged in an accompanying editorial in which it is stated that toxicity is a known problem with INH and correct adherence to protocol will result in the safe use of INH [78]. It is important to note that the amount of hepatic damage associated with INH may be severe enough to necessitate liver transplantation as shown in a CDC report of 10 patients [79].

In considering these potential problems with the use of INH in prophylaxis against the development of active TB, the CDC has made recommendations for preventive therapy [80] (Table 12.8). For a detailed discussion on the procedures required to determine tuberculin test status, refer to Chapter 8.

### 12.7.1 Asymptomatic close contacts of infected persons

Since household contacts have a significant (2–4%) risk of developing active TB in the first year after exposure [81], there is strong rationale to treat this group. The CDC recommends that close contacts of newly diagnosed persons with TB who have a tuberculin skin test of over 5 mm induration, but no active disease, should receive INH prophylaxis. In addition, close contacts who are children and adolescents, particularly children under 2 years of age, should be treated even if they have a negative skin test. The tuberculin test should be repeated 12 weeks later. Should it remain negative, the prophylaxis can be stopped. If, however, the skin test converts to positive, then INH should be continued for a total of 6–9 months [80]. The reason why these individuals should be treated initially, irrespective of their PPD status, is the high risk of early disseminated disease [74,82]. This risk is significant compared with the low risk of INH toxicity in this age group. Some European countries (e.g. the UK) routinely provide BCG vaccination to neonates of infected mothers. BCG vaccination is reported to provide protection both against the development of pulmonary and to a greater extent, extrapulmonary, especially miliary, disease [83,84]. BCG is discussed in more detail in Chapter 9.

### 12.7.2 Asymptomatic tuberculin positive persons

Persons in whom the tuberculin test is positive but who are not known or suspected to have been negative in the past 2 years with no known risk

**Table 12.8** Situations in which the CDC recommends prophylaxis with isoniazid

| Situation | Comments |
|---|---|
| • Asymptomatic close contacts of infectious persons | • Adults with tuberculin reaction of > 5 mm |
| | • All children irrespective of tuberculin status. If negative, repeat at 3 months and stop isoniazid if tuberculin test remains negative |
| | • ? BCG vaccination for neonates (UK) |
| • Asymptomatic tuberculin positive persons (for risk factors, see Chapter 8) | • High risk factor +, treat if tuberculin test > 5 mm |
| | • Moderate risk factor, treat if tuberculin test > 10 mm |
| | • No risk factor, (low prevalence group), treat if tuberculin test > 15 mm |
| • Recent tuberculin converter (in last 2 years) | • Treat, irrespective of age |
| • Persons with positive tuberculin test and chest X-ray compatible with quiescent TB | • If not previously treated |

factors for increased acquisition of TB are treated with INH if aged less than 35 years. There are data to suggest that 6 months of therapy is as efficacious as 12 months [85,86]. HIV-infected persons should receive 12 months' therapy [80]. Persons aged over 35 years without additional risk factors should be carefully monitored for the development of TB but not routinely treated because of an increased incidence of INH-induced hepatotoxicity.

### 12.7.3 Recent tuberculin converters

Persons documented to have converted from a negative to a positive tuberculin status within the last 2 years should be treated with preventive INH therapy [80]. The issue of skin test conversion following exposure to a patient with drug-resistant *M. tuberculosis* is discussed in Chapter 13.

### 12.7.4 Persons with chest X-rays compatible with old, healed tuberculosis

Preventive therapy is indicated for persons with positive tuberculin skin tests, chest X-ray findings compatible with old TB, negative sputum cultures and no history of prior anti-TB therapy [80]. Such patients have an increased risk of developing active disease, compared with those with normal X-rays, if they remain untreated. This risk remains for the patient's lifetime, though it may diminish with time.

### 12.7.5 Persons with underlying medical conditions

The presence of a positive tuberculin skin test in a patient with one or more of the conditions listed and discussed in detail in Chapter 8 mandates the initiation of a course of anti-TB prophylaxis [80]. The reason for this recommendation is the increased risk for the reactivation of TB compared with similar persons without these immunomodulating conditions.

### 12.7.6 Special social situations

Persons with no risk factors for the enhanced virulence of *M. tuberculosis* who are less than 35 years of age and have a tuberculin skin test greater than 10 mm should be treated prophylactically with INH in the settings of those born in countries with high prevalence of TB infection [87]; medically disenfranchised, low income populations, especially, in the USA, Blacks, Hispanics and native Americans [80]; and migrant workers [88]. This is based on the higher potential for transmission should reactivation develop.

### 12.7.7 Health care workers

Although no special recommendations apply to health care workers *per se*, it is worth highlighting their risk of nosocomial acquisition of infection with *M. tuberculosis*. Many studies have demonstrated the risk run by health care providers in caring for patients with pulmonary TB [88–90].

In a retrospective analysis of physicians who graduated from the University of Illinois, 66 cases of active TB occurred in 4575 physicians who graduated between 1938 and 1981 [89]. Two-thirds of the cases occurred within 6 years of finishing medical school. The risk of acquiring TB was 140 per 100 000 person years within 6 years of graduation. Interestingly, in that group of physicians who received BCG vaccination, there were 40% fewer cases of TB than in comparable unvaccinated persons.

Barret-Connor [90] reported a study involving a questionnaire mailed to 6425 persons listed on the rosters of seven California medical schools. A total of 146 physicians had been treated for active TB with 75% occurring within 10 years of starting medical school. A total of 1642 physicians stated that they had a positive tuberculin skin test, and of these, 166 (about 10%) had taken some form of TB chemoprophylaxis. Of known recent tuberculin skin test converters, 56% elected not to take INH prophylaxis. Of those beginning INH prophylaxis, 25% did not complete the prescribed course. Again, BCG recipients developed significantly fewer cases of active TB than their unvaccinated counterparts.

Recent epidemiologic data from Puerto Rico suggests that the problem remains a very significant one in the hospital setting. Nurses working on an HIV unit caring for patients with both TB and HIV disease, as well as nurses working on a general medical ward, had a statistically greater likelihood of having a positive tuberculin skin test than other hospital personnel such as ward clerks (skin tests were positive in nine of 19 nurses on the HIV unit, 45 of 90 nurses on the general medical ward and 35 of 188 clerical personnel) [91].

Thus, health care workers are at significant risk for the occupational acquisition of *M. tuberculosis* infection. They do not appear to be a very compliant group with respect to preventive INH therapy, even when indicated. Greater educational efforts will be required to improve compliance among physicians and other health care providers requiring INH therapy. This will benefit both the individuals involved as well as the patients they care for.

### 12.7.8 Alternatives to isoniazid

Alternatives to INH for preventive therapy should be considered in individuals who are intolerant of INH or who have been exposed to INH-resistant organisms. A study in Chinese men with silicosis found that rifampin was as effective as INH in a 5 year follow-up study [92]. Importantly, the rifampin group in the study was associated with no more hepatotoxicity than the placebo group. Using a mouse model, in which the animals develop a stable, non-progressive TB infection, rifabutin and rifapentine were comparable to rifampin. The half life of rifapentine makes it an excellent candidate for clinical studies [93]. This limited size, stable bacillary infection had been previously used by Lecoeur and colleagues to study chemopreventive regimens [94]. This group found that 3 months of rifampin or 2 months of rifampin and PZA were more effective than 6 months of INH treatment. As pointed out by Iseman, if a twice weekly rifampin/PZA regimen is effective, such a 2 month, intermittent dose DOT would consist of a total of 10 doses and could substantially aid in increasing the compliance of chemoprevention.

### 12.8 CONCLUDING COMMENTS

Tremendous progress has been made in TB treatment. What often used to be a fatal infection is now, in most cases, readily treatable. It has also been clearly demonstrated that in appropriate settings, prophylactic chemotherapy with INH decreases the incidence of subsequent clinically apparent TB in asymptomatically infected individuals. Recent clinical trials have demonstrated the efficacy of 6 month, intermittent therapy regimens for the treatment of non-drug-resistant pulmonary TB. The major challenges remaining in this field include the prevention of emergence of drug-resistant strains of *M. tuberculosis* and ensuring compliance in patients who are often disenfranchised from the medical community. The increased efforts of the public health authorities toward funding more DOT programs should, if successful, help prevent either of these issues from becoming too great a problem for the community.

## REFERENCES

1. Des Prez, R.M. and Heim, C.R. (1990) *Mycobacterium tuberculosis*, in *Principles and Practice of Infectious Diseases* (eds G.L. Mandell, R.G. Douglas and J.E. Bennett), Churchill-Livingstone, New York, pp. 1877–906.
2. Brudney, K. and Dobkin, J. (1991) Resurgent tuberculosis in New York City: human immunodeficiency virus, homelessness, and the decline of tuberculosis control programs. *Am Rev Respir Dis*, **144**, 745–9.
3. Wolinsky, E. (1993) Statement of the tuberculosis committee of the Infectious Diseases Society of America. *Clin Infect Dis*, **16**, 627–8.
4. Watson, J.M. (1993) Tuberculosis in Britain today: notifications are no longer falling. *Brit Med J*, **306**, 221–2.
5. Joseph, S. (1993) Tuberculosis, again. *Am J Publ Hlth*, **83**, 647–8.
6. Collison, G., Hindle, R., Kennedy, M. *et al.* (1993) Tuberculosis in Northland. *N Z Med J*, **106**, 43–4.
7. Reichman, L.B. (1993) Fear, embarrassment and grief: the tuberculosis epidemic and public health. *Am J Publ Hlth*, **83**, 639–40.
8. Bloom, B.R. and Murray, C.J.L. (1992) Tuberculosis: commentary on a re-emergent killer. *Science*, **257**, 1055–64.
9. McName, D. (1993) United against TB. *Lancet*, **341**, 1145.
10. Dooley, S.W., Jarvis, W.R., Marton, W.J. and Snider, D.E. (1992) Multidrug-resistant tuberculosis. *Ann Intern Med*, **117**, 257–9.
11. Small, P.M., Shafer, R.W., Hopewell, P.C. *et al.* (1993) Exogenous reinfection with multidrug-resistant *Mycobacterium tuberculosis* in patients with advanced HIV infection. *N Engl J Med*, **328**, 1137–44.
12. Nitta, A.T., Iseman, M.D., Newell, J.D. *et al.* (1993) Ten year experience with artificial pneumoperitoneum for end stage, drug resistant pulmonary tuberculosis. *Clin Infect Dis*, 16, 219–22.
13. Peloquin, C.A. (1992) Shortages of anti-mycobacterial drugs. *N Engl J Med,* **326**, 714.
14. American Thoracic Society (1986) Treatment of tuberculosis and tuberculosis infection in adults and children. *Am Rev Respir Dis,* **134**, 355–63.
14a.Jindani, A., Aber, V.R., Edwards, E.A. and Mitchison, D.A. (1980) The early bactericidal activity of drugs in patients with pulmonary tuberculosis. *Am Rev Respir Dis*, **121**, 939–49.
15. Centers for Disease Control and Prevention (1993) Initial therapy for tuberculosis in the era of multidrug resistance. Recommendations of the Advisory Council for the Elimination of Tuberculosis. *MMWR*, 42 (RR-7), 1–8.
16. Wolinsky, E. (1991) Antimycobacterial drugs, in *Infectious Diseases* (eds S.L. Gorbach, J.G. Bartlett and N. Blacklow), W.B. Saunders, Philadelphia, pp. 313–19.
17. Bobrowitz, I.D. and Robins, D.E. (1967) Ethambutol–isoniazid versus PAS–isoniazid in original treatment of pulmonary tuberculosis. *Am Rev Respir Dis*, **96**, 428–38.
18. Second East African/British Medical Research Council (1974) Controlled clinical trial of our 6 month regimens of chemotherapy for pulmonary tuberculosis. *Lancet*, **2**, 1100–4.
19. Fox, W. and Mitchison, D.C. (1975) Short course chemotherapy for tuberculosis. *Am Rev Respir Dis*, **111**, 325–53.

20. Snider, D.E., Graszyk, J., Bek, E. and Rogowski, J. (1984) Supervised six months treatment of newly diagnosed pulmonary tuberculosis using isoniazid, rifampin and pyrazinamide with and without streptomycin. *Am Rev Respir Dis,* **130**, 1091–4.

21. Cohn, D.H., Catlin, R.J., Peterson, K.L. *et al.* (1990) A 62-dose, 6 month therapy for pulmonary and extrapulmonary tuberculosis. *Ann Intern Med,* **112**, 407–15.

22. Hong Kong Chest Service/British Medical Research Council (1991) Controlled trial of 2, 4, and 6 months of pyrazinamide in 6 months, three times weekly regimens for smear positive pulmonary tuberculosis, including an assessment of a combined preparation of isoniazid, rifampin and pyrazinamide. *Am Rev Respir Dis,* **143**, 700–6.

23. Singapore Tuberculosis Service/British Medical Research Council (1988) Five year follow-up of a clinical trial of three 6 months regimens of chemotherapy given intermittently in the continuation phase in the treatment of pulmonary tuberculosis. Am Rev Respir Dis, **137**, 1147–50.

24. British Thoracic Society (1984) A controlled trial for six months chemotherapy in pulmonary tuberculosis: results during the 36 months after the end of chemotherapy and beyond. *Br J Dis Chest,* **78**, 330–6.

25. Hong Kong Chest Service/British Medical Research Council (1987) Five year follow-up of a controlled trial of five 6 month regimens of chemotherapy for pulmonary tuberculosis. *Am Rev Respir Dis,* **136**, 1339–42.

26. Prabhaker, R. (1982) Fully intermittent six month regimens for pulmonary tuberculosis in South India. *Bull Int Union Tuberc,* **62**, 21–3.

27. Anastasatu, C., Bercea, O. and Corlan, E. (1982) Pilot study of short course 3 plus 3 intermittent chemotherapy in previously untreated smear positive tuberculosis. *Bull Int Union Tuberc,* **52**, 1–19.

28. Singapore Tuberculosis Service/British Medical Research Council (1991) Assessment of a daily combined preparation of isoniazid, rifampin and pyrazinamide in a controlled trial of three 6 month regimens for smear-positive pulmonary tuberculosis. Am Rev Repir Dis, **143**, 707–12.

29. Combs, D.L., O'Brien, R.J. and Geiter, L.J. (1990) USPHS tuberculosis short course chemotherapy trial 21: Effectiveness, toxicity and acceptibility. *Ann Intern Med,* **112**, 397–406.

30. Snider, D.E., Zierski, M., Graczyk, J. *et al.* (1986) Short course tuberculosis chemotherapy studies conducted in Poland during the past decade. *Eur J Respir Dis,* **68**, 12–18.

31. Bobrowitz, I.D. (1980) Ethambutol compared to rifampin in original treatment of pulmonary tuberculosis. *Lung,* **157**, 117–25.

32. Davidson, P.T. and Le, H.Q. (1992) Drug treatment of tuberculosis – 1992. *Drugs,* **43**, 653–71.

33. Weissler, J.C. (1993) Tuberculosis – immunopathogenesis and therapy. *Am J Med Sci,* **305**, 52–65.

34. Weinberger, S.E. (1993) Recent advances in pulmonary medicine. *N Engl J Med,* **328**, 1462–70.

35. Sumartojo, E. (1993) When tuberculosis treatment fails: a social behavioral account of patient adherence. *Am Rev Respir Dis,* **147**, 1311–20.

36. Sbarbaro, J.A. and Johnson, S. (1968) Tuberculosis chemotherapy for recalcitrant outpatients administered twice weekly. *Am Rev Respir Dis,* **96**, 895–902.

37. Samarasinghe, D., Hawken, M. and Harrison, A.C. (1992) Intermittent supervised treatment of tuberculosis at Green Lane Hospital, 1987–8. *N Z J Med,* **105**, 243–5.

38. McDonald, R.J., Memon, A.M. and Reichman, L.B. (1982) Successful supervised ambulatory management of tuberculosis treatment failures. *Ann Intern Med,* **96**, 297–303.

39. Centers for Disease Control (1993) Approaches to improving adherence to antituberculous therapy – South Carolina and New York 1986–1991. *MMWR,* **42**, 74–6.

40. Iseman, M.D., Cohn, D.L. and Sbarbaro, J.A. (1993) Directly observed treatment of tuberculosis: we can't afford not to try it. *N Engl J Med,* **328**, 576–8.

41. American Thoracic Society/CDC (1992) Control of tuberculosis in the United States. *Am Rev Respir Dis,* **146**, 1623–33.

42. Gostin, L.O. (1993) Controlling the resurgent tuberculosis epidemic: 50 state survey of TB statutes and proposals for reform. *JAMA,* **269**, 255–61.

43. Annas, G.J. (1993) Control of tuberculosis – the law and the public's health. *N Engl J Med,* **328**, 585–8.

44. Berning, S.E., Huitt, G.A., Iseman, M.D. and Peloquin, C.A. (1992) Malabsorption of antituberculous medication by a patient with AIDS. *N Engl J Med,* **327**, 1817–18.

45. Glassroth, J., Robins, A.G. and Snider, D.E. (1980) Tuberculosis in the 1980's. *N Engl J Med,* **302**, 1441–50.

46. McGowan, J.E., Chesney, P.J., Crossley, K.R. and LaForce, F.M. (1992) Guidelines for the use of systemic glucocorticosteroids in the management of selected infections. *J Infect Dis,* **165**, 1–13.

47. Strang, J.I.G., Gibson, D.G., Nunn, A.J. *et al.* (1987) Controlled trial of prednisolone as adjuvant in treatment of tuberculous constrictive pericarditis. *Lancet,* **2**, 1418–22.

48. O'Toole, R.D., Thornton, G.F., Mukherjee, M.K. and Nath, R.L. (1969) Dexamethasone in tuberculous meningitis: relationship of cerebrospinal fluid effects to therapeutic efficacy. *Ann Intern Med,* **70**, 39–48.

49. Alzeer, A.H. and FitzGerald, J.M. (1993) Corticosteroids and tuberculosis: risks and use as adjunct therapy. *Tubercle,* **74**, 6–11.

50. Snider, D.E., Layde, R.M., Johnson, M.W. and Lyle, M.A. (1980) Treatment of tuberculosis during pregnancy. *Am Rev Respir Dis,* **122**, 65–73.

51. Snider, D.E. and Powell, K.E. (1984) Should women taking anti-tuberculous drugs breast feed? *Arch Intern Med,* **144**, 589–92.

52. Rieder, H.L., Snider, D.E. and Cauthen, G.M. (1990) Extrapulmonary tuberculosis in the United States. *Am Rev Respir Dis,* **141**, 347–51.

53. Daley, C.L., Small, P.M., Schechter, G.F. *et al.* (1992) An outbreak of tuberculosis with accelerated progression among persons infected with the human immunodeficiency virus: an analysis using restriction-fragment-length polymorphisms. *N Engl J Med,* **326**, 231–35.

54. Rich, A.R. and McCordock, H.A. (1933) Pathogenesis of tuberculous meningitis. *Bull Johns Hopkins Hosp,* **52**, 5–37.

55. Jacobs, R.F., Sunakorn, P., Chotpitayasunonah, T. *et al.* (1992) Intensive short course chemotherapy for tuberculous meningitis. *Ped Infect Dis J,* **11**, 194–8.

56. Lam, K.S.L., Sham, M.M.K., Tam, S.C.F. *et al.* (1993) Hypopituitarism after tuberculous meningitis in childhood. *Ann Intern Med,* **118**, 701–6.

57. Chambers, S.T., Record, C., Hendrickse, W.A. *et al.* (1984) Paradoxic expansion of intracranial tuberculomas during chemotherapy. *Lancet*, **2**, 181–3.

58. Teoh, R., Humphries, M.J. and O'Mahony, S.G. (1987) Symptomatic intracranial tuberculoma developing during treatment of tuberculosis: A report of 10 patients and review of the literature. *Quart J Med*, **63**, 449–60.

59. Malone, J.L., Paparello, S., Rickman, L.S. *et al.* (1990) Intracranial tuberculoma developing during therapy for tuberculous meningitis. *West J Med*, **152**, 188–90.

60. Watson, J.D.G., Shnier, R.C. and Seale, J.P. (1993) Central nervous system tuberculosis in Australia: A report of 22 cases. *Med J Aust*, **158**, 408–13.

61. Harder, E., Al-Kawzi, M.Z. and Carney, P. (1983) Intracranial tuberculoma: conservative management. *Am J Med*, **74**, 570–6.

62. MacDonell, A.H., Baird, R.W. and Bronze, M.S. (1990) Intramedullary tuberculomas of the spinal cord: case report and review. *Rev Infect Dis*, **12**, 432–9.

63. Munt, P.W. (1972) Miliary tuberculosis in the chemotherapy era: A clinical review in 69 American adults. *Medicine*, **51**, 139–55.

64. Epstein, D.M., Klein, L.R. and Albelda, S.M. (1987) Tuberculous pleural effusions. *Chest*, **91**, 106–9.

65. Fancourt, G.J., Ebden, P., Garner, P. *et al.* (1986) Bone tuberculosis: results and experience in Leicestershire. *Br J Dis Chest*, **80**, 265–72.

66. Gow, J.G. (1971) Genitourinary tuberculosis. A study of the disease in one unit over a period of 24 years. *Ann R Coll Surg Engl*, **49**, 50–70.

67. Simon, H.B., Weinstein, A.J., Pasternak, M.S. *et al.* (1977) Genitourinary tuberculosis. Clinical features in a general hospital population. *Am J Med,* **63**, 410–20.

68. Singh, M.M., Bhargava, A.N. and Jair, K.P. (1969) Tuberculous peritonitis. An evaluation of pathogenic mechanisms, diagnostic procedures and therapeutic measures. *N Engl J Med*, **281**, 1091–4.

69. Bastani, B., Shariatzadeh, M.R. and Dehdashti, F. (1985) Tuberculous peritonitis – report of 30 cases and review of the literature. *Quart J Med*, **56**, 549–57.

70. Summers, G.D. and McNicol, M.W. (1980) Tuberculosis of superficial lymph nodes. *Br J Dis Chest*, **74**, 369–73.

71. Menitove, S. and Harris, H.W. (1987) Miliary tuberculosis, in *Tuberculosis* (ed. D. Schlossberg), Springer Verlag, New York, pp. 179–91.

72. Nayyar, V., Ramakrishna, B., Mathew G. *et al.* (1993) Response to antituberculous chemotherapy after splenectomy. *J Int Med*, **233**, 81–3.

73. Kim, J.H., Langston, A.A. and Gallis, H.A. (1990) Miliary tuberculosis: Epidemiology, clinical manifestations, diagnosis and outcome. *Rev Infect Dis*, **12**, 583–90.

74. Styblo, K. (1980) Recent advances in epidemiological research in tuberculosis. *Adv Tuberc Res*, **20**, 1–63.

75. Rose, D.N., Schecter, C.B., Fahs, M.C. and Silver, A.L. (1988) Tuberculosis prevention: cost-effectiveness analysis of isoniazid chemoprophylaxis. *Am J Prev Med*, **4**, 102–9.

76. Ferebee, S.H. (1970) Controlled chemoprophylaxis trials in tuberculosis: A general review. *Adv Tuberc Res*, **17**, 28–106.

77. Moulding, T.S., Redeker, A.G. and Kanel, G.C. (1989) Twenty isoniazid-associated deaths in one state. *Am Rev Respir Dis*, **140**, 700–5.

78. Iseman, M.D. and Miller, B. (1989) If a tree falls in the middle of a forest: isoniazid and hepatitis. *Am Rev Respir Dis,* **140**, 575–6.

79. Centers for Disease Control (1993) Severe INH-associated hepatitis – New

York, 1991–1993. *MMWR*, **43**, 545–7.

80. Centers for Disease Control (1990) Screening for tuberculosis and tuberculous infection in high-risk populations, and the use of preventive therapy for tuberculous infection in the United States: Recommendation of the Advisory Committee for Elimination of Tuberculosis. *MMWR*, **39** (**RR-8**), 9–12.

81. Ferebee, S.H. and Mount, F.W. (1962) Tuberculosis morbidity in a controlled trial of the prophylactic use of isoniazid among household contacts. *Am Rev Respir Dis*, **85**, 490–521.

82. Comstock, G.W., Livesay, V.T. and Woolpert, S.F. (1974) The prognosis of a positive tuberculin reaction in childhood and adolescence. *Am J Epidemiol*, **99**, 131–8.

83. Anonymous (1990) Perinatal prophylaxis of tuberculosis. *Lancet*, **2**, 1479–80.

84. Curtis, H.M., Leck, I. and Bamford, F.N. (1984) Incidence of childhood tuberculosis after neonatal BCG vaccination. *Lancet*, **1**, 145–8.

85. International Union Against Tuberculosis (1982) Efficacy of various durations of isoniazid preventive therapy for tuberculosis: five years of follow-up in the IUAT trial. *Bull WHO*, **60**, 555–64.

86. Snider, D.E., Caras, C.F. and Koplan, J.P. (1986) Preventive therapy with isoniazid. Cost effectiveness of different duration therapy. *JAMA*, **255**, 1579–83.

87. Byrd, R.B., Fisk, D.E., Roethe, R.A. *et al.* (1979) Tuberculosis in oriental immigrants: a study in military dependents. *Chest*, **76**, 136–9.

88. Centers for Disease Control (1992) Prevention and control of tuberculosis in migrant farm workers, recommendations of the Advisory Council for the Elimination of Tuberculosis. *MMWR*, **41** (RR-10), 9–11.

89. Geisler, P.J., Nelson, K.E., Cristen, R.G. and Moses, V.K. (1986) Tuberculosis in physicians: a continuing problem. *Am Rev Respir Dis*, **133**, 773–8.

90. Barret-Connor, E. (1979) The epidemiology of tuberculosis in physicians. *JAMA*, **241**, 33–8.

91. Dooley, S.W., Villarino, M.E., Lawrence, M. *et al.* (1992) Nosocomial transmission of tuberculosis in a hospital unit for HIV-infected patients. *JAMA*, **267**, 2631–5.

92. Hong Kong Chest Service/British Medical Research Council (1992) A double-blind placebo-controlled clinical trial of three antituberculosis chemoprophylaxis regimens in patients with silicosis in Hong Kong. *Am Rev Respir Dis,* **145**, 36–41.

93. Ji, B., Truffot-Pernot, C., Lacroix, C. *et al.* (1993) Effectiveness of rifampin, rifabutin, and rifapentine for preventive therapy of tuberculosis in mice. *Am Rev Respir Dis*, 148, 1541–8.

94. Lecoeur, H.F., Truffot-Pernot, C. and Grosset, J.H. (1989) Experimental short-course preventive therapy of tuberculosis with rifampin and pyrazinamide. *Am Rev Respir Dis*, **140**, 1189–93.

# Treatment of multi-drug-resistant tuberculosis

**13**

Livette S. Johnson, Kent A. Sepkowitz

## 13.1 INTRODUCTION

Tuberculosis (TB) infections were chronicled by ancient Greek physicians as phthisis in describing the cough, fever and wasting character of this disease. TB did not become a major problem until the industrial revolution when urban overcrowding led to an increase in cases [1].

Cases of drug-resistant TB have been described since the introduction of effective antibiotic therapy. However, in recent years, cases of both single drug and multi-drug resistance in TB have been increasingly reported throughout the world. This had been the case in developing countries and is now occurring in the USA. Treatment regimens for drug-resistant TB tend to be less effective, more expensive and much more prolonged than therapy for sensitive TB. It is, therefore, an urgent public health priority to assure that the spread of resistant TB is interrupted. To achieve this goal, current cases of resistant TB must be identified and treated to completion, and effective prophylaxis must be developed for persons latently infected with drug-resistant TB. In addition, persons with sensitive TB must also be identified and treated to completion, to prevent further development of resistant strains. This chapter will review the currently available literature on the pathogenesis, epidemiology and treatment of resistant TB.

## 13.2 PATHOGENESIS

Streptomycin was the first effective antibiotic introduced for the treatment of TB. Resistance to this drug was quickly described soon after its initial use in 1944. Persons with pulmonary, miliary or meningeal TB treated with streptomycin alone showed an initially good response [2]. In some cases, however, this was followed within months by clinical and bacteriologic relapse due to the emergence of streptomycin-resistant organisms [3].

To investigate this clinical finding, studies were conducted that have been pivotal in understanding how and why resistant TB occurs. *Mycobacterium tuberculosis* from sputum in patients who had never received streptomycin was inoculated on media with various concentrations of the drug. Colonies appeared in media containing concentrations of 5–10 μg/ml streptomycin, which should have been inhibitory, revealing that drug resistance could be present naturally (so called wild type or primary resistance) in an untreated individual [4]. Additional experiments demonstrated that the larger the inoculum of acid-fast bacillus (AFB), the higher the likelihood that resistant bacilli would be found [5].

Primary drug resistance to isoniazid (INH) is found in 1 in $10^6$ organisms, to rifampin in 1 in $10^8$ organisms, to ethambutol in 1 in $10^6$ organisms and to streptomycin in 1 in $10^5$ organisms. The chance of resistance of one organism to any two drugs is the product of the individual probabilities of the drugs [6]. It is estimated that the number of bacilli commonly found within lung cavities of 2.5 cm in diameter is 100 million ($10^8$). It is expected, therefore, that wild strain resistance to more than one drug in a single bacillus is unlikely. However, inadequate chemotherapeutic regimens or patient noncompliance may lead to the unchecked growth of resistant TB and ultimately to a case of drug-resistant TB. At particular risk for this phenomenon are patients with high bacillary burdens, such as those with cavitary lung diseases in contrast, people with, for example, TB pleural infection, have a low bacterial load.

The influence of drug therapy on the susceptibility of *M. tuberculosis* in sputum samples collected serially is well studied. In one report, sputum from patients treated with streptomycin alone for 12 weeks was inoculated onto media containing streptomycin. The number of colonies recovered approached the number of colonies in media containing no streptomycin. *In vitro* resistance had developed within 12 weeks [5].

The results of these experiments led to a distinction between primary and secondary or acquired drug resistance. Primary drug resistance is that encountered in patients who have never had any chemotherapy, arising either from a mixed population of both sensitive and resistant organisms in, for example, a large lung cavity, or in someone whose initial infection was with an already resistant organism. Secondary resistance is the result of inadequate drug therapy, either because insufficient drugs were used, or because they were incompletely administered.

Because of the rapid emergence of drug resistance to therapy with a single drug, the practice of using multiple drugs to treat TB quickly became routine. From 1947 to 1952, streptomycin was used in combination with para-aminosalicylic acid (PAS). In the early 1950s, INH was introduced.

Soon, double and triple drug initial therapy, to accomplish faster sterilization and to retard or prevent the emergence of resistance, became standard care. Within a few years, previously used treatment modalities with variable effectiveness, such as surgical resection, collapse therapy and prolonged bed rest became unnecessary and TB sanatoria were gradually closed.

However, because of noncompliance [6], incorrectly selected regimens and an increasing number of susceptible patients, the development of almost a dozen effective agents did not successfully lead to the complete eradication of TB. Rather it has resulted in the emergence of multi-drug-resistant (MDR) infection, a disease that, in some ways, is as difficult to treat as sensitive TB was a century ago.

Thus, widespread drug resistance is the result of 40 years of effective antibiotics that have been ineffectively administered. Over time, drug-resistant organisms have been systematically selected for, so that now, the occurrence of strains resistant to as many as seven anti-TB drugs is increasingly common. In addition, the particular propensity of HIV-infected persons to develop active infectious TB can amplify exponentially a resistant strain from a single index case, further increasing the number of cases of resistant disease.

## 13.3 EPIDEMIOLOGY

In the 1950s, primary drug resistance in the USA was 1–2% [7,8]. Over the next decade resistance to INH, PAS and streptomycin remained constant at about 3% [7,8]. During the 1970s, primary drug resistance to at least one drug had increased to 8.6% [9]. Some populations and areas of the country were found to have a much higher incidence of resistant disease. Byrd *et al.* [10] found drug resistance above 50% in the Oriental wives of US servicemen from Southeast Asia. Another report from the late 1970s found Asian and Hispanic US populations with resistance rates as high as 15–20% [9].

A survey from Centers for Disease Control (CDC) sentinel hospitals throughout the USA in the early 1980s found primary resistance to one or more drugs to be approximately 7% [11], with ranges from 4.9% in a White non-Hispanic population to 14.8% in Asians [11]. In 31 health departments across the USA, a 1991 CDC surveillance study found a primary drug resistance rate of 9% to at least one drug and a 22.8% rate of secondary resistance [12]. A 1987 southern California report found a stable high rate of resistance among isolates from 1969 to 1984. Twenty-three per cent of patients who had never been treated and 59% of previously treated patients were resistant to at least one drug [13]. A review of 355 cases among children at Kings County Hospital in Brooklyn from 1961 to 1980 found a rate of resistant TB of 15.8% [14].

The rate was even higher in a 1991 survey of 465 cases from New York City where 33% were resistant to at least one drug and 19% were resistant to both INH and rifampin [15]. Primary resistance to one drug was found in 23%, and secondary resistance in 44% [15]. Numerous nosocomial outbreaks of MDR TB were occurring in New York City at this time and contributed to this startlingly high rate of resistance. Over the 4 year period between 1988 and 1991, a Rochester, New York report found that the percentage of TB isolates resistant to any drug rose from 5% to 21%, INH and rifampin resistance rose from 0% to 12% and five-drug resistance rose from 0% to 3% [16]. Surveys from other parts of the country have also demonstrated increasing rates of resistance. During the first three months of 1991, 14.4% of TB cases throughout the USA were resistant to at least one drug and 3.3% were resistant to both INH and rifampin [17].

Outside the USA, drug resistance is and has been a significant problem for many more years. During the late 1970s and 1980s, primary drug resistance in India was 20% and over 30% in Pakistan [18]. A report covering a 12-month period from 1988 to 1989 showed a 22% drug resistance rate in Central Haiti [19]. In Asia, a Taiwanese study found an 11.4% resistance rate to INH and streptomycin in combination as far back as 1976 [18]. A 1983 report from Turkey found a 9.4% resistance rate to the combination of INH and streptomycin [18]. In Europe, the rates of resistance have not been as high but 13% resistance to any one drug was reported in Spain from 1966 to 1975, while France had an 8.9% resistance rate to at least one medication [18]. Worldwide, the highest reported rate of resistant TB is in sub-Saharan Africa [18]. Parts of Africa experienced a 35% resistance rate to INH alone and a 33.3% rate to streptomycin in 1980 [18]. A city in the Horn of Africa from 1985 to 1992 had a 36% resistance rate to all first line drugs and a 78% resistance rate to at least two first line drugs [20].

## 13.4 DRUG THERAPY FOR RESISTANT TUBERCULOSIS

In general, patients with TB that is resistant to both INH and rifampin have a much worse prognosis than those patients who have TB that is sensitive to either or both of these two drugs. Treatment of TB resistant to any single first line drug is accomplished by using other first line agents to which the organism is sensitive, including INH, rifampin, pyrazinamide (PZA), ethambutol and streptomycin. If the organism is resistant to either INH or streptomycin alone, a 94–96% success rate has been reported, even with short course therapy [21]. When the organism is rifampin resistant, the outcome of therapy is less successful and second line drugs may be recommended [22].

A review of available second line drugs is given in Chapter 12. Some comments regarding these agents in the treatment of drug resistant disease are found below.

### 13.4.1 Intramuscular drugs: kanamycin, amikacin and capreomycin

Although similar in their toxicity profiles, the aminoglycosides (strepto-mycin, kanamycin and amikacin) differ in structure from the cyclic polypeptide, capreomycin. Capreomycin has, additionally, no uniform cross resistance with the aminoglycosides [23]. In persons who are not hospitalized and in whom a 7 day dosing schedule is not practical, a 3–5 day/week regimen is acceptable. The dose limiting problem with these medications is often the lack of venous access, particularly in cachectic patients who do not have the available muscle mass to receive repeated intramuscular injections.

Duration of therapy depends on the susceptibility of the organism, but in general is about 2 months, pending stabilization of the patient. In some cases of resistance to six or seven drugs, however, therapy must be extended for as long as the patient can tolerate it. Occasionally, in such cases, the use of capreomycin with an aminoglycoside is required (assuming the strain is susceptible to both types of injectables). The expected toxicities of renal and ototoxicity occur more rapidly, and doctors and patients are occasionally confronted with the dilemma of choosing between continuing effective therapy with the possibility of loss of hearing, or risking less effective therapy in an attempt to preserve hearing. Other than streptomycin, these drugs are not FDA approved for the treatment of TB.

### 13.4.2 Fluoroquinolones

In TB chemotherapy, either ciprofloxacin or ofloxacin can be used for drug-resistant disease. Ofloxacin, and its L-isomer, levofloxacin, are better studied. Since the replication time of mycobacteria is slower than that of other bacteria, once daily dosing is acceptable [24]. Persons who develop fever and rash with ciprofloxacin may tolerate ofloxacin and the reverse is also true. Neither drug is FDA approved for the treatment of TB.

### 13.4.3 Ethionamide

Ethionamide is chemically related to INH and pyrazinamide. Many experts consider that INH resistance predicts ethionamide resistance, regardless of *in vitro* testing results, but there is no clear consensus for this. It is one of the more efficacious of the second line drugs.

The most common problem associated with ethionamide is gastro-intestinal distress which is often intolerable to the patient. The intolerance can be decreased by gradually introducing progressively higher doses of the drug, starting at 250 mg/day and increasing 250 mg every week, up to 1000 mg/day. Dividing the doses may also lead to better tolerance, as well as the use of premedication with anti-emetic agents. Some experts recommend the concurrent administration of pyridoxine (50–150 mg/day) to reduce potential side effects. The efficacy of this practice is undetermined.

### 13.4.4 Cycloserine

Cycloserine is a tuberculostatic drug that is highly alkaline and rapidly destroyed when exposed to neutral or acidic environments [25]. The most consistent and problematic side effects are seen in the central nervous system. Symptoms ranging from somnolence, headache, tremor and vertigo to confusion, psychosis and seizures are well described. Because of these effects, all patients on cycloserine should have their blood levels monitored. These side effects are thought to be dose related but may be seen in individuals with normal blood levels [26].

The effects usually occur in the first weeks of therapy and disappear after withdrawal of the drug. Reinstitution of a lower dose of the drug after the resolution of side effects may be necessary and is usually well tolerated. However, patients who develop seizures while on cycloserine should not have the drug restarted. The addition of pyridoxine at a dose of 100–150 mg/day may decrease side effects. In addition, cycloserine may have additive CNS effects when used with ofloxacin [27].

### 13.4.5 Para-aminosalicylic acid

PAS was developed at the same time as streptomycin by the Swedish chemist Lehmann who also discovered the anticoagulant effects of coumadin. Side effects include nausea, vomiting, diarrhea, hepatitis, hypothyroidism and hemolytic anemia in glucose-6-phosphate dehydrogenase deficient persons. Many people find the size and number of the pills onerous and this contributes to noncompliance. Sodium overload may also occur. Persons with a history of congestive heart failure, liver disease with ascites or renal failure should be closely monitored while on this drug.

### 13.4.6 Clofazimine

Clofazimine is a phenazine dye initially used in the treatment of leprosy. It has recently been used for the treatment of TB at a daily dose of 100–200 mg. Major side effects include orange–brown skin discoloration and gastrointestinal upset. Pruritus has also been seen and is associated with skin deposition of the drug. Clofazimine has been much less well studied than the other second line agents. It should only be used in MDR strains of TB when no better options are available.

## 13.5 TREATMENT OF DRUG-RESISTANT TUBERCULOSIS

Treatment of drug-resistant TB remains one of the most difficult challenges for the infectious disease or pulmonary specialist. Some patients may be asked to take over 20 pills per day for up to 2 years. Despite this, with persistence and adherence to basic principles, stabilization and even cure of persons with MDR TB is possible. If rifampin can be used in the treatment regimen with at least one other first line drug, treatment in immunocompetent individuals with limited disease may be completed in as little as 6–9 months [28]. Sensitivity to INH without rifampin necessitates a 12–18 month course of therapy with high success rates. However, when no first line agents are susceptible, therapy for more than 24 months may be required. Potential regimens and suggested duration are listed in Table 13.1 [28].

### 13.5.1 Multi-drug-resistant infection in HIV-negative patients

The results of drug therapy in HIV-negative patients with MDR TB have been disappointing. Reports from Denver National Jewish Hospital have described the results of therapy of MDR TB in 134 patients from 1973 to 1983 [29,30]. The patients were resistant to a median of six drugs. Despite the excellence of the facility and the treating physicians, only about 50% were medically cured. An additional 25% were surgically cured and the other 25% were treatment failures. The results reflect how difficult this disease can be to cure, even in an optimal setting.

### 13.5.2 Multi-drug-resistant infection in HIV-positive patients

Initial reports describing the outcome of individuals (including health care workers) with MDR TB and AIDS has stressed its extremely high and rapid mortality. Most studies place survival after diagnosis at 1–3 months, with an overall mortality of more than 85% [31–34]. Fischl *et al.* [35] found that patients with HIV infection but not AIDS who developed this infection fared as well as persons with AIDS and sensitive TB. What is most notable in all of these studies is that, because drug-resistant TB was not anticipated, few patients who were subsequently found to have this infection had been receiving effective therapy for their infection. In a sense, these results demonstrate the natural history of untreated drug-resistant TB in persons with AIDS.

Since these early dismal reports, some of the hospitals that had experienced outbreaks of resistant infection began to use a six or seven drug regimen as initial therapy with relatively encouraging results [36,37]. Edlin *et al.* [36] reported that patients treated during an outbreak of MDR TB who had received at least two drugs to which their isolate was ultimately found to be sensitive had better survival than those who received fewer than two active drugs (13/21 (62%) compared with 4/12 (33%)). An update of this data suggested that, not surprisingly, even better results were found in individuals who had received at least three agents to which their isolate was ultimately found to be sensitive. Lockhart *et al.* [37] examined the effect of an initial five or six drug regimen on survival of patients with MDR infection. Of 12 patients, seven were alive a median of 5 months

**Table 13.1** Potential regimens for patients with tuberculosis and various patterns of drug resistance [28][a]

| Resistance | Suggested regimen | Duration of therapy | Comments |
|---|---|---|---|
| Isoniazid and streptomycin | Rifampin, pyrazinamide, ethambutol, amikacin[b] | 6–9 months | Anticipate 100% response rate and less than 5% relapse rate [29] |
| Isoniazid and ethambutol (± streptomycin) | Rifampin, pyrazinamide, ofloxacin or ciprofloxacin, amikacin[b] | 6–12 months | Efficacy should be comparable to above regimen |
| Isoniazid and rifampin (± streptomycin) | Pyrazinamide, ethambutol, ofloxacin or ciprofloxacin, amikacin[b] | 18–24 months | Consider surgery |
| Isoniazid, rifampin and ethambutol (± streptomycin) | Pyrazinamide, ofloxacin or ciprofloxacin, amikacin[b] Plus 2[c] | 24 months after conversion | Consider surgery |
| Isoniazid, rifampin and pyrazinamide (± streptomycin) | Ethambutol, ofloxacin or ciprofloxacin, amikacin[b] Plus 2[c] | 24 months after conversion | Consider surgery |
| Isoniazid, rifampin, pyrazinamide and ethambutol (± streptomycin) | Ofloxacin or ciprofloxacin, amikacin[b] Plus 3[c] | 24 months after conversion | Surgery, if possible |

[a]   Reproduced with permission from the *New England Journal of Medicine*, **329**, 784–91, 1993, and the Massachusetts Medical Society.

[b]   If there is resistance to amikacin, kanamycin and streptomycin, capreomycin is a good alternative. Injectable agents are usually continued for 4–6 months if toxicity does not intervene. All the injectable drugs are given daily (or twice or thrice weekly) and may be administered intravenously or intramuscularly.

[c]   Potential agents from which to choose: ethionamide, cycloserine or aminosalicylic acid. Others that are potentially useful but of unproved utility include clofazimine and amoxicillin-clavulanate. Clarithromycin, azithromycin and rifabutin are unlikely to be active.

after diagnosis, while median survival for the remaining five patients was 6–7 months. The median CD4 cell count in this group was 50 (range 0–160), indicating that all were severely immunocompromised.

This data demonstrates that the key determinant in survival for patients with this infection and AIDS is prompt selection of an effective regimen. Even patients with a severely compromised immune system may respond if treated with appropriate drugs. The selection of specific empiric regimens will necessarily depend on the local pattern of susceptibility at a given medical center. Compiling such resistance patterns, therefore, will aid significantly in the choice of an empiric regimen awaiting sensitivities. Rapid techniques for isolation and drug sensitivities (Chapter 7) become more valuable in this situation. One regimen used in New York City to treat persons suspected of having an increasingly common seven drug resistant strain includes INH, rifampin, PZA, ofloxacin, cycloserine and capreomycin.

Although these results are promising, two future areas of concern must be considered. First, adding a six or seven drug regimen, usually with several toxic second line agents, to patients with AIDS who are often already receiving five to ten other medicines requires extreme diligence on the part of the treating physician, as well as a willing patient. Common toxicities such as rash, fever or hepatitis are very difficult to ascribe to a specific agent until all suspected drugs have been stopped and then re-added, often one per week. In addition, the impact of administering a relatively toxic polydrug regimen to patients who turn out to have either sensitive TB or who do not have TB at all must be considered. There is currently, however, no reliable way to anticipate who will have resistant TB. Historical features, such as past therapy or contact with persons with known resistant TB, either at home, at a shelter, a prison or in a hospital are useful to suggest the diagnosis but in no way verify it. Until rapid tests to determine susceptibility are obtainable, care deliverers who treat large numbers of patients with resistant TB will need to continue to treat all cases of potentially resistant TB with awkward six or seven drug regimens, pending culture results.

A second area of concern is the ultimate disposition of patients with MDR infection and AIDS who survive and are well enough to be discharged from hospital. Many, if not most of these patients, remain intermittently smear and culture positive for 12–18 months into therapy, despite such clinical responses as defervescence, weight gain and normalization of chest X-ray. Many such patients had previously lived in congregate housing, prisons or with HIV infected family members. Because there may be no suitable place for them to live, many remain hospitalized, resulting in a tragic loss of personal dignity as well as enormous hospital expense. As the number of patients with AIDS and MDR TB that is controlled but not eradicated grows, this may become a greater concern. In such hospitalized patients, it appears that the enforcement of the readily implementable control measures in TB management (Chapter 9) can interrupt the transmission of MDR TB to health care workers [38,39].

### 13.5.3 Surgical therapy

In some adherent patients with localized pulmonary disease who are failing to improve with treatment after a minimum of 3 months, adjunctive surgical therapy has been utilized. Results from Denver's National Jewish Center for Immunology and Respiratory Medicine have been encouraging. At that center between August 1985 and October 1990, 42 patients with drug-resistant infection had a pulmonary resection. Complications of surgery included wound infection, respiratory failure, Horner's syndrome, bleeding and bronchopleural fistula. One patient died intraoperatively, and six patients died at a later date. Only two deaths were considered to be related to TB. Of these 42 patients, 38 (90%) were considered cured [29].

## 13.6 PREVENTIVE THERAPY FOR MULTI-DRUG-RESISTANT *M. TUBERCULOSIS*

To reduce the risk of active disease, it is recommended that tuberculin skin test convertors, some high risk tuberculin reactors and close contacts of infectious cases receive INH preventive therapy [40–43]. Contacts of persons with MDR TB who are at risk for infection should be assessed regarding the likelihood of infection with an MDR strain. The infectiousness of the source case is one crucial variable. A patient with a cough and a positive sputum AFB smear is more likely to be infectious. Other factors to consider are the closeness and intensity of the exposure and the likelihood of infection from another potential source with a drug susceptible strain.

In patients newly infected with strains of *M. tuberculosis* resistant to INH but sensitive to rifampin, rifampin prophylaxis is effective, while INH is not [44]. However, if the strain is multi-drug-resistant, treatment options are limited and no studies have demonstrated efficacy [45]. Drug susceptibility testing from the source case is the primary consideration in selecting preventive therapy. If neither INH or rifampin can be used, preventive therapy should include at least two drugs to which the index organism is sensitive. Alternative regimens for preventive therapy include pyrazinamide, 25–30 mg/kg and ethambutol, 15–25 mg/kg.

Studies in a mouse model suggest that PZA enhances the efficacy of other bacteriocidal drugs, since the combination of pyrazinamide and rifampin is more effective than rifampin alone [46]. Ethambutol at a dose of 25 mg/kg is bacteriocidal, but at 15 mg/kg it is bacteriostatic [47]. If the higher dose is used, the patient is at risk for increased toxicity especially ocular toxicity (Chapter 11). This dose should not be used in children. Another potential regimen for this prophylaxis is PZA and a fluoroquinolone. Ofloxacin at 400 mg twice a day or ciprofloxacin at 750 mg twice a day along with pyrazinamide is suggested. These drugs have a similar efficacy *in vitro* [48]. The suggested duration of preventive therapy is 6–12 months, although this regimen has been difficult to tolerate [49].

To control MDR TB, cases must be identified and treated to completion, and latently infected individuals must be given effective prophylaxis. In addition, patients being treated for sensitive TB must be treated to completion so that they do not, over time, develop resistant disease. Aggressive education of health care workers about infection control should be conducted [50]. Although costly, effective TB treatment programs have been instituted in countries of modest means [51]. Preventing the spread of MDR TB to other patients and hospital staff [52–59], as well as avoiding the cost of treating a case of MDR TB, more than compensates for the cost of developing and implementing an effective program of TB control.

## REFERENCES

1. Des Prez, R.M. and Heim, C.R. (1990) Mycobacterium tuberculosis, in *Principles and Practices of Infectious Diseases* (eds G.L. Mandell, R.D. Douglas and J.E. Bennett), Churchill Livingstone, New York, pp. 1877–906.
2. Holmberg, S.D. (1990) The rise of tuberculosis in America before 1820. *Am Rev Respir Dis*, **142**, 1228–32.
3. Youmans, G.P., Williston, E.H., Feldman, W.H. and Hinshaw, H.L. (1946) Increase in resistance of tubercle bacilli to streptomycin: Preliminary report. *Proc Staff Meet Mayo Clinic*, **21**, 126–7.
4. Pyle, M.M. (1947) Relative numbers of resistant tubercle bacilli in sputa of patients before and after treatment with streptomycin. *Proc Staff Meet Mayo Clinic*, **22**, 465–73.
5. Toman, K. (1979) Chemotherapy, in *Tuberculosis Case-Finding and Chemotherapy*, World Health Organization, Geneva, pp. 75–93.
6. Brudney, K. and Dobkin, J. (1991) Resurgent tuberculosis in New York City: human immunodeficiency virus, homelessness and the decline of tuberculosis control programs. *Am Rev Respir Dis*, **144**, 745–9.
7. Doster, B.D., Casas, G.J. and Snider, D.E. (1976) A continuing survey of primary drug resistance in tuberculosis, 1961 to 1968. *Am Rev Respir Dis*, **113**, 419–25.
8. Zeidberg, L.D., Gass, R.S., Dillion, A. *et al.* (1963) The Williamson County tuberculosis study. A twenty-four-year epidemiologic study. *Am Rev Respir Dis*, **87**, 1–88.
9. Kopanoff, D.E., Kilburn, J.O., Glassroth, J.L. *et al.* (1978) A continuing survey of primary drug resistance in the United States: March 1975 to November 1977. *Am Rev Respir Dis*, **118**, 835–42.
10. Byrd, R.B., Fisk, D.E., Roethe, R.A. *et al.* (1979) Tuberculosis in Oriental immigrants: A study in military dependents. *Chest*, **76**, 136–9.
11. Centers for Disease Control (1983) Primary resistance to antituberculosis drugs – United States. *MMWR*, **32**, 521–3.
12. Snider, D.E., Cauthen, G.M., Farer, L.S. *et al.* (1991) Drug-resistant tuberculosis. *Am Rev Respir Dis*, **144**, 732.

13. Ben-Dov, I. and Mason, G.R. (1987) Drug-resistant tuberculosis in a Southern California hospital. Trends from 1969 to 1984. *Am Rev Respir Dis*, **135**, 1307–10.

14. Steiner, P., Rao, M., Victoria, M.S. *et al.* (1983) A continuing study of primary drug-resistant tuberculosis among children observed at Kings County Hospital Medical Center between the years 1961 and 1980. *Am Rev Respir Dis*, **128**, 425–8.

15. Freiden, T.R., Sterling, T., Ariel, P.M. *et al.* (1993) The emergence of drug-resistant tuberculosis in New York City. *N Engl J Med*, **328**, 521–6.

16. Weymouth, L.A., Kaminski, D.A., Vonbuskirk, R.L. and Hyde, R.W. (1992) *Change in drug resistance patterns of Mycobacterium tuberculosis in Rochester, New York*. Interscience Conference on Antimicrobial Agents and Chemotherapy, Anaheim, CA, American Society for Microbiology.

17. Centers for Disease Control (1990) Tuberculosis morbidity in the United States: final data. *MMWR*, **40 (SS-3)**, 23–7.

18. Kleeberg, H. and Oliver, M. (1984) *A World Atlas of Initial Drug Resistance*, Tuberculosis Research Institute of the South African Medical Research Council (MRC), Pretoria, South Africa.

19. Scalicini, M., Carre, G., Jean-Daptisue, M. *et al.* (1990) Antituberculous drug resistance in Central Haiti. *Am Rev Respir Dis*, **142**, 508–11.

20. Rodier, G., Gravier, P., Sevre, J. *et al.* (1993) Multidrug-resistant tuberculosis in the Horn of Africa. *J Infect Dis*, **168**, 523–4.

21. Hong Kong Chest Service/British Medical Research Council (1987) Five-year follow-up of a controlled trial of five 6 month regimes of chemotherapy for pulmonary tuberculosis. *Am Rev Respir Dis*, **136**, 1339–42.

22. Mitchison, D. and Nunn, A. (1986) Influence of initial drug resistance on the response to short-course chemotherapy of pulmonary tuberculosis. *Am Rev Respir Dis*, **133**, 423–30.

23. McClatchy, J.K., Kane, S.W., Davidson, P.R. *et al.* (1977) Cross-resistance in *M. tuberculosis* to kanamycin, capreomycin and viomycin. *Tubercle*, **58**, 29–34.

24. Simone, P.M. and Iseman, M.D. (1992) Drug-resistant tuberculosis: A deadly-and-growing-danger. *J Respir Dis*, **13**, 960–71.

25. Stead, W.W., To, T., Harrison, R.W. and Abraham, J.H. (1987) Benefit–risk considerations in preventive treatment for tuberculosis in elderly persons. *Ann Intern Med*, **107**, 843–5.

26. Mandell, G.L. and Sande, M.A. (1990) Drugs used in the chemotherapy of tuberculosis and leprosy, in *Goodman and Gilman's The Pharmacologic Basis of Therapeutics* (eds A.G. Gilman, T.W. Rall, A.S. Nies and P. Taylor), Pergamon Press, New York, pp. 1146–62.

27. Yew, W.W., Wong, C.F., Wong, P.C. *et al.* (1993) Adverse neurological reactions in patients with multidrug-resistant pulmonary tuberculosis after coadministration of cycloserine and ofloxacin. *Clin Infect Dis*, **17**, 288–9.

28. Iseman, M.D. (1993) Treatment of multidrug-resistant tuberculosis. *New Engl J Med*, **329**, 784–91.

29. Iseman, M.D., Madsen, L., Goble, M. and Pomerantz, M. (1990) Surgical intervention in the treatment of pulmonary disease caused by drug-resistant *Mycobacterium tuberculosis*. *Am Rev Respir Dis*, **141**, 623–5.

30. Goble, M.J., Iseman, M., Madsen, L.A. *et al.* (1993) Treatment of 171 patients with pulmonary tuberculosis resistant to isoniazid and rifampin. *New Engl J Med*, **328**, 527–32.

31. Di Perri, G., Crucian, M., Danz, M.C. *et al.* (1989) Nosocomial epidemic of active tuberculosis among HIV-infected patients. *Lancet*, **2**, 1502–4.

32. Fischl, M.A., Uttamchandani, R.B., Daikos, G.L. *et al.* (1992) An outbreak of tuberculosis caused by multiple-drug-resistant tubercle bacilli among patients with HIV infection. *Ann Intern Med*, **117**, 177–83.

33. Daley, C.L., Small, P.M., Schecter, G.F. *et al.* (1992) An outbreak of tuberculosis with accelerated progression among persons infected with human immuno-deficiency virus. An analysis using restriction-fragment-length polymorphisms. *N Engl J Med*, **326**, 231–5.

34. Centers for Disease Control (1991) Tuberculosis outbreak among persons in a residential facility for HIV-infected persons – San Francisco. *MMWR*, **40**, 649–52.

35. Fischl, M.A., Daikos, G.L., Uttamchandani, R.B. *et al.* (1992) Clinical presentation and outcome of patients with HIV infection and tuberculosis caused by multiple drug-resistant bacilli. *Ann Intern Med*, **117**, 184–90.

36. *Edlin, B.R., Attoe, L.S., Grieco, M.H. et al. (1993) Recognition and treatment of primary multidrug-resistant tuberculosis (MDRTB) in HIV-infected patients.* IXth International Conference on AIDS, Berlin, World Health Organization.

37. Lockhart, B., Sharp, V., Squires, K. *et al.* (1993) *Improved outcome of MDR-TB in patients receiving a five or more drug initial therapy.* IXth International Conference on AIDS, Berlin, World Health Organization.

38. Stroud, L., Tokars, J., Grieco, M. *et al.* (1993) *Interrruption of Nosocomial Transmission of Multi-drug Resistant Mycobacterium tuberculosis in a New York City Hospital.* Society of Hospital Epidemiologists of America, Chicago, IL.

39. Wenger, P., Beck-Sague, C., Otten, J. *et al.* (1993) *Efficacy of Control Measures in Preventing Nosocomial Transmission of Multi-drug Resistant Mycobacterium tuberculosis among Patients and Health Care Workers.* Society of Hospital Epidemiologists of America, Chicago, IL.

40. Ferebee, S.H. (1970) Controlled chemoprophylaxis trials in tuberculosis: A general review. *Adv Tuberc Res*, **17**, 28–106.

41. American Thoracic Society/CDC (1986) Treatment of tuberculosis and tuberculosis infection in adults and children. *Am Rev Respir Dis*, **134**, 355–63.

42. Comstock, G.W., Liversay, V.T. and Woolpert, S.F. (1974) The prognosis of a positive tuberculin reaction in childhood and adolescence. *Am J Epidemiol*, **99**, 131–8.

43. International Union Against Tuberculosis, Committee on Prophylaxis (1982) Efficacy of various durations of isoniazid preventive therapy for tuberculosis: Five years of follow-up in the IUAT trial. *Bull WHO*, **60**, 555–64.

44. Fairshter, R.D., Randazzo, G.P., Garlin, J. and Wilson, A.F. (1975) Failure of isoniazid prophylaxis after exposure to isoniazid-resistant tuberculosis. *Am Rev Respir Dis*, **112**, 37–43.

45. Centers for Disease Control (1992) National action plan to combat multidrug-resistant tuberculosis. *MMWR*, **41 (RR-11)**, 1–45.

46. Lecoeur, H.F., Truffot-Pernot, C. and Grosset, J.H. (1989) Experimental short course preventive therapy of tuberculosis with rifampin and pyrazinamide. *Am Rev Respir Dis*, **140**, 1189–93.

47. Croule, A.J., Sbarbaro, J.A., Judson, F.N. and May, M.H. (1985) The effect of ethambutol on tubercle bacilli within cultured human macrophages. *Am Rev Respir Dis*, **132**, 742–5.

48. Gorzynski, E.A., Gutman, S.I. and Allen, W. (1989) Comparative antimycobacterial activities of difloxacin, temafloxacin, enoxacin, perfloxacin, reference fluoroquinolones, and a new macrolide clarithromycin. *Antimicrob Agents Chemother*, **33**, 591–2.

49. Horn, D.L., Hewlett, D., Alfalla, C. *et al.* (1994) Limited tolerance of ofloxacin and pyrazinamide prophylaxis against tuberculosis. *N Engl J Med*, **330**, 1241.

50. Dooley, S.W., Jarvis, W.R., Martone, W.J. and Snider, D.E. (1992) Multidrug-resistant tuberculosis. *Ann Intern Med*, 117, 257–8.

51. Brudney, K. and Dobkin, J. (1991) A tale of two cities: Tuberculosis control in Nicaragua and New York City. *Semin Resp Infect*, **6**, 261–72.

52. Pearson, M.L., Jereb, J.A., Frieden, T.R. *et al.* (1992) Nosocomial transmission of multidrug-resistant *Mycobacterium tuberculosis*: a risk to patients and health care workers. *Ann Intern Med*, **117**, 191–6.

53. Centers for Disease Control (1990) Nosocomial transmission of multidrug-resistant tuberculosis to the health care workers and HIV-infected patients in an urban hospital – Florida. *MMWR*, **39**, 718–22.

54. Centers for Disease Control (1991) Nosocomial transmission of multidrug-resistant tuberculosis among HIV-infected persons – Florida and New York, 1988–1991. *MMWR*, **40**, 585–91.

55. Edlin, B.R., Tokars, J.I., Grieco, M.H. *et al.* (1992) Nosocomial transmission of multidrug-resistant tuberculosis among AIDS patients: Epidemiologic studies and restriction fragment length polymorphism analysis. *N Engl J Med*, **326**, 1514–21.

56. Reves, R., Blakey, D., Snider, D.E. and Farer, L.S. (1981) Transmission of multiple drug-resistant tuberculosis: report of a school and community outbreak. *Am J Epidemiol*, **113**, 423–35.

57. Centers for Disease Control (1987) Outbreak of multidrug-resistant tuberculosis – North Carolina. *MMWR*, **35**, 785–7.

58. Centers for Disease Control (1990) Outbreak of multidrug-resistant tuberculosis – Texas, California, and Pennsylvania. *MMWR*, **39**, 369–72.

59. Nardell, E., McInnis, B., Thomas, B. and Weidhass, D. (1986) Exogenous reinfection with tuberculosis in a shelter for the homeless. *N Engl J Med*, **315**, 1570–5.

# Non-tuberculous mycobacterial infections

**14**

Edward K. Chapnick

## 14.1 INTRODUCTION

Non-tuberculous mycobacteria (NTM) are increasingly appreciated as human pathogens. Often isolated from the environment, it may be difficult to determine their pathogenicity in a clinical specimen. Therefore, it is essential to be aware of the epidemiology and presentations of disease caused by NTM in order to interpret culture results.

## 14.2 CLASSIFICATION

Using differences in growth characteristics, especially pigment production, Runyon described a useful classification system for NTM [1]. Group I, the photochromogens, are organisms which produce little or no pigment in the dark, but bright yellow, orange or red pigment when grown in light. Important members include *Mycobacterium kansasii*, *M. marinum* and *M. simiae*. The scotochromogens (Group II) produce yellow or orange pigment when grown in the dark. Members include *M. scrofulaceum*, *M. szulgai* and *M. gordonae*. Group III, the nonphotochromogens, includes *M. avium-intracellulare* ("Battey bacillus'), *M. xenopi*, *M. malmoense* and *M. ulcerans*. Finally, Group IV, the rapid growers, are distinguished by growth within 48 hours. This group includes *M. fortuitum*, *M. chelonae* and *M. smegmatis*.

## 14.3 EPIDEMIOLOGY

While the origin of NTM in a patient is invariably undetermined, environmental isolation of these organisms is common. Many NTM are ubiquitous and have been isolated from soil [2], pasteurized milk [3] and water [4]. In the latter report [4], contamination of a hospital water supply with NTM caused a pseudoepidemic, with falsely positive bronchoscopy specimens for acid-fast bacilli (AFB). Person-to-person transmission of these pathogens is felt to be rare. Most cases are likely to be due to environmental organisms acquired by inhalation, ingestion or inoculation [5].

The incidence and prevalence of NTM in the USA has been surveyed [6]. With isolates of NTM from over 5000 patients, *M. avium-intracellulare* was found to be the most common, accounting for over 50% of cases of disease. It was followed by *M. kansasii, M. fortuitum, M. scrofulaceum* and *M. chelonae*. Over 90% of the isolates were from respiratory specimens. The data is summarized in Table 14.1.

For patients with AIDS, *M. avium-intracellulare* is the most frequent NTM pathogen, accounting for 96% of cases of disseminated NTM infection [7,8].

## 14.4 DIAGNOSIS

Since NTM are found in the environment, isolation in a clinical specimen may represent contamination or colonization of the host. A thorough knowledge of clinical presentation and epidemiology is mandatory to decide if a given isolate is causing disease. While unique features for each pathogen exist, certain generalizations apply. The newer cultural techniques for TB (Chapter 7) can also be used for NTM. Certain organisms causing cutaneous infection, such as *M. chelonae, M. marinum* and *M. haemophilum* grow better at 28–32°C for primary isolation. *Mycobacterium xenopi* is thermophilic growing best at 42–43°C.

Pulmonary disease is the most common presentation of NTM, with systemic symptoms less common and less severe than those found with TB. X-ray manifestations are nonspecific. A miliary pattern is uncommon and the apical and posterior segments of the upper lobes are most often affected [9]. While cavitation occurs in a minority of patients with NTM pulmonary disease, when present the cavities are small and thin walled, compared with larger (over 5 cm) thick walled cavities in TB [9]. These findings are not diagnostic of NTM. Skin testing using antigens from NTM has not generally been helpful diagnostically [5,10]. In children with cervical lymphadenopathy, however, some NTM skin tests have been reported to be useful [11,12].

Specific criteria for the diagnosis of pulmonary disease due to NTM have been derived. In the presence of a cavitary infiltrate, NTM disease may be diagnosed when two or more sputa (or one sputum and a bronchial washing) are AFB smear positive and/or result in moderate to heavy growth of NTM on culture, and other reasonable causes for the disease process have been excluded [5]. If a noncavitary infiltrate is present, the

**Table 14.1** NTM surveillance reports received October 1981–September 1983 representing disease by species and source

| | M. avium | M. kansasii | M. fortuitum | M. scrofulaceum | M. chelonae | M. xenopi | M. simiae | M. marinum | M. szulgai | M. hemophilum | Total | (%) |
|---|---|---|---|---|---|---|---|---|---|---|---|---|
| Sputum | 967 | 417 | 60 | 22 | 36 | 7 | 9 | 2 | 4 | 0 | 1524 | (72.7) |
| Bronchial washing | 91 | 30 | 5 | 0 | 3 | 2 | 2 | 0 | 0 | 0 | 133 | (6.3) |
| Gastric aspirate | 5 | 2 | 0 | 0 | 1 | 0 | 0 | 3 | 0 | 0 | 11 | (0.5) |
| Lung tissue | 27 | 1 | 1 | 1 | 1 | 0 | 0 | 0 | 0 | 0 | 31 | (1.5) |
| Skin | 7 | 5 | 2 | 1 | 3 | 0 | 0 | 19 | 1 | 1 | 39 | (1.9) |
| Lymph nodes | 97 | 11 | 6 | 18 | 0 | 2 | 1 | 5 | 0 | 0 | 140 | (6.7) |
| Urine | 3 | 0 | 0 | 0 | 0 | 1 | 0 | 0 | 0 | 0 | 4 | (0.2) |
| Other tissue | 73 | 25 | 10 | 4 | 15 | 6 | 1 | 20 | 1 | 0 | 155 | (7.4) |
| Other fluid | 21 | 8 | 12 | 1 | 8 | 0 | 1 | 4 | 2 | 0 | 57 | (2.7) |
| Unknown | 2 | 1 | 0 | 0 | 0 | 0 | 0 | 0 | 0 | 0 | 3 | (0.1) |
| Total | 1293 | 500 | 96 | 47 | 67 | 18 | 14 | 53 | 8 | 1 | 2097 | |
| (%) | (61.7) | (23.8) | (4.6) | (2.2) | (3.2) | (0.9) | (0.7) | (2.5) | (0.4) | (0.0) | | |

Reproduced from [6] with permission of American Lung Association, copyright 1987.

diagnostic criteria are: two or more sputa (or one sputum and a bronchial washing) are AFB smear positive and/or result in moderate to heavy growth on culture; failure of the sputum cultures to convert to negative with either bronchial hygiene or 2 weeks of specific drug therapy; and other reasonable causes for disease have been excluded [5].

Although pleural fluid is regarded as normally sterile, isolation of NTM does not necessarily indicate pathogenicity. In one study of 22 patients with NTM in the pleural fluid, only three were felt to be pathogens [13]. One can only diagnose NTM in these cases if there is evidence of disease due to the same organism at other sites. Gribetz *et al.* [13] postulated that the NTM may multiply in a pleural effusion of another etiology without causing pathology.

Definitive diagnosis in areas such as lymph nodes, skin and bones requires isolation of the causative organism. While a lymph node with caseating granulomata in a patient with a negative tuberculin test suggests NTM as the cause [5], histopathology alone does not distinguish TB from NTM-induced lesions in pulmonary or lymphatic tissue [14].

### 14.5 *MYCOBACTERIUM KANSASII*

#### 14.5.1 Epidemiology

*Mycobacterium kansasii* is the second most common pathogenic NTM in the USA [6]. When isolated from clinical specimens, it has been classified as a pathogen in 75% [6]. It is also the second most common cause of NTM infection in AIDS patients, accounting for 2.9% of disseminated cases [7]. *Mycobacterium kansasii* has a definite distribution in the USA, with most cases from California, Texas, Louisiana, Illinois and Florida [15]. Humans seem to acquire it from the environment, without person-to-person transmission [16] with water being an important environmental source [17].

#### 14.5.2 Clinical syndromes reported

Pulmonary infection is the most common form of *M. kansasii* disease occurring mostly in patients with chronic pulmonary disease. In 47 cases of *M. kansasii* pulmonary disease, 72% had underlying lung disease, and chest X-rays were similar to those found in pulmonary TB [16]. Symptoms are also similar to TB, and can include chronic cough, fever, weight loss, night sweats and hemoptysis. Sputum AFB smears are positive in about 25% of cases, with cultures positive in 75% [16]. Slowly progressive or intermittent disease has persisted for up to 14 years in some untreated cases [18].

Tendon sheath infection and/or hand osteomyelitis may occur secondary to trauma [19] or steroid injections [20] in non-immunocompromised hosts. Osteomyelitis in other locations has been reported [21].

Cutaneous infection occurs from direct inoculation or hematogenous spread and can appear as a sporotrichoid pattern [22], cellulitis [23] or multiple plaque-like lesions [24]. AFB are usually seen in biopsy specimens or purulent drainage.

Cervical lymphadenitis in children occurs rarely [25]. Disseminated disease is extremely uncommon. Presentation includes fever, hepatospleno-megaly and leukopenia, with occasional lymphatic, bone, skin, genitourinary or gastrointestinal involvement [16]. Most cases occur in compromised hosts, with the prognosis related to their underlying disease [16].

### 14.5.3 Treatment

The treatment in non-HIV patients is uncomplicated, with the use of isoni-azid (INH), rifampin and ethambutol for 18 months [5,26]. *Mycobacterium kansasii* is less susceptible than *M. tuberculosis* to most drugs used in susceptibility testing [27], and may be reported as resistant when it is sensitive to levels only slightly higher than the cut off used for TB. Therefore, INH and streptomycin, when indicated, should be used as part of a rifampin containing regimen, even if resistance is reported [5]. Data from Great Britain suggest that treatment with rifampin and ethambutol, with or without INH, for only 9 months is effective [28]. Response to therapy is generally good.

Failure to respond can be due to resistance to rifampin. Ahn *et al.* treated nine patients who had failed other treatments with sulfameth-oxazole, high dose INH and ethambutol and 2–3 months of streptomycin, with success in eight of them [27]. Most strains are sensitive to ciprofloxacin and clarithromycin [26] and resistant to para-aminosalicylic acid (PAS), capreomycin and pyrazinamide (PZA). A follow-up 1994 report suggested the use of high dose INH (900 mg/day), streptomycin and clarithromycin for rifampin-resistant strains [28a].

### 14.5.4 Disease in patients with HIV

*Mycobacterium kansasii* had not been thought to be a common pathogen in AIDS patients. Of 1100 HIV-infected patients from Dallas, only 9 (less than 1%) were found to have *M. kansasii* compared with 160 with *M. avium-intracellulare* [29]. HIV-infected patients account for many cases of disseminated *M. kansasii*. Valainis, Cardona and Greer found that six of seven cases of disseminated disease were co-infected with HIV [30].

The infrequent occurrence of *M. kansasii* in HIV patients was questioned in a recent report [31]. Of 19 patients with *M. kansasii*, 17 had pulmonary involvement alone. It was found that the patients had CD4 counts greater than 200/mm$^3$ and nine had positive AFB sputum smears. Chest X-rays showed diffuse infiltrates in nine and upper lobe infiltrates in eight. Treatment was associated with improvement. *Mycobacterium kansasii* resembled TB clinically but occurred at later stages of HIV disease.

It may also cause disseminated disease in HIV patients, with involvement of the gastrointestinal tract [31], blood [29,30], lymph nodes [29, 31], CNS [29,32,33], liver [29] and bone [31]. Since these cases occur in severely compromised hosts, often with multiple opportunistic infections, the contribution of *M. kansasii* to the outcome can be difficult to assess.

The proper treatment for *M. kansasii* in patients with HIV infection has not been determined. While some feel that the organism should always be treated when isolated from an HIV-infected patient [30], others state that treatment is only indicated if invasive disease is present [34].

## 14.6 *MYCOBACTERIUM MARINUM*

### 14.6.1 Epidemiology

*Mycobacterium marinum* is a photochromogenic organism which grows best at cooler temperatures (31–33°C). It was described as a human pathogen in 1951 [35], after isolation from skin lesions associated with swimming pool exposure. It has caused skin infections linked to aquaria [36] or to salt or brackish water [37,38]. The organism has been referred to as *M. platypoecilus* and *M. balnei* in older literature. In the USA, *M. marinum* has been reported to cause 2.5% of NTM infections [6]. About 75% of isolates are from skin or soft tissue, reflecting temperature-related growth characteristics.

### 14.6.2 Clinical syndromes reported

*Mycobacterium marinum* skin and soft tissue lesions may present as verrucous granulomas, draining sinuses, sporotrichoid nodules, tenosynovitis, bursitis or arthritis [37]. The incubation period after trauma or exposure averages 2 weeks. Most lesions are asymptomatic and not associated with lymphadenopathy. Histology reveals nonspecific inflammation early in disease, followed by granulomas, with AFB stains usually negative [36,38]. The most commonly involved sites are the fingers, hands and knees.

Disseminated cutaneous disease has been reported in immunocompromised patients [39,40]. In the latter case [40], the illness was exacerbated by steroids and occurred 2 years after a puffer fish sting. Disseminated cutaneous disease in immunologically normal hosts has been reported [41,42]. In one case [42], the affected infant had been bathed in a tub in which her father had cleaned an aquarium.

Visceral involvement with *M. marinum* is extremely uncommon. A case of disseminated cutaneous *M. marinum* with presumed involvement of the liver and lung has been reported [43]. Sclerokeratitis associated with topical steroid use has been reported [44]. *Mycobacterium marinum* can cause septic bursitis, often linked to corticosteroid injections and/or water contact. Of 50 joint isolates of NTM, *M. marinum* was the most frequently isolated species (40%) [45]. Osteomyelitis and synovitis have also been described [46].

### 14.6.3 Treatment

*In vitro* susceptibility testing has shown *M. marinum* to be susceptible to amikacin and the tetracyclines [47,48]. Rifampin and ethambutol have variable activity [47] and resistance has been reported to gentamicin [48], quinolones [47] and to INH and PAS [47]. Variable sensitivity has been reported to trimethoprim/sulfamethoxazole [47,48].

Response to treatment for *M. marinum* infections is generally good. Successful results have been obtained with minocycline [49], tetracycline [50], trimethoprim/sulfamethoxazole [5], ciprofloxacin [26] or clarithromycin [50a] for cutaneous disease. In cases of treatment failure or more serious infection, rifampin alone or combined with INH or ethambutol has been effective [51]. Treatment should be continued for at least 2–3 months [5,50,52].

While medical treatment alone is effective for superficial skin infections, the role of surgery in deeper infections, usually of the hand, is controversial. In 24 cases of infection of the deep structures of the hand, only 10 required surgical debridement [52]. Surgery was used only in patients who failed to respond to medical treatment (rifampin and ethambutol) or who had persistent pain, a discharging sinus, or a previous local steroid injection. Others recommend debridement and medical treatment (minocycline) for all cases of *M. marinum* infections of the deep structures of the hand [53]. Surgery may prolong healing in superficial disease [36,53].

### 14.6.4 Disease in HIV patients

*Mycobacterium marinum* is generally not mentioned as an opportunistic infection in HIV patients. It has been reported to cause disseminated cutaneous disease which responded to INH, rifampin and ethambutol [54], and disseminated infection including skin, blood, bone marrow and bronchial washings, which did not respond to treatment with clofazimine, ciprofloxacin and ethionamide [55]. There are insufficient data to make treatment recommendations.

## 14.7 *MYCOBACTERIUM GORDONAE*

### 14.7.1 Epidemiology

*Mycobacterium gordonae* is also known as *M. aquae*. It has been referred to as the 'tap water bacillus', and is found in aquarium water [56]. It is, therefore, not surprising that pseudoepidemics of this organism have been associated with cleaning bronchoscopes with contaminated water [57]. Since it is commonly found in the environment and rarely documented to cause disease, *M. gordonae* is generally considered to be a contaminant or colonizer when isolated from clinical specimens. One report [58] noted that two of 14 isolates of *M. gordonae* were pathogenic. In an extensive review of NTM [6], *M. gordonae* is not listed as a pathogen.

### 14.7.2 Clinical syndromes reported

*Mycobacterium gordonae* may be associated with chronic cavitary pulmonary disease similar to TB. The illness most often occurs in patients with pre-existing lung disease, involving the upper lobes [59]. Since most isolates do not represent disease, care must be taken to evaluate their significance critically. Localized infections are similarly uncommon. Keratitis has been reported to occur after ocular surgery and topical steroid therapy [60] and after trauma [61]. Peritonitis in a patient receiving continuous ambulatory peritoneal dialysis [62] and synovitis [63] have also been reported.

Disseminated infection has occurred, most often affecting immunocompromised patients, including disease involving the liver and peritoneum [64] and the lung, liver, CSF and kidney [65]. Biopsy specimens in both cases showed noncaseating granulomas. Disseminated disease involving the liver and bone marrow associated with prosthetic valve endocarditis has been found in a normal host [66]. Additionally, cases of disseminated infection involving the lung, urine and liver [67] and lung and bone marrow [68] in immunologically normal hosts have been reported.

### 14.7.3 Treatment

Based on anecdotal reports [57–65], *M. gordonae* has been generally found to be sensitive to rifampin, ethambutol and aminoglycosides and resistant to INH. The organism also appears to be sensitive to clarithromycin [69]. Response to therapy has been good in individual reports, when INH, rifampin and ethambutol, with or without an aminoglycoside, were used. Valve replacement was needed for cure of prosthetic valve endocarditis [66] and removal of the peritoneal dialysis catheter seemed to result in improvement of peritonitis [62]. Topical amikacin with surgery was effective for keratitis [60,61], and surgical debridement with medical therapy resulted in resolution of synovitis [63]. Disseminated disease has responded to chemotherapy [59]. Owing to the small number of cases, the optimal therapeutic regimen and length of therapy are unknown.

### 14.7.4 Disease in HIV patients

*Mycobacterium gordonae* may be responsible for disseminated disease in patients with AIDS, accounting for 0.6% of 1984 cases of disseminated NTM disease [7]. Three of five respiratory isolates of *M. gordonae* in patients with HIV infection represented disease [68]. Two had AFB on sputum stain, and all three responded to combination therapy. When isolated from pulmonary secretions of HIV patients, especially those with AIDS, *M. gordonae* appears to be more likely to be a pathogen and should be treated if there is any evidence of lung disease.

## 14.8 *MYCOBACTERIUM SCROFULACEUM*

### 14.8.1 Epidemiology

*Mycobacterium scrofulaceum* is the fourth most common NTM isolated in the USA, with 22% of isolates representing disease [6]. The organism, which has some genetic similarities with the *M. avium-intracellulare* complex has been found in water [56] and household dust [70], suggesting a significant environmental presence. Individuals with *M. scrofulaceum* lung disease are more likely to have occupational dust exposure than those with infections due to other NTM [71].

### 14.8.2 Clinical syndromes reported

The most common manifestation of *M. scrofulaceum* is cervical lymphadenitis in children [72]. Occurring most often in children 1–5 years of age, it is usually painless and without systemic symptoms. Histopathology of involved lymph nodes does not reliably distinguish between NTM and TB [73].

In adults, the most common presentation is pulmonary, with a clinical illness similar to TB [74]. The majority of sputum isolates of *M. scrofulaceum* do not represent disease. In one study [74], the organism was felt to be a pathogen in only one of 71 patients, while another study [6] showed *M. scrofulaceum* to be pathogenic in 22 of 175 pulmonary isolates (12.6%). It has also been reported to cause chronic soft tissue infection [75], and deeper infections involving tendons, joints and bursae [76]. Many of the musculoskeletal cases were preceded by local steroid injections. A case of granulomatous hepatitis in a healthy man has also been reported [77].

Disseminated disease may also occur. As with other NTM, this tends to occur in compromised hosts. Examples include documented hepatic involvement in a patient on chemotherapy [78] and *M. scrofulaceum* found in the lung, liver, bone marrow, urine and aural discharge in a steroid-treated patient [79]. In both cases, noncaseating granulomas were seen in the involved organs.

### 14.8.3 Treatment

For cervical lymphadenitis caused by *M. scrofulaceum*, excision alone is the recommended treatment [80]. Incisional or needle biopsy should be avoided because of the possibility of chronic sinus tract formation.

*In vitro* testing generally shows the organism to be resistant to INH, streptomycin, ethambutol and PAS [15] and to cefoxitin and amikacin [81]. It has been found to be sensitive to cycloserine [77,78], erythromycin [82] and clarithromycin [69].

With a dearth of available clinical data, it is impossible to determine the optimal regimen. Wolinsky [26] recommends treatment as for *M. avium-intracellulare*, with INH, rifampin, ethambutol and an aminoglycoside. Clinical success has been reported with INH, rifampin and cycloserine for granulomatous hepatitis [77] and with INH, ethambutol and streptomycin for disseminated disease [78]. In the latter case, treatment success was obtained despite *in vitro* resistance to all agents used. Resection may be needed for refractory pulmonary disease [74].

Based on the above, it seems reasonable to treat infection (except cervical adenitis) with combination therapy using INH, ethambutol, cycloserine and/or a macrolide agent.

### 14.8.4 Disease in the HIV patients

Patients infected with HIV may be more prone to disseminated infection with *M. scrofulaceum*. Both patients with disseminated *M. scrofulaceum* infection in one series [83] had AIDS.

## 14.9 *MYCOBACTERIUM AVIUM-INTRACELLULARE*

Human disease due to *M. avium* was described in 1943 [84]. Because of clinical and microbiologic similarities between *M. avium* and *M. intracellulare*, they are usually not differentiated, and are reported as *M. avium-intracellulare* (MAI). Newer diagnostic testing using gene probes provides the tools to distinguish these organisms [85].

### 14.9.1 Epidemiology

MAI is the most common NTM isolate in the USA, representing about 50% of the total [6]. As with most NTM, MAI is ubiquitous in the environment and has been found in house dust [70], as well as in water from taps, lakes, rivers and ponds [56]. In nature, it is found in higher numbers in swamps in the southeastern USA with higher temperature, lower pH and lower oxygen content [86]. Water may be the source of nosocomial infections with MAI. The organism has been found in hospital water taps, especially hot water and those that produce aerosols (i.e. showers) [87].

### 14.9.2 Clinical syndromes reported

The most common presentation of MAI is pulmonary infection. Many isolates, however, still represent colonization rather than disease. Patients with thoracic disease are at higher risk of being colonized or infected with MAI. Patients with MAI pulmonary infection are significantly more likely than the general population to have pectus excavatum (27% *versus* 2.4%) or scoliosis (52% *versus* 1%) [88]. In a 1991 series of patients with MAI pulmonary disease [89], 12 of 29 had pre-existing chronic lung disease. An indolent productive cough was common, but fever and constitutional symptoms may not occur. Patients without underlying lung disease, more commonly women, are more likely to have nodular infiltrates and less likely to have cavitation [90].

While most mycobacterial lymphadenitis in adults is caused by TB, MAI has eclipsed *M. scrofulaceum* as the most common cause in children [91]. As is true for *M. scrofulaceum*, lymphadenitis due to MAI is indistinguishable histologically from other mycobacteria [92]. It is not accompanied by systemic symptoms and is generally cured by excision alone [80].

Other localized infections due to MAI are uncommon, but varied. Skin involvement may be chronic and localized [93] or generalized [94]. In the latter case, bone involvement was also present in an otherwise healthy patient. Chronic meningitis with a mass lesion due to MAI has been reported in an immunologically normal adult, which may have been related to a ventricular shunt [95]. MAI has also been reported to cause mastoiditis [96] and a corneal ulcer [97]. Reported cardiac disease due to MAI has included endocarditis in an intravenous drug user [98] and pacemaker infection in an apparently healthy, but malnourished woman [99]. Disease involving the gastrointestinal and genitourinary tracts has also been reported, manifesting as a gastric ulcer [100] and as granulomatous prostatitis [101]. Tenosynovitis due to this organism has been reviewed [102]. All reported cases have involved the hand, suggesting direct inoculation. Disseminated osteomyelitis with or without lung involvement may also occur [103,104].

MAI is the most common cause of disseminated NTM infection. In a review of 37 cases in non-AIDS patients [105], 20 were immunosuppressed. Symptoms included fever, weight loss, night sweats, chills and anorexia. Examination most often revealed fever, nodular skin lesions or rash, hepatosplenomegaly and lymphadenopathy. Chest X-rays were usually abnormal but non-specific. The most commonly involved sites were bone marrow, lung, bone, liver and lymph nodes, with granulomas, usually non-caseating, seen in most. AFB were generally not seen. In children, disseminated MAI disease is uncommon, with 36% of reported cases occurring in immunocompromised hosts [106]. Some cases of disseminated infection with MAI occur in patients with idiopathic CD4 and T-lymphocytopenia and others have been described in families [106a].

### 14.9.3 Treatment

In lung disease, the decision whether to treat must be based on the condition of the patient. If treatment is planned, it may be with the intent to cure or merely to halt its progression. Treatment may be withheld because of advanced age, slowly or nonprogressive disease, paucity of symptoms or concurrent medical illness [89]. Treatment with intent to suppress may be used in those judged to be too frail to tolerate a multiple drug regimen.

*In vitro*, MAI is generally resistant to INH, PAS and aminoglycosides, with variable sensitivity to ethambutol, rifampin, ethionamide, cycloserine and clofazimine [107], as well as to erythromycin [82]. It is sensitive to clarithromycin [69]. Response to multi-drug therapy for pulmonary disease has nonetheless been good. In one report, 15 of 16 patients treated with intent to cure responded, and only one of these relapsed [89]. Another report [107] found that 50 of 75 patients treated with six drugs responded to treatment, with responders having received more medications to which their isolate was susceptible. Empiric treatment was suggested, with regimens based on sensitivity only for relapses or for patients with life threatening disease. A favorable response to four drug treatment (INH, rifampin, ethambutol and streptomycin) in 42 of 46 patients has been shown [108]. These authors recommend at least 24 months of therapy, with streptomycin for the first 6 months.

For pulmonary disease due to MAI, the American Thoracic Society (ATS) recommends the use of INH, rifampin and ethambutol with streptomycin for the first 3–6 months, regardless of susceptibility testing results [5]. If intolerance occurs, cycloserine or ethionamide can be substituted. For treatment failures, multiple drug regimens including cycloserine, ethionamide and/or streptomycin may be used. Clofazimine or ciprofloxacin have also been utilized. For localized pulmonary disease which does not respond to medical therapy, cure may be achieved with lung resection [109]. If a solitary pulmonary nodule is removed and found to be due to MAI, no further therapy is recommended [110].

There has been only anecdotal experience with other localized disease due to MAI. In addition to appropriate chemotherapy, surgical debridement is recommended for mastoiditis [96], prostatitis [101] and tenosynovitis [102]. Replacement of an infected aortic valve [98] and removal of an infected pacemaker [99] were also needed for cure.

For disseminated disease, treatment regimens identical to those used for pulmonary disease are recommended [5]. In one series [105], 24 of 33 treated patients responded, with a better outcome in patients receiving cycloserine or clofazimine. A recommendation was made for initial therapy with INH, ethambutol, cycloserine, clofazimine and ethionamide. A 1994 report [106a] suggested that interferon gamma can be useful in some cases of disseminated disease refractory to standard therapy.

### 14.9.4 Disease in HIV patients

Disseminated infection with MAI was noted in homosexual men and intravenous drug users before AIDS was well described [111]. The incidence of disseminated MAI in AIDS patients in the USA and Europe has been increasing, as survival lengthens [112]. However, it appears to be less common in African AIDS patients for unclear reasons, despite frequent environmental isolation of the organism [113]. The clinical characteristics of AIDS patients with MAI have been well described [114]. Those with MAI were more likely to have weight loss, abdominal pain, diarrhea, a normal pulmonary examination and lower CD4 cell counts. Granuloma formation was poor or absent. The best diagnostic test was blood culture which had an 86% yield. In another study, disseminated MAI was found almost exclusively in individuals with less than 100 CD4 cells/mm$^3$ and was significantly associated with an elevated serum alkaline phosphatase level [112].

In HIV patients, it is important to distinguish TB from MAI when AFB are found. *Mycobacterium tuberculosis* infection is more likely to be the first manifestation of HIV disease and MAI tends to present later. In addition, most MAI-infected patients have had a prior opportunistic infection. Compared with patients with TB, those with MAI are less likely to have localized lymphadenopathy or pulmonary disease, have a lower CD4 count and are more likely to be bacteremic [115]. Cavitary infiltrates are uncommon in both entities.

Cutaneous manifestations of MAI may occur, including ulcers in the perianal area [115,116] and at intravenous sites [116]. Purple colored lesions [117] can appear similar to Kaposi's sarcoma or bacillary epithelioid angiomatosis and underscores the importance of biopsy for diagnosis.

Treatment regimens for AIDS patients with disseminated MAI are changing. Early studies showed that combination therapy including rifabutin and clofazimine was ineffective [118]. In 1990, however, two separate studies [119,120] found sustained decreases or elimination of MAI bacteremia and symptomatic improvement for up to 22 weeks using four drug regimens. Chin *et al.* [119] used ethambutol, rifampin and ciprofloxacin, with amikacin for the first 4 weeks. Roy *et al.* [120] used INH, rifabutin, clofazimine and ethambutol.

More recently, clarithromycin [69] and azithromycin [121] have been shown to be effective *in vitro* for MAI. Because of the high intracellular levels of these drugs, organisms resistant *in vitro* to serum levels often respond well to therapy. A controlled study showed clarithromycin to reduce MAI bacteremia in AIDS patients [122]. Additionally, rifabutin has been shown to be effective in delaying or preventing MAI bacteremia in AIDS patients [123].

MAI may become resistant to monotherapy with clarithromycin [124]. Therefore, this agent is often combined with ethambutol and/or clofazimine, with very promising results [125]. Serious infections should be treated with a four drug regimen [119,120] with a macrolide-based treatment for less severe disease.

### 14.10 *MYCOBACTERIUM XENOPI*

#### 14.10.1 Epidemiology

*Mycobacterium xenopi* was isolated from toads in 1959 [126]. It is an unusual US isolate, accounting for 2.7% of NTM, with 25% of isolates representing disease [6]. Europe and Canada, however, have a higher incidence. *Mycobacterium xenopi* is the second most common NTM isolate in England [127] and Ontario, Canada [128].

As is true for many NTM, *M. xenopi* can be found in the environment, and has been isolated from hospital and residential water taps [129], being thermophilic it is more common in hot water taps.

#### 14.10.2 Clinical syndromes reported

The most common site of infection is the lung. Since optimal growth occurs at 42–43°C, it should be suspected in patients with AFB on sputum smears, but no growth at 37°C. Simor, Salit and Vellend [128] reported 28 patients from Toronto with positive cultures of which nine were pathogenic. The eight cases of pulmonary infection presented as a chronic, indolent illness with pre-existing pulmonary disease and cavitation on chest X-ray. Nosocomial pulmonary disease can occur [130]. Of note, 17 of 19 patients had pre-existing lung disease and seven were asymptomatic.

#### 14.10.3 Treatment

*In vitro* testing can show the organism to be sensitive to most agents, including INH, rifampin, ethambutol, PAS and aminoglycosides [81,128, 131]. Some, however, found resistance to ethambutol in 100%, and to rifampin in 80% of strains tested [130]. Response to treatment of pulmonary disease is moderate, with most patients responding symptomatically and with sputum conversion. In the series from Ontario with a higher rate of resistance, however, five of seven treated patients relapsed after therapy [128]. Another series from Ontario also found a high rate of resistance (over 50% of strains) to primary anti-TB medications and a 29% sputum conversion rate (10 of 34) [132].

Treatment for *M. xenopi* is controversial. ATS [5] and Wolinsky [26] recommend INH, rifampin and ethambutol, with or without the initial use of streptomycin. The Canadian group, however, suggests the use of ethambutol, ethionamide and streptomycin, with or without rifampin [128]. In the USA, where there is lower incidence of resistance, the former seems reasonable. Treatment should be continued for at least 18 months. For refractory or relapsing disease, the use of cycloserine and/or clarithromycin may be considered [26].

### 14.10.4 Disease in HIV patients

*Mycobacterium xenopi* has rarely been reported as a pathogen in HIV patients, but colonization does occur. In a series from Brooklyn, New York, 23 of 33 isolates of *M. xenopi* were from patients infected with HIV [83]. Pulmonary disease due to *M. xenopi* has been described as a first manifestation of HIV infection [133].

Disseminated disease is rare. Of 1984 disseminated NTM infections in US AIDS patients, none were due to *M. xenopi* [7]. A case of pulmonary *M. xenopi* was reported with hepatic granulomas in an AIDS patient whose disease responded to treatment with INH, rifampin and PZA [134]. Two cases of nosocomial disseminated *M. xenopi* in AIDS patients occurred, with concurrent growth of the organism from the hospital hot water [135].

## 14.11 *MYCOBACTERIUM ULCERANS*

### 14.11.1 Epidemiology

First described in Australia [136], it has subsequently been found to occur in Equatorial Africa, New Guinea, Mexico, French Guyana and Malaysia [137]. Infection is most common in individuals who live near a body of water [138]. The mode of acquisition is unknown. Attempts to isolate the organism from environmental water sources have been unsuccessful [138]. Infection with *M. ulcerans* acquired in the USA or Europe has not been reported, but it may first present in an immigrant from an endemic area after arrival [139].

### 14.11.2 Clinical syndromes reported

Infection with *M. ulcerans* involves the skin and adjacent structures [140], beginning with a subcutaneous swelling or nodule. Most common on the extremities, the lesions are rarely painful but may be pruritic, are usually single and not accompanied by a systemic illness. Histopathology usually shows AFB without granulomas [140]. The overlying skin then desquamates, loses pigmentation and ulcerates. More aggressive lesions, involving large areas, may not be preceded by a subcutaneous nodule [140].

With progression to ulceration, involvement proceeds to the deep fascia, but does not involve muscle [137]. AFB can be seen in clumps, with the greatest concentration at the center of the lesions [141].

Owing to the lack of medical facilities in endemic areas, the diagnosis is usually clinical. Suggested criteria include ulcer edges which are widely undermined, subcutaneous tissue necrosis and shiny hyperpigmented skin surrounding the ulcer [142].

Osteomyelitis due to *M. ulcerans* has been reported from West Africa [143]. Bone specimens revealed AFB and the organism was identified by DNA amplification and gene probe.

### 14.11.3 Treatment

The mainstay of treatment is surgery with simple excision curative at the pre-ulcerative stage [140]. For later stages, excision with repeated skin grafting is needed. Chemotherapy alone is not indicated [15,141]. Trimethoprim/sulfamethoxazole has been reported to be both effective [138] and ineffective [142], and clofazimine may be of minimal benefit [138]. Streptomycin and dapsone, with or without ethambutol, for at least 2 weeks after healing of the surgical wound has been recommended [15]. Osteomyelitis responded to therapy with INH, rifampin, ethambutol and PZA followed by clarithromycin and trimethoprim/sulfamethoxazole [142].

### 14.11.4 Disease in HIV patients

Several AIDS patients have been reported to have indolent leg ulcers due to *M. ulcerans* [8,143a]. The lesion responded to treatment with rifabutin and amikacin in one case and rifampin/clarithromycin in another.

## 14.12 *MYCOBACTERIUM FORTUITUM-CHELONAE* COMPLEX

Owing to similarities between *M. fortuitum* and *M. chelonae*, they are discussed together as *M. fortuitum-chelonae* complex (MFC). Both grow on routine bacteriologic media, as well as those specific for mycobacteria, in 7 days or less. The species *M. fortuitum* has three biovariants: *fortuitum, peregrinum,* and an unnamed third biovariant. *Mycobacterium chelonae* may be divided into three subspecies: *chelonae, abscessus* and '*M. chelonae*-like'. While the groups have similar clinical presentations, antibiotic susceptibility and therapy differ. *Mycobacterium chelonae* subsp. *absessus* is called *M. absessus* by some.

### 14.12.1 Epidemiology

*Mycobacterium fortuitum* and *M. chelonae* account for 14% of NTM isolates in the USA, with 23% representing disease [6]. In a review of 125 cases of infection, the skin (59%) was the most common site, followed by lung (14%), disseminated disease (7%), eye (4%), prosthetic heart valve (3%) and cervical lymph node (3%) [144].

Nosocomial epidemics and pseudoepidemics of MFC are not uncommon. MFC is found in water and has been responsible for pseudoepidemics from contaminated water used to clean bronchoscopes [57]. Thirty patients developed sputum colonization with *M. fortuitum* in one hospital ward, which was traced to a contaminated ice machine [145]. Post-surgical infections have been reported from a variety of procedures. Instruments cleaned with tap water containing *M. chelonae* have been implicated in outbreaks of otitis media [146] and post-rhinoplasty nasal cellulitis [147].

Three cases of *M. chelonae* keratitis were reported in patients treated in one private office [148], with no clear source.

The most common surgical procedures to be associated with MFC are augmentation mammaplasty and cardiac surgery. In the USA, MFC sternal wound infections are more likely to be due to *M. fortuitum* and to occur in the Southern coastal states [149]. Local environmental contamination is felt to occur. Each reported outbreak has been with a distinctive strain [149]. In 1977, eight of 16 porcine heart valves were retrospectively found to be contaminated with *M. chelonae* [150], but none of the patients receiving the valves developed endocarditis. Other reports have included *M. chelonae* bacteremia associated with hemodialysis [151] and soft tissue infections from electromyography electrodes rinsed with contaminated tap water [152]. Soft tissue infections associated with plastic surgery have been traced to a gentian violet skin marking solution contaminated with *M. chelonae* [153]. All of the outbreaks abated when cleaning procedures were changed to avoid or sterilize the water supply involved.

### 14.12.2 Clinical syndromes reported

*Mycobacterium chelonae* is a more common cause of pulmonary disease than *M. fortuitum* [144]. Patients may not have underlying disease, with only five of 24 in one series having pre-existing pulmonary abnormalities [144]. Most patients have unilateral patchy infiltrates without cavitation [144]. *Mycobacterium fortuitum* has presented as an enlarging lung nodule with a negative bronchoalveolar lavage [154].

Mineral oil aspiration [155] and achalasia [156] have been reported to predispose to infection with MFC. In the former, routine AFB smears may be negative because the bacilli are lost with the oil during preparation. Contact smears of lung tissue may be necessary. In achalasia, the retained food in the esophagus could provide a medium for the growth of MFC. Patients with cystic fibrosis may also develop infection with MFC [157].

MFC cutaneous disease may be local or disseminated. Local disease is often due to trauma or surgical wounds. The most common presentation is a localized abscess or cellulitis, with no systemic symptoms, pulmonary involvement or underlying medical illness. AFB are seen in wound drainage or biopsy specimens. Most patients have a history of injury with soil or water contact. MFC subcutaneous abscesses have been found at immunization sites [158]. Cutaneous infection with a sporotrichoid pattern has also been described [159].

*Mycobacterium fortuitum* is more frequent than *M. chelonae* as a cause of surgical wound infection [144,160]. Median sternotomy wound infections present with failure to heal or wound breakdown with serous drainage containing AFB on stain. Infections of mammaplasty wounds present with pain and swelling without significant systemic symptoms. While the source is likely to be environmental, the finding of a spontaneous nontraumatic MFC abscess suggests that MFC may be part of the normal flora of the nipple or breast [160].

As with most NTM, disseminated disease, often presenting as nodular skin lesions, occurs mostly in immunocompromised hosts. One reported case also had involvement of the bone, with granulomas on biopsy [161]. Disseminated disease may also occur in the immunocompetent host [162]. *Mycobacterium chelonae* is responsible for most cases of disseminated MFC disease [144,163]. Infection related to intravenous catheters occurs most often in patients receiving chemotherapy. In these cases, either *M. fortuitum* or *M. chelonei* may be responsible, and skin lesions are uncommon [164].

Bacteremia due to MFC may also occur secondary to endocarditis. Cases have been reported with both species and may involve bioprosthetic [165], metallic [166] or native [167] heart valves. Virtually all reported cases have been fatal.

In addition to disease associated with hemodialysis, MFC may cause peritonitis with peritoneal dialysis. Since no cases of spontaneous MFC peritonitis have been reported, it is likely due to catheter or site contamination [168]. *Mycobacterium fortuitum* is a more frequent cause than *M. chelonae* [169]. Clinical findings include a predominance of neutrophils in the fluid, a positive AFB stain and granulomas on peritoneal biopsy [169]. The diagnosis may be missed unless the laboratory is instructed to hold the specimen for more than 48 hours.

### 14.12.3 Treatment

Before treating MFC, it is important to verify its identification. MFC may appear Gram positive and be dismissed as 'diphtheroids'. In addition, the bacilli may appear as chains and be confused with *Nocardia* sp. This has occurred in the author's personal experience, when a patient with bacteremia due to *M. fortuitum* was initially diagnosed and treated for nocardiosis. It has also been reported in the literature [170].

MFC susceptibility testing is reliable in predicting clinical efficacy. In one study [171], 68 of 76 patients with *M. fortuitum* (90%) and 34 of 47 patients with *M. chelonei* (72%) responded to such therapy. In general, *M. fortuitum* is more sensitive than *M. chelonae*. In a study of susceptibility of 300 strains of MFC to ß-lactam agents, most strains were moderately susceptible to cefoxitin but neither cefoxitin nor cefmetazole had any activity against *M. chelonae* subsp. *chelonae*. Amoxicillin/clavulanic acid was only active against *M. fortuitum* and imipenem was the most active ß-lactam and the only one to inhibit *M. chelonae* subsp. *chelonae* (39% of isolates were sensitive) [172]. Amikacin is active against all strains of both organisms [173], doxycycline inhibits some strains of *M. fortuitum* (56%) and *M. chelonae* (23%) [173], and sulfamethoxazole is active against *M. fortuitum* but not *M. chelonae* [26]. The quinolones have good activity against

*M. fortuitum*, but are poor for *M. chelonae* [174]. The newer macrolides have good activity against both *M. fortuitum* and *M. chelonae*, with clarithromycin the most effective *in vitro* [175].

For lung disease, treatment may be withheld if the illness is minimally or not progressive [5]. With progressive disease, a regimen of amikacin and cefoxitin is used, with consideration of tobramycin rather than amikacin for *M. chelonae* subsp. *chelonae* [26]. Quinolone monotherapy has been anecdotally shown to be effective for *M. fortuitum* lung disease [176] and prolonged treatment with trimethoprim/sulfamethoxazole can be used for sensitive strains [177]. Imipenem alone may be used for *M. chelonae* [176]. Length of treatment is not well established, but should be at least 8 weeks.

Surgical treatment may be indicated for localized disease due to *M. chelonae* [178], although most patients respond to chemotherapy [179]. If the lesions do not respond to incision and drainage, wide excision is indicated, with antibiotic therapy for at least 3 months [180]. Debridement and antibiotic therapy are indicated for surgical wound infections, with one report of success in two of three patients treated with ofloxacin for 3–4 months after sternal debridement [181]. In addition to appropriate antibiotic therapy, removal of prosthetic devices infected with MFC is necessary [164,165,168,169]. In catheter-related infections, removal alone is sufficient if bacteremia is not present [164].

In disseminated disease, the results of treatment depend on the underlying medical condition. Patients with lesser degrees of immunosuppression have a survival rate of 90%, but those with more immunosuppressive illnesses have a 10% survival [163].

### 14.12.4 Disease in HIV patients

MFC caused 10 of 1984 cases (0.5%) of disseminated NTM infection in AIDS patients [7]. Case reports of MFC infection in AIDS patients are uncommon. One case of relapsing *M. fortuitum* pneumonia was reported which was cured surgically [182]. Another case of disseminated disease involving skin and bone was successfully treated with cefoxitin and amikacin followed by ciprofloxacin and doxycycline [183].

## 14.13 INFREQUENTLY ISOLATED NTM SPECIES

### 14.13.1 *Mycobacterium simiae*

*(a) Epidemiology*

*Mycobacterium simiae* was isolated from monkeys in 1965 [184]. It has been infrequently reported as a human pathogen, with the mode of transmission to humans unknown. The organism has, however, been isolated from hospital tap water [25]. *M. simiae* has been reported to cause 0.9% of

NTM disease in the USA, with virtually all cases involving the lung and 21% of isolates classified as causing disease [6].

### (b) Clinical syndromes reported

The largest series of clinical isolates of *M. simiae* was reported in 1983 [185]. Five patients with underlying diseases and definite or probable *M. simiae* pulmonary disease are described, with isolates from 19 patients not felt to be pathogenic. When obtained, lung tissue showed caseating granulomas. Two cases of disseminated disease have been reported [186]. One was a co-infection with *M. kansasii* of kidney and bone marrow which improved with eradication of *M. kansasii*; the other was isolated from bone and stabilized without specific treatment.

### (c) Treatment

Owing to the small number of reported cases, the optimal regimen is not known. The organism is often resistant *in vitro* to all anti-TB drugs except ethionamide and cycloserine [15]. It is one of only two species of NTM to be resistant *in vitro* to clarithromycin [69]. Response to treatment has generally been poor [185]. In a case of mixed infection with MAI in an AIDS patient [187], *M. simiae* was eradicated from the blood with ethionamide and cycloserine.

### (d) Disease in HIV patients

In a large series of cases of NTM infection in AIDS patients [7], no cases of *M. simiae* were reported. There have been two reports of mixed infection with *M. avium-intracellulare* and *M. simiae* [187,188]. One was lost to follow-up [188] and the other died with progressive MAI disease despite eradication of *M. simiae* from the blood [187].

### 14.13.2 *Mycobacterium szulgai*

#### (a) Epidemiology

*Mycobacterium szulgai* has been reported to cause 0.4% of US cases of NTM disease, with 57% of isolates classified as pathogenic [6]. Most isolates have been from the respiratory tract.

#### (b) Clinical syndromes reported

*Mycobacterium szulgai* was reported as a human pathogen in 1973 [189]. The report described five cases of pulmonary disease, three with chronic, productive cough and cavitary infiltrates and four with smears positive for AFB. None had pre-existing lung disease.

Involvement of other organs is rare. Olecranon bursitis [190], cervical adenitis [191], tenosynovitis [192] and cellulitis [193] have been reported. There has been one reported case of disseminated disease, with involvement of skin, lymph nodes and bone in an otherwise healthy male [194].

### (c) Treatment

With small numbers of cases, it is difficult to define treatment. In the largest *in vitro* study (23 strains) more than 50% of isolates were susceptible to streptomycin, capreomycin, INH and rifampin, with less sensitivity to ethambutol, cycloserine, PAS and PZA [195]. *Mycobacterium szulgai* appears to be susceptible to clarithromycin *in vitro* [69]. With the exception of the case of disseminated disease, in which lesions progressed despite five medications [194], response to therapy has been good.

Treatment should include at least three drugs to which the isolate is susceptible, with INH, rifampin and ethambutol being a reasonable initial regimen [15,32,190]. The proper length of treatment is unclear, but therapy should be continued for at least 9–12 months after sputum cultures become negative [190] or until disease resolves at extrapulmonary sites. If therapy fails or is poorly tolerated, amikacin and cefoxitin may be tried [81].

### (d) Disease in HIV patients

Two isolates of *M. szulgai* have been reported from patients with AIDS [196]. Clinical details were not provided.

### 14.13.3 *Mycobacterium malmoense*

### (a) Epidemiology

In a study of US NTM isolates, only four of 5469 were *M. malmoense*, none of which was classified as a pathogen [6]. However, one review found over 180 reported cases of human infection due to this organism [197] since it was described in 1977 [198]. Found mostly in northern Europe, it is second only to MAI as a cause of non-TB mycobacterial infection in Sweden [198a]. Unlike most NTM, *M. malmoense* has not been easily found in inanimate environmental sources [198a]. It has been found in armadillos in Louisiana [199], but the route of human acquisition is unknown.

### (b) Clinical syndromes reported

Pulmonary disease has been described in Europe [200] and in the USA [201]. Cases have often occurred with a history of lung disease and/or smoking but 19% of Swedish cases had no predisposing illness [198a].

Presentation is indistinguishable from TB, with chronic fever, cough, weight loss and cavitary upper lobe infiltrates. The most common extra-pulmonary manifestation is cervical lymphadenitis in children [202], which is cured by excision. Tenosynovitis [203,204], urinary tract infection [198a] and disseminated disease [198a,205] may occur.

### (c) Treatment

In vitro susceptibility testing generally shows M. malmoense to be resistant to INH, rifampin and PAS, sensitive to ethionamide, cycloserine and kanamycin, and variably sensitive to streptomycin and ethambutol [205]. A case report [197] showed sensitivity to clofazimine and resistance to quinolones. The paucity of cases makes it difficult to determine the optimal regimen. One report had best results using INH, rifampin and ethambutol for 18–24 months [206]. Other authorities [5,26] recommend treatment as for MAI with the above drugs plus streptomycin.

### (d) Disease in HIV patients

The organism was reported as a pathogen in AIDS patients in 1991 [207]. Two patients with advanced HIV disease and M. malmoense pulmonary disease who were treated with four anti-TB drugs were described. Another case of M. malmoense lung infection in an AIDS patient, with concurrent isolation from the stool, has been described [197]. This illness responded to treatment with INH, rifabutin, clofazimine and ethambutol. Based on this information, the optimal regimen for M. malmoense in AIDS patients is uncertain but the inclusion of clofazimine in a multi-drug regimen may be reasonable. Despite its frequency in Sweden, it is rare in local AIDS patients [198a]. This paucity of cases may be related to the lack of stimulation of intracellular growth of M. malmoense by HIV compared with MAI [207a].

### 14.13.4 *Mycobacterium smegmatis*

*Mycobacterium smegmatis* was the first mycobacterium to be identified after M. tuberculosis. Despite its name, it has not been isolated from the genitourinary tract in modern times. In a review, nine of 5469 isolates of NTM in the USA were M. smegmatis, but none was felt to be causing disease [6]. As is true for other NTM, M. smegmatis is likely to have an environmental source [208]. Clinical disease is similar to that caused by MFC. Reported cases include pneumonia, sternotomy wound infections and soft tissue infections, which are most often related to trauma [208,209]. *Mycobacterium smegmatis* has not been reported as a pathogen in patients with HIV infection.

Most isolates have been sensitive to ethambutol, imipenem, doxycycline, sulfa, amikacin and ciprofloxacin, and moderately susceptible to cefoxitin [208]. There are insufficient data to recommend empiric treatment and therapy should be based on the susceptibility pattern of the infecting strain. Response to treatment is good. Soft tissue infections may require extensive surgical debridement [209].

### 14.13.5 *Mycobacterium bovis*

*Mycobacterium bovis*, a member of the *M. tuberculosis* complex, is found in animals, especially cattle. It was a common cause of TB in the USA prior to the institution of eradication programs in cattle and milk pasteurization. Humans may acquire the disease by ingestion or by the airborne route, the latter suggested by cases in zookeepers caring for a sick rhinoceros [210]. While human disease is rare in developed countries, a series of 73 cases during a 12 year period in San Diego was recently reviewed [211], mostly from Mexico.

Disease in children often presents as cervical lymphadenitis after ingestion of unpasteurized dairy products. In adults, reactivation pulmonary disease is most frequent, with extrapulmonary disease involving lymph nodes, genitourinary tract, pleura, bones and joints, meninges and peritoneum.

Treatment is similar to that for *M. tuberculosis*, with the important caveat that *M. bovis* is intrinsically resistant to PZA. Therefore, rapid sterilization regimens containing PZA should be used with caution.

## 14.14 RECENTLY DESCRIBED NTM SPECIES

### 14.14.1 *Mycobacterium haemophilum*

*Mycobacterium haemophilum* has been infrequently reported to cause skin lesions in immunocompromised individuals, especially transplant recipients [212]. Cases have been reported from the USA, Canada, Australia and France. The lesions may be nodular, ulcerated and/or necrotic, often clustering over joints, and AFB are seen on biopsy. The lesions may take months to years to heal, and the rapidity of healing is more related to the underlying immune status than to specific therapy [213]. *In vitro* susceptibility results have been variable and rifampin, ethambutol and INH have been used with surgical debridement [15]. A report of 13 cases from New York found ciprofloxacin, clarithromycin, cycloserine and rifabutin to be the most active [214].

The paucity of reports of infection due to *M. haemophilum* may be due to the need for culture at 30°C for 10 weeks in media supplemented with ferric ammonium citrate or hemin [212].

### 14.14.2 *Mycobacterium genavense*

*Mycobacterium genavense* is similar to *M. simiae* and has been reported as a pathogen in patients with AIDS [215,216]. Clinical illness is similar to MAI, occurring in patients with CD4 counts less than 50/mm$^3$, and presenting with fever, diarrhea, abdominal pain, weight loss and hepatosplenomegaly [215]. The organism is slow growing and blood cultures should be held for 8 weeks for growth [216]. Appropriate treatment is unknown, but seven of 19 patients responded to treatment with regimens used for MAI in one study [215], and such treatment prolonged survival from 2.5 to 8 months in another [216].

### 14.15 SUMMARY

Some of the information presented in this chapter is summarized in tabular form. Table 14.2 shows the clinical syndromes which have been reported from NTM. The most common presentations, as well as those which have only been described as single case reports, are noted. *In vitro* antimicrobial susceptibilities are summarized in Table 14.3, and suggested treatment regimens are given in Table 14.4. When antimicrobial susceptibility information is available, it should guide treatment and supersede the regimens suggested.

**Table 14.2** Clinical manifestations.

| Organism | Most common | Others |
|---|---|---|
| *M. kansasii* | Pulmonary | Musculoskeletal<br>Cutaneous<br>Cervical lymphadenitis[a]<br>Disseminated |
| *M. marinum* | Cutaneous | Bursitis[b]<br>Sclerokeratitis[b]<br>Osteomyelitis[b]<br>Disseminated[b] |
| *M. gordonae* | Pulmonary | Keratitis<br>Peritonitis<br>Synovitis[b]<br>Disseminated |
| *M. scrofulaceum* | Cervical lymphadenitis[a]<br>Pulmonary[c] | Tenosynovitis[b]<br>Hepatitis[b]<br>Meningitis<br>Disseminated |
| *M. avium-intracellulare* | Pulmonary | Lymphadenitis<br>Cutaneous |

*cont'd*

**Table 14.2** *continued*

| Organism | Most common | Others |
|---|---|---|
| | | Meningitis[b] |
| | | Mastoiditis[b] |
| | | Corneal ulcer[b] |
| | | Endocarditis[b] |
| | | Gastric ulcer[b] |
| | | Prostatitis[b] |
| | | Tenosynovitis |
| | | Osteomyelitis |
| | | Disseminated |
| *M. xenopi* | Pulmonary | |
| *M. ulcerans* | Cutaneous | Disseminated[a,b] |
| *M. fortuitum-chelonae* | Cutaneous[d] | Pulmonary |
| | | Disseminated |
| | | Ocular |
| | | Endocarditis |
| | | Lymphadenitis |
| | | Otitis |
| | | Peritonitis |
| | | Prostheses |
| | | Urinary tract |
| *M. simiae* | Pulmonary | Disseminated |
| *M. szulgai* | Pulmonary | Bursitis[b] |
| | | Cervical lymphadenitis[a,b] |
| | | Disseminated[b] |
| *M. malmoense* | Pulmonary | Lymphadenitis[a] |
| | | Tenosynovitis |
| | | Disseminated |
| *M. smegmatis* | Pulmonary | |
| | Cutaneous[d] | |
| *M. haemophilum* | Cutaneous | |
| *M. genavense* | Disseminated[e] | |

[a] Pediatrics only.
[b] One reported case.
[c] Adults.
[d] Associated with trauma or surgery.
[e] Only reported in patients with AIDS.

**Table 14.3** Drug susceptibilities of mycobacterial isolates reported by CDC between 1980 and 1984*[a]

| Mycobacterium species | No. of strains | Percentage of strains susceptible[b] | | | | | | | | | | | | |
|---|---|---|---|---|---|---|---|---|---|---|---|---|---|---|
| | | CAP-10 | SM-2 | SM-10 | INH-0.2 | INH-1 | INH-5 | PAS-2 | RIF-1 | THA-5 | KM-5 | PZA-25 | CS-30 | EMB-5 |
| tuberculosis | 592 | 97 | 82 | 88 | 71 | 76 | 84 | 89 | 84 | 88 | 96 | 85 | 96 | 89 |
| bovis | 38 | 97 | 97 | 100 | 84 | 89 | 100 | 87 | 97 | 76 | 100 | 16 | 87 | 89 |
| bovis-BCG | 22 | 100 | 100 | 100 | 77 | 91 | 95 | 100 | 91 | 41 | 100 | 21 | 82 | 100 |
| kansasii | 71 | 48 | 11 | 77 | 6 | 45 | 93 | 13 | 82 | 68 | 14 | 2 | 83 | 42 |
| marinum | 33 | 91 | 33 | 97 | 3 | 6 | 24 | 30 | 100 | 70 | 97 | <1 | 94 | 91 |
| simiae | 28 | 4 | <1 | 14 | <1 | <1 | 4 | 4 | 4 | <1 | 7 | <1 | 57 | <1 |
| asiaticum | 10 | 20 | <1 | 70 | <1 | 10 | 40 | 10 | <1 | <1 | 70 | <1 | 70 | 20 |
| scrofulaceum | 51 | 29 | 25 | 71 | 2 | 4 | 14 | 8 | 49 | 24 | 55 | <1 | 47 | 14 |
| szulgai | 23 | 70 | 39 | 87 | 13 | 30 | 61 | 22 | 61 | 13 | 70 | <1 | 30 | 39 |
| xenopi | 25 | 100 | 100 | 100 | 64 | 92 | 96 | 72 | 92 | 92 | 100 | 13 | 72 | 64 |
| gordonae | 141 | 75 | 18 | 71 | 1 | 4 | 46 | 20 | 79 | 10 | 89 | <1 | 51 | 57 |
| flavescens | 15 | 93 | 80 | 80 | 20 | 67 | 80 | <1 | 13 | 7 | 93 | <1 | 40 | 73 |
| avium complex | 713 | 9 | 8 | 40 | <1 | 1 | 25 | 4 | 14 | 5 | 24 | <1 | 26 | 13 |
| malmoense | 47 | 47 | 38 | 68 | <1 | 2 | 43 | 17 | 60 | 53 | 64 | 2 | 62 | 21 |
| terrae complex | 64 | 45 | 25 | 59 | <1 | 2 | 19 | 2 | 31 | 8 | 34 | 3 | 22 | 69 |
| triviale | 2 | 50 | 100 | 100 | <1 | <1 | <1 | <1 | 100 | 50 | 100 | <1 | 50 | <1 |
| gastri | 4 | 75 | 75 | 75 | <1 | 5 | 100 | <1 | 75 | 75 | 75 | <1 | 50 | 25 |
| fortuitum | 198 | 49 | 1 | 4 | <1 | 1 | 14 | <1 | 2 | <1 | 13 | <1 | 2 | 3 |
| chelonae | 170 | 2 | 2 | 4 | <1 | <1 | 1 | <1 | <1 | <1 | 3 | <1 | <1 | 5 |

\* Reprinted by permission of the publisher from Good, R.C., Silcox, V.A., Kilburn, J.O. and Plikaytis, B.D. (1985) *Identification and Drug Susceptibility Test Results for Mycobacterium spp.* copyright by Elsevier Science Publishing Co., Inc.

[a] All identification and drug susceptibility tests were performed in CDC laboratories.

[b] CAP, capreomycin; SM, streptomycin; INH, isoniazid; PAS, para-aminosalicylic acid; RIF, rifampin; THA, ethionamide; KM, kanamycin; PZA, pyrazinamide; CS, cycloserine; EMB, ethambutol.

**Table 14.4** Treatment

| Organism | Suggested treatments[a] |
|---|---|
| M. kansasii | INH/RIF/EMB |
| M. marinum | TCN<br>RIF/EMB[b] |
| M. gordonae | INH/RIF/EMB[c] |
| M. scrofulaceum | Lymph node excision<br>INH/EMB/CS/CLA[d] |
| M. avium-intracellulare | INH/RIF/EMB/SM/CLO[e]<br>CLA/CLO/EMB[f]<br>EMB/RIF/CIP/AK[b,f] |
| M. xenopi | INH/RIF/EMB/SM |
| M. ulcerans | Surgery |
| M. fortuitum-chelonei | AK/CEF |
| M. simiae | ETH/CS[c] |
| M. szulgai | INH/RIF/EMB |
| M. malmonense | INH/RIF/EMB/SM |
| M. smegmatis | Insufficient data |
| M. haemophilum | INH/RIF/EMB[c] |
| M. genavense | As for MAI[c] |

[a] INH, isoniazid; RIF, rifampin; EMB, ethambutol; ETH, ethionamide; SM, streptomycin; CS, cycloserine; AK, amikacin; TCN, tetracycline; CLA, clarithromycin; CLO, clofazimine; CIP, ciprofloxacin; CEF, cefoxitin.
[b] For more serious infections.
[c] Based on very limited information.
[d] For all except adenitis.
[e] For disseminated disease.
[f] Alternative for AIDS patients.

## REFERENCES

1. Runyon, E.H. (1959) Anonymous mycobacteria in pulmonary disease. *Med Clin North Am*, **43**, 273–90.
2. Wolinsky, E. and Rynearson, T.K. (1968) Mycobacteria in soil and their relation to disease-associated stains. *Am Rev Respir Dis*, **97**, 1032–37.
3. Chapman, J.S. and Speight, M. (1968) Isolation of atypical mycobacteria from pasteurized milk. *Am Rev Respir Dis*, **98**, 1052–4.
4. Stine, T.M., Harris, A.A., Levin, S. *et al.* (1987) A pseudoepidemic due to atypical mycobacteria in a hospital water supply. *JAMA*, **258**, 809–11.
5. Wallace, R.J., O'Brien, R., Glassroth, J. *et al.* (1990) Diagnosis and treatment of disease caused by nontuberculous mycobacteria. *Am Rev Respir Dis*, **142**, 940–53.
6. O'Brien, R.J., Geiter, L.J. and Snider, D.E. (1987) The epidemiology of nontuberculous mycobacterial disease in the United States. *Am Rev Respir Dis*, **135**, 1007–14.

7. Horsburgh, C.R. and Selik, R.M. (1989) The epidemiology of disseminated nontuberculous mycobacterial infection in the acquired immunodeficiency syndrome (AIDS). *Am Rev Respir Dis*, **139**, 4–7.

8. Helbert, M., Robinson, D., Buchanan, D. *et al.* (1990) Mycobacterial infection in patients infected with the human immunodeficiency virus. *Thorax*, **45**, 45–8.

9. Woodring, J.H. and Vandiviere, H.M. (1990) Pulmonary disease caused by nontuberculous mycobacteria. *J Thoracic Imaging*, **5**, 64–76.

10. Huebner, R.E., Schein, M.F., Cauthen, G.M. *et al.* (1992) Evaluation of the clinical usefulness of mycobacterial skin test antigens in adults with pulmonary mycobacterioses. *Am Rev Respir Dis,* **148**, 1160–6.

11. Huebner, R.E., Schein, M.F., Cauthen, G.M. *et al.* (1992) Usefulness of skin testing with mycobacterial antigens in children with cervical lymphadenopathy. *Pediatr Infect Dis J*, **11**, 450–6.

12. Margileth, A.M., Chandra, R. and Altman, P. (1984) Chronic lymphadenopathy due to mycobacterial infection. *Am J Dis Child*, **138**, 917–22.

13. Gribetz, A.R., Damsker, B., Morchevsky, A. and Bottone, E.J. (1985) Nontuberculous mycobacteria in pleural fluid. *Chest*, **87**, 495–7.

14. Merckx, J.J., Soule, E.H. and Karlson, A.G. (1964) The histopathology of lesions caused by infection with unclassified acid-fast bacteria in man. *Am J Clin Path*, **41**, 244–55.

15. Woods, G.L. and Washington, J.A. (1987) Mycobacteria other than *Mycobacterium tuberculosis*: review of microbiologic and clinical aspects. *Rev Infect Dis*, **9**, 275–94.

16. Lillo, M., Orengo, S., Cernoch, P. and Harris, R.L. (1990) Pulmonary and disseminated infection due to *Mycobacterium kansasii*: a decade of experience. *Rev Infect Dis*, **12**, 760–7.

17. Steadham, J.E. (1980) High-catalase strains of *Mycobacterium kansasii* isolated from water in Texas. *J Clin Microbiol*, **11**, 496–8.

18. Francis, P.B., Jay, S.J. and Johanson, W.G. (1975) The course of untreated *Mycobacterium kansasii* disease. *Am Rev Respir Dis*, **111**, 477–87.

19. Dillon, J., Millson, C. and Morris, I. (1989) *Mycobacterium kansasii* infection of the wrist and hand. *Br J Rheumatol*, **29**, 150–3.

20. Minkin, B.I., Mills, C.L., Bullock, D.W. and Burke, F.D. (1987) *Mycobacterium kansasii* osteomyelitis of the scaphoid. *J Hand Surg*, **12A**, 1092–4.

21. Watanakunakorn, C. and Trott, A. (1972) Vertebral osteomyelitis due to *Mycobacterium kansasii*. *Am Rev Respir Dis*, **107**, 846–50.

22. Owens, D.W. and McBride, M.E. (1969) Sporotrichoid cutaneous infection with *Mycobacterium kansasii*. *Arch Dermatol*, **100**, 54–8.

23. Fraser, D.W., Buxton, A.E., Barker C.F. *et al.* (1975) Disseminated *Mycobacterium kansasii* infection presenting as cellulitis in a recipient of a renal homograft. *Am Rev Respir Dis*, **112**, 125–9.

24. Hanke, C.W., Temofeew, R.K. and Slama, S.L. (1987) *Mycobacterium kansasii* infection with multiple cutaneous lesions. *J Am Acad Dermatol*, **16**, 1122–8.

25. Wolinsky, E. (1979) Nontuberculous mycobacteria and associated diseases. *Am Rev Respir Dis*, **119**, 107–59.

26. Wolinsky, E. (1992) Mycobacterial diseases other than tuberculosis. *Clin Infect Dis*, **15**, 1–12.

27. Ahn, C.H., Wallace, R.J., Steele, L.C. and Murphy, D.T. (1987) Sulfonamide-

containing regimens for disease caused by rifampin-resistant *Mycobacterium kansasii*. *Am Rev Respir Dis*, **135**, 10–16.

28. Banks, J. (1989) Treatment of pulmonary disease caused by opportunistic mycobacteria. *Thorax*, **44**, 449–54.

28a. Wallace, R.J., Dunbar, D., Brown, B.A. *et al.* (1994) Rifampin-resistant *Mycobacterium kansasii*. *Clin Infect Dis*, **18**, 736–43.

29. Carpenter, J.L. and Parks, J.M. (1991) *Mycobacterium kansasii* infections in patients positive for human immunodeficiency virus. *Rev Infect Dis*, **13**, 789–96.

30. Valainis, G.T., Cardona, L.M. and Greer, D.L. (1991) The spectrum of *Mycobacterium kansasii* disease associated with HIV-1 infected patients. *J AIDS*, **4**, 516–20.

31. Levine, B. and Chaisson, R.E. (1991) *Mycobacterium kansasii*: a cause of treatable pulmonary disease associated with advanced Human Immunodeficiency Virus (HIV) infection. *Ann Intern Med*, **114**, 861–8.

32. Gordon, S.M. and Blumberg, H.M. (1992) *Mycobacterium kansasii* brain abscess in a patient with AIDS. *Clin Infect Dis*, **14**, 789–90.

33. Bergen, G.A., Yangco, B.G. and Adelman, H.M. (1993) Central nervous system infection with *Mycobacterium kansasii*. *Ann Intern Med*, **118**, 396.

34. Valainis, G.T. (1991) *Mycobacterium kansasii* infection (letter). *Ann Intern Med*, **115**, 496.

35. Norden, A. and Linell, F. (1951) A new type of pathogenic mycobacterium. *Nature*, **168**, 826.

36. Huminer, D., Pitlik, S.D., Block, C. *et al.* (1986) Aquarium-borne *Mycobacterium marinum* skin infection. *Arch Dermatol*, **122**, 698–703.

37. Holly, H.W. and Seabury, J.H. (1972) Infections with *Mycobacterium marinum*. *Arch Dermatol*, **106**, 32–6.

38. Iredell, J., Whitby, M. and Blacklock, Z. (1992) *Mycobacterium marinum* infection: epidemiology and presentation in Queensland 1971–1990. *Med J Aust*, **157**, 596–8.

39. Gombert, M.E., Goldstein, E.J.C., Corrado, M.L. *et al.* (1981) Disseminated *Mycobacterium marinum* infection after renal transplantation. *Ann Intern Med*, **94**, 486–7.

40. Enzenauer, R.J., McKoy, J., Vincent, D. and Gates, R. (1990) Disseminated cutaneous and synovial *Mycobacterium marinum* infection in a patient with systemic lupus erythematosus. *South Med J*, **83**, 471–4.

41. Gould, W.M., McMeekin, D.R. and Bright, R.D. (1968) *Mycobacterium marinum* (balnei) infection: report of a case with cutaneous and laryngeal lesions. *Arch Dermatol*, **97**, 159–62.

42. King, A.J., Fairley, J.A. and Rasmussen, J.E. (1983) Disseminated cutaneous *Mycobacterium marinum* infection. *Arch Dermatol*, **119**, 268–70.

43. Lacaille, F., Blanche, S., Bodemer, C. *et al.* (1990) Persistent *Mycobacterium marinum* infection in a child with probable visceral involvement. *Pediatr Infect Dis J*, **9**, 58–60.

44. Schonherr, U., Naumann, G.O.H., Lang, G.K. and Bialasiewicz, A.A. (1989) Sclerokeratitis caused by *Mycobacterium marinum*. *Am J Ophthalmol*, **108**, 607–8.

45. Winter, F.E. and Runyon, E.H. (1965) Prepatellar bursitis caused by *Mycobacterium marinum (balnei)*. *J Bone Joint Surg*, **47A**, 375–9.

46. Clark, R.B., Spector, H., Friedman, D.M. *et al.* (1990) Osteomyelitis and

synovitis produced by *Mycobacterium marinum* in a fisherman. *J Clin Microbiol*, **28**, 2570–2.

47.  Arai, H., Nakajima, H. and Kaminaga, Y. (1990) In vitro susceptibility of *Mycobacterium marinum* to dihydromycoplanecin A and ten other antimicrobial agents. *J Dermatol*, **17**, 370–4.

48.  Sanders, W.J. and Wolinsky, E. (1980) In vitro susceptibility of *Mycobacterium marinum* to eight antimicrobial agents. *Antimicrob Agents Chemother*, **18**, 529–31.

49.  Loria, P.R. (1976) Minocycline hydrochloride for atypical acid-fast infection. *Arch Dermatol*, **112**, 517–9.

50.  Izumi, A.K., Hanke, W. and Higaki, M. (1977) *Mycobacterium marinum* infections treated with tetracycline. *Arch Dermatol*, **113**, 1067–8.

50a. Bonnet, E., Debal-Zoguereh, D., Fetit, N. *et al.* (1994) Clarithromycin: a potent agent against infections due to *Mycobacterium marinum*. *Clin Infect Dis*, **18**, 664–6.

51.  Donta, S.T., Smith, P.W., Levitz, R.E. and Quintiliani, R. (1986) Therapy of *Mycobacterium marinum* infections. *Arch Intern Med*, **146**, 902–4.

52.  Chow, S.P., Ip, F.K., Lau, J.H.K. *et al.* (1987) *Mycobacterium marinum* infection of the hand and wrist. *J Bone Joint Surg*, **69A**, 1161–8.

53.  Hurst, L.C., Amadio, P.C., Badalamente, M.A. *et al.* (1987) *Mycobacterium marinum* infections of the hand. *J Hand Surg*, **12A**, 428–35.

54.  Ries, K.M., White, G.L. and Murdock, R.T. (1990) Atypical mycobacterial infection caused by *Mycobacterium marinum*. *N Engl J Med*, **322**, 633.

55.  Tchornobay, A.M., Claudy, A.L., Perrot, J.L. *et al.* (1992) Fatal disseminated *Mycobacterium marinum* infection. *Int J Dermatol*, **31**, 286–7.

56.  Goslee, S. and Wolinsky, E. (1976) Water as a source of potentially pathogenic mycobacteria. *Am Rev Respir Dis*, **113**, 287–92.

57.  Gubler, J.G.H., Salfinger, M. and von Graevenitz, A. (1992) Pseudoepidemic of nontuberculous mycobacteria due to a contaminated bronchoscope cleaning machine. *Chest*, **101**, 1245–9.

58.  Douglas, J.G., Calder, M.A., Choo-Kang, Y.F.J. and Leitch, A.G. (1986) *Mycobacterium gordonae*: a new pathogen? *Thorax*, **41**, 152–3.

59.  Weinberger, M., Berg, S.L., Feuerstein, I.M. *et al.* (1992) Disseminated infection with *Mycobacterium gordonae*: report of a case and critical review of the literature. *Clin Infect Dis*, **14**, 1229–39.

60.  Sossi, N., Feldman, R.N., Feldman, S.T. *et al.* (1991) *Mycobacterium gordonae* keratitis after penetrating keratoplasty. *Arch Ophthalmol*, **109**, 1064–5.

61.  Moore, M.B., Newton, C. and Kaufman, H.E. (1986) Chronic keratitis caused by *Mycobacterium gordonae*. *Am J Ophthalmol*, **102**, 516–21.

62.  London, R.D., Damsker, B., Neibart, E.P. *et al.* (1988) *Mycobacterium gordonae*: an unusual peritoneal pathogen in a patient undergoing continuous ambulatory peritoneal dialysis. *Am J Med*, **85**, 703–4.

63.  Berman, L.B. (1983) Infection of synovial tissue by *Mycobacterium gordonae*. *Can Med Assoc J*, **129**, 1078–9.

64.  Kurnik, P.B., Padmanabh, U., Bonatsos, C. and Cynamon, M.H. (1983) *Mycobacterium gordonae* as a human hepato-peritoneal pathogen, with a review of the literature. *Am J Med Sci*, **285**, 45–8.

65.  Turner, D.M., Ramsey, P.G., Ojemann, G.A. and Ralph, D.D. (1985) Disseminated *Mycobacterium gordonae* infection associated with glomerulonephritis. *West J Med*, **142**, 391–3.

66. Lohr, D.C., Goeken, J.A., Doty, D.B. and Donta, S.T. (1978) *Mycobacterium gordonae* infection of a prosthetic aortic valve. *JAMA*, **239**, 1528–30.

67. Jarikre, L.N. (1991) Disseminated *Mycobacterium gordonae* infection in a non-immunocompromised host. *Am J Med Sci*, **302**, 383–4.

68. Barber, T.W., Craven, D.E. and Farber, H.W. (1991) *Mycobacterium gordonae*: a possible opportunistic respiratory tract pathogen in patients with advanced Human Immunodeficiency Virus, Type I infection. *Chest*, **100**, 716–20.

69. Brown, B.A., Wallace, R.J. and Onyi, G.O. (1992) Activities of clarithromycin against eight slowly growing species of nontuberculous mycobacteria, determined by using a broth microdilution MIC system. *Antimicrob Agents Chemother*, **36**, 1987–90.

70. Reznikov, M., Leggo, J.H. and Dawson, D.J. (1971) Investigation by seroagglutination of strains of the *Mycobacterium intracellulare – M. scrofulaceum* group from house dusts and sputum in southeastern Queensland. *Am Rev Respir Dis*, **104**, 951–3.

71. Yamamoto, M., Sudo, K., Taga, M. and Hibino, S. (1967) A study of diseases caused by atypical mycobacteria in Japan. *Am Rev Respir Dis*, **96**, 779–87.

72. Prissick, F.H. and Masson, A.M. (1956) Cervical lymphadenitis in children casued by chromogenic mycobacteria. *Can Med Assoc J*, **75**, 798–803.

73. Reid, J.D. and Wolinsky, E. (1969) Histopathology of lymphadenitis caused by atypical mycobacteria. *Am Rev Respir Dis*, **99**, 8–12.

74. Gracey, D.R. and Byrd, R.B. (1970) Scotochromogens and pulmonary disease. *Am Rev Respir Dis*, **101**, 959–63.

75. Cohen, M.J., Matz, L.R. and Elphick, H.R. (1970) Infection of the soft tissues of the ankle by a group II atypical mycobacterium (scotochromogens). *Med J Austr*, **2**, 679–82.

76. Kelly, P.J., Weed, L.A. and Lipscomb, P.R. (1963) Infection of tendon sheaths, bursae, joints and soft tissues by acid fast bacilli other than tubercle bacilli. *J Bone Joint Surg*, **45A**, 327–36

77. Patel, K.M. (1981) Granulomatous hepatitis due to *Mycobacterium scrofulaceum*: report of a case. *Gastroenterology*, **81**, 156–8.

78. McNutt, D.R. and Fudenberg, H.H. (1971) Disseminated scotochromogen infection and unusual myeloproliferative disorder. *Ann Intern Med*, **75**, 737–44.

79. Joos, H.A., Hilty, L.B., Courington, D. *et al.* (1967) Fatal disseminated scotochromogenic mycobacteriosis in a child. *Am Rev Respir Dis*, **96**, 795–801.

80. Taha, A.M., Davidson, P.T. and Bailey, W.C. (1985) Surgical treatment of atypical mycobacterial lymphadenitis in children. *Pediatr Infect Dis J*, **4**, 664–7.

81. Haas, H., Michel, J. and Sacks, T.G. (1982) In vitro susceptibility of mycobacteria species other than *Mycobacterium tuberculosis* to amikacin, cephalosporins, and cefoxitin. *Chemotherapy*, **28**, 1–5.

82. Molavi, A. and Weinstein, L. (1971) In-vitro activity of erythromycin against atypical mycobacteria. *J Infect Dis*, **123**, 216–9.

83. Shafer, R.W. and Sierra, M.F. (1992) *Mycobacterium xenopi, Mycobacterium fortuitum, Mycobacterium kansasii* and other nontuberculous mycobacteria in an area of endemicity for AIDS. *Clin Infect Dis*, **15**, 161–2.

84. Feldman, W.H., Davis, R., Moses, H.E. and Andberg, W. (1943) An unusual *Mycobacterium* isolated from sputum of a man suffering from pulmonary disease of long duration. *Am Rev Tuberc*, **48**, 82–93.

85. Drake, T.A., Hindler, J.A., Berlin, G.W. and Bruckner, D.A. (1987) Rapid identification of *Mycobacterium avium* complex in culture using DNA probes. *J Clin Microbiol*, **25**, 1442–5.

86. Kirschner, R.A., Parker, B.C. and Falkingham, J.O. (1992) Epidemiology of infection by nontuberculous mycobacteria. *Am Rev Respir Dis*, **145**, 271–5.

87. Du Molin, G.C., Stottmeier, K.D., Pelletier, P.A. *et al.* (1988) Concentration of *Mycobacterium avium* by hospital hot water systems. *JAMA*, **260**, 1599–1601.

88. Iseman, M.D., Buschman, D.L. and Ackerson, L.M. (1991) Pectus excavatum and scoliosis. Thoracic anomalies associated with pulmonary disease caued by *Mycobacterium avium* complex. *Am Rev Respir Dis*, **144**, 914–6.

89. Reich, J.M. and Johnson, R.E. (1991) *Mycobacterium avium* complex pulmonary disease. *Am Rev Respir Dis*, **143**, 1381–5.

90. Prince, D.S., Peterson, D.D., Steiner, R.M. *et al.* (1989) Infection with *Mycobacterium avium* complex in patients without predisposing conditions. *N Engl J Med*, **321**, 863–8.

91. Lai, K.K., Stottmeier, K.D., Sherman, I.H. and McCabe, W.R. (1984) Mycobacterial cervical lymphadenopathy. *JAMA*, **251**, 1286–8.

92. Corpe, R.F. and Stergus, I. (1963) Is the histopathology of nonphotochromogenic mycobacterial infections distinguishable from that caused by *Mycobacterium tuberculosis*? *Am Rev Respir Dis*, **87**, 289–91.

93. Cox, S.K. and Strausbaugh, L.J. (1981) Chronic cutaneous infection caused by *Mycobacterium intracellulare*. *Arch Dermatol*, **117**, 794–6.

94. Lugo-Janer, G., Cruz, A. and Sanchez, J.L. (1990) Disseminated cutaneous infection caued by *Mycobacterium avium* complex. *Arch Dermatol*, **126**, 1108–10.

95. Uldry, P.A., Bogousslavsky, J., Regli, F. *et al.* (1992) Chronic *Mycobacterium avium* complex infection of the central nervous system in a nonimmunosuppressed woman. *Eur Neurol*, **32**, 285–8.

96. Kinsella, J.P., Grossman, M. and Black, S. (1986) Otomastoiditis caused by *Mycobacterium avium-intracellulare*. *Pediatr Infect Dis J*, **5**, 704–6.

97. Knapp, A., Stern, G.A. and Hood, C.I. (1987) *Mycobacterium avium-intracellulare* corneal ulcer. *Cornea*, **6**, 175.

98. Landymore, R.W., Murphy, D.A., Marrie, T.J. and Johnston, B.L. (1992) *Mycobacterium avium-intracellulare* endocarditis causing rupture: replacement and repair with aortic homograft. *Can J Cardiol*, **8**, 729–32.

99. Amin, M., Gross, J., Andrews, C. and Furman, S. (1990) Pacemaker infection with *Mycobacterium avium* complex. *Pace*, **14**, 152–4.

100. Cappell, M.S. and Taunk, J.L. (1991) A chronic gastric ulcer refractory to conventional antiulcer therapy associated with localized gastric *Mycobacterium avium-intracellulare* infection. *Am J Gastroenterol*, **86**, 654.

101. Mikolich, D.J. and Mates, S.M. (1992) Granulomatous prostatitis due to *Mycobacterium avium* complex. *Clin Infect Dis*, **14**, 589–91.

102. Eggelmeijer, F., Kroon, F.P., Zeeman, R.J. *et al.* (1992) Tenosynovitis due to *Mycobacterium avium-intracellulare*: case report and a review of the literature. *Clin Exp Rheumatol*, **10**, 169–71.

103. Kwong, J.S., Munk, P.L., Conwell, D.G. and Gianoulis, M.E. (1991) Disseminated *Mycobacterium avium-intracellulare* osteomyelitis. *Skeletal Radiol*, **20**, 458–62.

104. Sato, Y., Tamura, K. and Seita, M. (1992) Multiple osteomyelitis due to

*Mycobacterium avium* with no pulmonary presentation in a patient of sarcoidosis. *Intern Med*, **31**, 489–92.

105. Horsburgh, C.R., Mason, U.G., Farhi, D.C. and Iseman, M.D. (1985) Disseminated infection with *Mycobacterium avium-intracellulare*. *Medicine*, **64**, 36–48.

106. Stone, A.B., Schelonka, R.L., Drehner, D.M. *et al.* (1992) Disseminated *Mycobacterium avium* complex in non-Human Immunodeficiency Virus-infected pediatric patients. *Pediatr Infect Dis J*, **11**, 960–4.

106a. Holland, S.M., Eisenstein, E.M., Kuhns, D.B. *et al.* (1994)Treatment of refractory disseminated nontuberculous mycobacterial infection with interferon gamma. *N Engl J Med*, **330**, 1348–55.

107. Horsburgh, C.R., Mason, U.G., Heifets, L.B. *et al.* (1987) Response to therapy of pulmonary *Mycobacterium avium-intracellulare* infection correlates with results of in vitro susceptibility testing. *Am Rev Respir Dis*, **135**, 418–23.

108. Ahn, C.H., Ahn, S.S., Anderson, R.A. *et al.* (1986) A four-drug regimen for the initial treatment of cavitary disease caused by *Mycobacterium avium* complex. *Am Rev Respir Dis*, **134**, 436–41.

109. Moran, J.F., Alexander, L.G., Staub E.W. *et al.* (1983) Long-term results of pulmonary resection for atypical mycobacterial disease. *Ann Thoracic Surg*, **35**, 597–604.

110. Gribetz, A.R., Damsker, B., Bottone, E.J. *et al.* (1981) Solitary pulmonary nodules due to nontuberculous mycobacterial infection. *Am J Med*, **70**, 39–43.

111. Greene, J.B., Sidhu, G.S., Lewin, S. *et al.* (1982) *Mycobacterium avium-intracellulare*: a cause of disseminated life-threatening infection in homosexuals and drug abusers. *Ann Intern Med*, **97**, 539–46.

112. Havlik, J.A., Horsburgh, C.R., Metchcock, G. *et al.* (1992) Disseminated *Mycobacterium avium* complex infections: clinical identification and epidemiologic trends. *J Infect Dis*, **165**, 577–80.

113. Benson, C.A. and Ellner, J.J. (1993) *Mycobacterium avium* complex infection and AIDS: advances in theory and practice. *Clin Infect Dis*, **17**, 7–20.

114. Wallace, J.M. and Hannah, J.B. (1988) *Mycobacterium avium* complex infection in patients with the Acquired Immunodeficiency Syndrome. *Chest*, **93**, 926–32.

115. Modilevsky, T., Sattler, F.R. and Barnes, P.F. (1989) Mycobacterial disease in patients with human immunodeficiency virus infection. *Arch Intern Med*, **149**, 2201–5.

116. Freed, J.A., Pervez, N.K., Chen, V. *et al.* (1987) Cutaneous mycobacteriosis: occurrence and significance in two patients with the acquired immunodeficiency syndrome. *Arch Dermatol*, **123**, 1601–3.

117. Clark, J.A. and Margolis, D.M. (1993) A cutaneous lesion in a patient with AIDS: an unusual presentation of infection due to *Mycobacterium avium* complex. *Clin Infect Dis*, **16**, 555–7.

118. Hawkins, C.C., Gold, J.W.M., Whimbey, E. *et al.* (1986) *Mycobacterium avium* complex infections in patients with the Acquired Immunodeficiency Syndrome. *Ann Intern Med*, **105**, 184–8.

119. Chin, J., Nussbaum, J., Bozzette, S. *et al.* (1990) Treatment of disseminated *Mycobacterium avium* complex infection in AIDS with amikacin, ethambutol, rifampin, and ciprofloxacin. *Ann Intern Med*, **113**, 358–61.

120. Roy, J., Mijch, A., Sandland, M. *et al.* (1990) Quadruple-drug therapy for

*Mycobacterium avium-intracellulare* bacteremia in AIDS patients. *J Infect Dis*, **161**, 801–5.

121. Inderlied, C.B., Kolonoski, P.T., Wu, M. and Young, L.S. (1989) In vitro and in vivo activity of azithromycin (CP 62,993) against the *Mycobacterium avium* complex. *J Infect Dis*, **159**, 994–7.

122. Dautzenberg, B., Truffot, C., Legris, S. *et al.* (1991) Activity of clarithromycin against *Mycobacterium avium* infection in patients with the Acquired Immune Deficiency Syndrome. *Am Rev Respir Dis*, **144**, 564–9.

123. Nightingale, S.D., Cameron, D.W., Gordin, F.M. *et al.* (1993) Two placebo controlled trials of rifabutin prophylaxis against *Mycobacterium avium* complex infection in AIDS patients. *N Engl J Med*, **329**, 828–33.

124. Dautzenberg, B., Saint Marc, T., Meyohas, M.C. *et al.* (1993) Clarithromycin and other antimicrobial agents in the treatment of disseminated *Mycobacterium avium* infections in patients with Acquired Immunodeficiency Syndrome. *Arch Intern Med*, **153**, 368–72.

125. Chaisson, R.E., Benson, C., Dube, M. *et al.* (1992) *Clarithromycin therapy for disseminated Mycobacterium avium complex in AIDS.* Interscience Conference on Antimicrobial Agents and Chemotherapy, Anaheim, CA, American Society for Microbiology.

126. Schwabacher, H. (1959) A strain of *Mycobacterium* isolated from skin lesions of a cold-blooded animal, *Xenopus laevis*, and its relation to atypical acid-fast bacilli occurring in man. *J Hyg*, **57**, 57–67.

127. Beck, A. and Stanford, J.L. (1968) *Mycobacterium xenopi*: a study of sixteen strains. *Tubercle*, **49**, 226–34.

128. Simor, A.E., Salit, I.E. and Vellend, H. (1984) The role of *Mycobacterium xenopi* in human disease. *Am Rev Respir Dis*, **129**, 435–8.

129. Bullin, C.H., Tanner, E.I. and Collins, C.H. (1970) Isolation of *Mycobacterium xenopi* from water taps. *J Hyg*, **68**, 97–100.

130. Costrini, A.M., Mahler, D.A., Gross, W.M. *et al.* (1981) Clinical and roentgenographic features of nosocomial pulmonary disease due to *Mycobacterium xenopi*. *Am Rev Respir Dis*, **123**, 104–8.

131. Sennesael, J.J., Maes, V.A., Pierard, D. *et al.* (1990) Streptomycin pharmacokinetics in relapsing *Mycobacterium xenopi* peritonitis. *Am J Nephrol*, **10**, 422–5.

132. Contreras, M.A., Cheung, O.T., Sanders, D.E. and Goldstein, R.J. (1988) Pulmonary infection with nontuberculous mycobacteria. *Am Rev Respir Dis*, **137**, 149–52.

133. Wilks, D., George, R.J.D. and Spiro, S.J.G. (1990) Pulmonary *Mycobacterium xenopi* infection as a first manifestation of HIV infection. *J Roy Soc Med*, **83**, 401–2.

134. Eng, R.H.K., Forrester, C., Smith, S.M. and Sobel, H. (1984) *Mycobacterium xenopi* infection in a patient with Acquired Immunodeficiency Syndrome. *Chest*, **86**, 145–7.

135. Ausina, V., Barrio, J., Luquin, M. *et al.* (1988) *Mycobacterium xenopi* infections in the Acquired Immunodeficiency Syndrome. *Ann Intern Med*, **109**, 461–2.

136. MacCallum, P., Tolhurst, J.C., Buckle, G. and Sissons, H.A. (1948) A new mycobacterial infection in man. *J Pathol Bacteriol*, **60**, 93–122.

137. Christie, M. (1987) Suspected *Mycobacterium ulcerans* disease in Kiribati. *Med J Austr*, **146**, 600–3.

138. Oluwasanmi, J.O., Solanke, T.F., Olurin, E.O. *et al.* (1976) *Mycobacterium ulcerans* (Buruli) skin ulceration in Nigeria. *Am J Trop Med Hyg*, **25**, 122–8.

139. Lindo, S.D. and Daniels, F. (1974) Buruli ulcer in New York City. *JAMA*, **228**, 1138–9.

140. Bradley, D.J., Hutt, M.S.R., Kiryabwire, J.W.M. *et al.* (1970) Clinical features and treatment of pre-ulcerative Buruli lesions. *Brit Med J*, **2**, 390–3.

141. Connor, D.H. and Lunn, H.F. (1966) Buruli ulceration. *Arch Pathol*, **81**, 183–9.

142. Muelder, K. and Nourou, A. (1990) Buruli ulcer in Benin. *Lancet*, **ii**, 1109–11.

143. Hofer, M., Hirschel, B., Kirschner, P. *et al.* (1993) Brief report: disseminated osteomyelitis from *Mycobacterium ulcerans* after a snakebite. *N Engl J Med*, **328**, 1007–9.

143a. Delaporte, E., Alfandari, S. and Piette, F. (1994) *Mycobacterium ulcerans* associated with infections due to the Human Immunodeficiency Virus. *Clin Infect Dis*, **18**, 839.

144. Wallace, R.J., Swenson, J.M., Silcox, V.A. *et al.* (1983) Spectrum of disease due to rapidly growing mycobacteria. *Rev Infect Dis*, **5**, 657–79.

145. Laussucq, S., Baltch, A.L., Smith, R.P. *et al.* (1988) Nosocomial *Mycobacterium fortuitum* colonization from a contaminated ice machine. *Am Rev Respir Dis*, **138**, 891–4.

146. Lowry, P.W., Jarvis, W.R., Oberle, A.D. *et al.* (1988) *Mycobacterium chelonae* causing otitis media in an ear-nose-and-throat practice. *N Engl J Med*, **319**, 978–82.

147. Soto, L.E., Bobadilla, M., Villalobos, Y. *et al.* (1991) Post-surgical nasal cellulitis outbreak due to *Mycobacterium chelonae*. *J Hosp Infect*, **19**, 99–106.

148. Newman, P.E., Goodman, R.A., Waring, G.O. *et al.* (1984) A cluster of cases of *Mycobacterium chelonae* keratitis associated with outpatient office procedures. *Am J Ophthalmol*, **97**, 344–8.

149. Wallace, R.J., Musser, J.M., Hull, S.I. *et al.* (1989) Diversity and sources of rapidly growing mycobacteria associated with infections following cardiac surgery. *J Infect Dis*, **159**, 708–16.

150. Laskowski, L.F., Marr, J.J., Spernoga, J.F. *et al.* (1977) Fastidious mycobacteria grown from porcine prosthetic-heart-valve cultures. *N Engl J Med*, **297**, 101–2.

151. Bolan, G., Reingold, A.L., Carson, L.A. *et al.* (1985) Infections with *Mycobacterium chelonae* in patients receiving dialysis and using processed hemodialyzers. *J Infect Dis*, **152**, 1013–9.

152. Nolan, C.M., Hashisaski, P.A. and Dundas, D.F. (1991) An outbreak of soft tissue infections due to *Mycobacterium fortuitum* associated with electromyography. *J Infect Dis*, **163**, 1150–3.

153. Safranek, T.J., Jarvis, W.R., Carson, L.A. *et al.* (1987) *Mycobacterium chelonae* wound infections after plastic surgery employing contaminated gentian violet skin-marking solution. *N Engl J Med*, **317**, 197–201.

154. Pesce, R.R., Fejka, S. and Colodny, S.M. (1991) *Mycobacterium fortuitum* presenting as an asymptomatic enlarging pulmonary nodule. *Am J Med*, **91**, 310–2.

155. Hutchins, G.M. and Boitnott, J.K. (1978) Atypical mycobacterial infection complicating mineral oil pneumonia. *JAMA*, **240**, 539–41.

156. Howard, R.S., Woodring, J.H., Vandiviere, H.M. and Dillon, M.L. (1991) *Mycobacterium fortuitum* pulmonary infection complicating achalasia. *South Med J*, **84**, 1391–3.

157. Kilby, J.M., Gilligan, P.H., Yankaskas, J.R. *et al.* (1992) Nontuberculous mycobacteria in adult patients with cystic fibrosis. *Chest*, **102**, 70–5.

158. Borghans, J.G.A. and Stanford, J.L. (1973) *Mycobacterium chelonei* in abscesses after injection of diphtheria-pertussis-tetanus-polio vaccine. *Am Rev Respir Dis*, **107**, 1–8.

159. Greer, K.E., Gross, G.P. and Martensen, S.H. (1979) Sporotrichoid cutaneous infections due to *Mycobacterium chelonei*. *Arch Dermatol*, **115**, 738–9.

160. Wallace, R.J., Steele, L.C., Labidi, A. and Silcox, V.A. (1989) Heterogeneity among isolates of rapidly growing mycobacteria responsible for infections following augmentation mammaplasty despite case clustering in Texas and other southern coastal states. *J Infect Dis*, **160**, 281–8.

161. Drabick, J.J., Duffy, P.E., Samlaska, C.P. and Scherbenske, J.M. (1990) Disseminated *Mycobacterium chelonae* subspecies chelonae infection with cutaneous and osseous manifestations. *Arch Dermatol*, **126**, 1064–7.

162. Nelson, B.R., Rapini, R.P., Wallace, R.J. and Tschen, J.A. (1989) Disseminated *Mycobacterium chelonae ssp. abscessus* in an immunocompetent host and with a known portal of entry. *J Am Acad Dermatol*, **20**, 909–12.

163. Ingram, C.W., Tanner, D.C., Durack, D.T. *et al.* (1993) Disseminated infection with rapidly growing mycobacteria. *Clin Infect Dis*, **16**, 463–71.

164. Raad, I.I., Vartivarian, S., Khan, A. and Bodey, G.P. (1991) Catheter-related infections caused by the *Mycobacterium fortuitum* complex: 15 cases and review. *Rev Infect Dis*, **13**, 1120–5.

165. Rumisek, J.D., Albus, R.A. and Clarke, J.S. (1985) Late *Mycobacterium chelonae* bioprosthetic valve endocarditis: activation of implanted contaminant. *Ann Thor Surg*, **39**, 277–9.

166. Altmann, G., Horowitz, A., Kaplinsky, N. and Frankl, O., (1975) Prosthetic valve endocarditis due to *Mycobacterium chelonei*. *J Clin Microbiol*, **1**, 531–3.

167. Singh, M., Bofinger, A., Cave, G. and Boyle, P. (1992) *Mycobacterium fortuitum* endocarditis in a patient with chronic renal failure on hemodialysis. *Pathology*, **24**, 197–200.

168. Dunmire, R.B. and Breyer, J.A. (1991) Nontuberculous mycobacterial peritonitis during continuous ambulatory peritoneal dialysis. *Am J Kidney Dis*, **18**, 126–30.

169. Hakim, A., Hisam, N. and Reuman, P.D. (1993) Environmental mycobacterial peritonitis complicating peritoneal dialysis: three cases and review. *Clin Infect Dis*, **16**, 426–31.

170. Paul, J., Baigrie, C. and Parums, D.V. (1992) Fatal case of disseminated infection with the turtle bacillus *Mycobacterium chelonae*. *J Clin Pathol*, **45**, 528–30.

171. Wallace, R.J., Swenson, J.M., Silcox, V.A. and Bullen, M.G. (1985) Treatment of nonpulmonary infections due to *Mycobacterium fortuitum* and *Mycobacterium chelonei* on the basis of in vitro susceptibilities. *J Infect Dis*, **152**, 500–14.

172. Wallace, R.J., Brown, B.A. and Onyi, G.O. (1991) Susceptibilities of *Mycobacterium fortuitum biovar. fortuitum* and the two subgroups of *Mycobacterium chelonei* to imipenem cefmetazole, cefoxitin, and amoxicillin-clavulanic acid. *Antimicrob Agents Chemother*, **35**, 773–5.

173. Dalovisio, J.R. and Pankey, G.A. (1978) In vitro susceptibility of *Mycobacterium fortuitum* and *Mycobacterium chelonei* to amikacin. *J Infect Dis*, **137**, 318–21.

174. Wallace, R.J., Bedsole, G., Sumter, G. *et al.* (1990) Activities of ciprofloxacin and ofloxacin against rapidly growing mycobacteria with demonstration of acquired resistance following single drug therapy. *Antimicrob Agents Chemother*, 34, 65–70.

175. Brown, B.A., Wallace, R.J., Onyi, G.O. *et al.* (1992) Activities of four macrolides including clarithromycin, against *Mycobacterium fortuitum*, *Mycobacterium chelonae* and *M. chelonae*-like organisms. *Antimicrob Agents Chemother*, **36**, 180–4.

176. Yew, W.W., Kwan, S.Y.L., Wong, P.C. and Lee, J. (1990) Ofloxacin and imipenem in the treatment of *Mycobacterium fortuitum* and *Mycobacterium chelonae* lung infections. *Tubercle*, **71**, 131–3.

177. Pacht, E.R. (1990) *Mycobacterium fortuitum* lung abscess: resolution with prolonged trimethoprim/sulfamethoxazole therapy. *Am Rev Respir Dis*, **141**, 1599–1601.

178. Trulock, E.P., Bolman, R.M. and Genton, R. (1989) Pulmonary disease caused by *Mycobacterium chelonae* in a heart-lung transplant recipient with obliterative bronchiolitis. *Am Rev Respir Dis*, **140**, 802–4.

179. Singh, N. and Yu, V.L. (1992) Successful treatment of pulmonary infection due to *Mycobacterium chelonae*: case report and review. *Clin Infect Dis*, **14**, 156–61.

180. Rappaport, W., Dunington, G., Norton, L. *et al.* (1990) The surgical management of atypical mycobacterial soft-tissue infections. *Surgery*, **108**, 36–9.

181. Yew, W.W., Kwan, S.Y.L., Ma, W.K. *et al.* (1989) Single daily dose ofloxacin monotherapy for *Mycobacterium fortuitum* sternotomy infection. *Chest*, **96**, 1150–2.

182. Lambert, G.W. and Baddour, L.M. (1992) Right middle lobe syndrome caued by *Mycobacterium fortuitum* in a patient with Human Immunodeficiency Virus infection. *South Med J*, **85**, 767–9.

183. Rodriquez-Barrados, M.C., Clarridge, J. and Darouiche, R. (1992) Disseminated *Mycobacterium fortuitum* disease in an AIDS patient. *Am J Med*, **93**, 473–4.

184. Karasseva, V., Weiszfeiler, J.G. and Krasznay, E. (1965) Occurrence of atypical mycobacteria in *Macacus rhesus*. *Acta Microbiol Acad Sci Hung*, **12**, 275–82.

185. Bell, R.C., Higuchi, J.H., Donovan, W.N. *et al.* (1983) *Mycobacterium simiae*. Clinical features and follow-up of twenty-four patients. *Am Rev Respir Dis*, **127**, 35–8.

186. Rose, H.D., Dorff, G.J., Lauwasser, M. and Sheth, N.K. (1982) Pulmonary and disseminated *Mycobacterium simiae* infection in humans. *Am Rev Respir Dis*, **126**, 1110–13.

187. Torres, R.A., Nord, J., Feldman, R. *et al.* (1991) Disseminated mixed *Mycobacterium simiae – Mycobacterium avium* complex infection in Acquired Immunodeficiency Syndrome. *J Infect Dis*, **164**, 432–3.

188. Levy-Frebault, V., Pangon, B., Bure, A. *et al.* (1987) *Mycobacterium simiae* and *Mycobacterium avium – M. intracellulare* mixed infection in Acquired Immunodeficiency Syndrome. *J Clin Microbiol*, **25**, 154–7.

189. Schaefer, W.B., Wolinsky, E., Jenkins, P.A. and Marks, J. (1973) *Mycobacterium szulgai* – a new pathogen. *Am Rev Respir Dis*, **108**, 1320–6.

190. Maloney, J.M., Gregg, C.R., Stephens, D.S. *et al.* (1987) Infections caused by *Mycobacterium szulgai* in humans. *Rev Infect Dis*, **9**, 1120–6.

191. Marks, J., Jenkins, P.A. and Tsukamura, M. (1972) *Mycobacterium szulgai*: a new pathogen. *Tubercle*, **53**, 210–4.

192. Stratton, C.W., Phelps, D.B. and Reller, L.B. (1978) Tuberculoid tenosynovitis and carpal tunnel syndrome caused by *Mycobacterium szulgai*. *Am J Med*, **65**, 349–51.

193. Cross, G.M., Guill, M.A. and Aton, J.K. (1985) Cutaneous *Mycobacterium szulgai* infection. *Arch Dermatol*, **121**, 247–9.

194. Gur, H., Porat, S., Haas, H. *et al.* (1984) Disseminated mycobacterial disease caused by *Mycobacterium szulgai*. *Arch Intern Med*, **144**, 1861–3.

195. Good, R.C., Silcox, V.A., Kilburn, J.D. and Plikaytis, B.D. (1985) Identification and drug susceptibility test results for *Mycobacterium spp. Clin Microbiol Newsl*, **7**, 133–6.

196. Good, R.C. (1985) Opportunistic pathogens in the genus Mycobacterium. *Ann Rev Microbiol*, **39**, 347–69.

197. Zaugg, M., Salfinger, M., Opravil, M. and Luthy, R. (1993) Extrapulmonary and disseminated infections due to *Mycobacterium malmoense*: case report and review. *Clin Infect Dis*, **16**, 540–9.

198. Schroder, K.H. and Juhlin, I. (1977) *Mycobacterium malmoense* sp. nov. *Int J Syst Bacteriol*, **27**, 241–6.

198a. Henriques, B., Hoffner, S.E., Petrini, B. *et al.* (1994) Infection with *Mycobacterium malmoense* in Sweden: Report of 221 cases. *Clin Infect Dis*, **18**, 596–600.

199. Portaels, F., Walsh, G.P., DeRidder, K. *et al.* (1987) Cultivable mycobacteria isolated from 32 newly captured wild armadillos (*Dasypus novemcinctus*) from Louisiana. *Twenty-Second Joint U.S.–Japan Leprosy Research Conference, Bethesda, Maryland*. National Institutes of Health, U.S. Government Printing Office, pp. 103–8.

200. Roberts, C., Clague, H. and Jenkins, P.A. (1985) Pulmonary infection with *Mycobacterium malmoense*. A report of 4 cases. *Tubercle*, **66**, 205–9.

201. Warren, N.G., Body, B.A., Silcox, V.A. and Matthews, J.H. (1984) Pulmonary disease due to *Mycobacterium malmoense*. *J Clin Microbiol*, **20**, 245–7.

202. White, M.P., Bangash, H., Goel, K.M. and Jenkins, P.A. (1986) Non-tuberculous mycobacterial lymphadenitis. *Arch Dis Child*, **61**, 368–71.

203. Elston, R.A. (1989) Missed diagnosis of mycobacterial infection. *Lancet*, **1**, 1144.

204. Prince, H., Ispahani, P. and Backer, M. (1988) A *Mycobacterium malmoense* infection of the hand presenting as carpal tunnel syndrome. *J Hand Surg*, **13**, 328–30.

205. Gannon, M., Otridge, B., Hone, R. *et al.* (1990) Cutaneous *Mycobacterium malmoense* infection in an immunocompromised patient. *Int J Dermatol*, **29**, 149–50.

206. Banks, J., Jenkins, P.A. and Smith, A.P. (1985) Pulmonary infection with *Mycobacterium malmoense* – a review of treatment and response. *Tubercle*, **66**, 197–203.

207. Claydon, E.J., Coker, R.J. and Harris, J.R.W. (1991) *Mycobacterium malmoense* infections in HIV positive patients. *J Infect*, **23**, 191–4.

207a. Källenius, G., Melles, H., Hoffner, S.E. and Svenson, S.B. (1993) Why *Mycobacterium avium* and not *M. malmoese*? Interscience Conference on Antimicrobial Agents and Chemotherapy, New Orleans, LA.

208. Wallace, R.J., Nash, D.R., Tsukamura M. *et al.* (1988) Human disease due to *Mycobacterium smegmatis. J Infect Dis*, **158**, 52–9.

209. Newton, J.A., Weiss, P.J., Bowler, W.A. and Oldfield, E.C. (1993) Soft tissue infection due to *Mycobacterium smegmatis*: report of two cases. *Clin Infect Dis*, **16**, 531–3.

210. Dalovisio, J.R., Stetter, M. and Mikota-Wells, S. (1992) Rhinoceros' rhinorhea: cause of an outbreak of infection due to airborne *Mycobacterium bovis* in zookeepers. *Clin Infect Dis*, **15**, 598–600.

211. Dankner, W.M., Waecker, N.J., Essey, M.A. *et al.* (1993) *Mycobacterium bovis* infections in San Diego: a clinico-epidemiologic study of 73 patients and a historical review of a forgotten pathogen. *Medicine*, **72**, 11–37.

212. Wayne, L.G. and Sramek, H.A. (1992) Agents of newly recognized or infrequently encountered mycobacterial diseases. *Clin Microbiol Rev*, **5**, 1–25.

213. Abbott, M.R. and Smith, D.D. (1981) Mycobacterial infections in immunosuppressed patients. *Med J Aust*, **1**, 351–3.

214. Straus, W.L., Ostroff, S.M., Jernigen, D.B. *et al.* (1994) Clinical and epidemiologic characteristics of *Mycobacterium haemophilum*, an emerging pathogen in immunocompromised patients. *Ann Intern Med*, **120**, 118–25.

215. Bottger, E.C., Teske, A., Kirschner, P. *et al.* (1992) Disseminated '*Mycobacterium genavense*' infection in patients with AIDS. *Lancet*, **i**, 76–80.

216. Wald, A., Coyle, M.B., Carlson, L.C. *et al.* (1992) Infection with a fastidious mycobacterium resembling *Mycobacterium simiae* in seven patients with AIDS. *Ann Intern Med*, **117**, 586–9.

# Index

Page numbers appearing in **bold** refer to figures and page numbers appearing in *italic* refer to tables.